Introduction to Pharmacology

In the ocean depths off Madagascar, obsolete fish keep their laggard appointments. In the depths of the human mind, obsolete assumptions go their daily rounds. And there is little difference between the two, except that the fish do no harm.

Robert Ardrey
African Genesis, 1967

That which in the beginning may be just like poison, but at the end is like nectar, and which awakens one to self-realization, is said to be happiness in the mode of goodness.

Bhagavad Gita

Nothing in life is to be feared, it is only to be understood.

Marie Curie

Introduction to Pharmacology

Second Edition

Mannfred A. Hollinger, Ph.D.

Professor Emeritus,
Department of Medical
Pharmacology and Toxicology
University of California, Davis

Taylor & Francis
Taylor & Francis Group

LONDON AND NEW YORK

First published 1997 by Taylor & Francis
Second edition published 2003 by Taylor & Francis
11 New Fetter Lane, London EC4P 4EE

Simultaneously published in the USA and Canada
by Taylor & Francis Inc,
29 West 35th Street, New York, NY 10001

Taylor & Francis is an imprint of the Taylor & Francis Group

© 1997, 2003 Taylor & Francis

Typeset in 10/12 pt Sabon by Graphicraft Limited, Hong Kong
Printed and bound in Great Britain by TJ International Ltd, Padstow, Cornwall

Every effort has been made to ensure that the advice and information in this
book is true and accurate at the time of going to press. However, neither the
publisher nor the authors can accept any legal responsibility or liability for any
errors or omissions that may be made. In the case of drug administration, any
medical procedure or the use of technical equipment mentioned within this
book, you are strongly advised to consult the manufacturer's guidelines.

British Library Cataloguing in Publication Data
A catalogue record for this book is available from the British Library

Library of Congress Cataloging in Publication Data
Hollinger, Mannfred A.
    Introduction to pharmacology / Mannfred A. Hollinger.—2nd ed.
        p.   cm.
    Includes bibliographical references and index.
    1. Pharmacology.   I. Title.
    [DNLM: 1. Pharmacology.   2. Pharmaceutical Preparations. QV 4 H74li
    2003]
    RM300 .H65 2003
    615′.1—dc21   2002072005

ISBN 0-415-28033-8 (hbk)
ISBN 0-415-28034-6 (pbk)

Contents

Acknowledgements

The author would like to express his thanks for the continuing support of his wife Georgia throughout this project. In addition, the always-present commiseration of sons Randy and Chris served as a never-ending source of insight and intellectual stimulation. The author would also like to acknowledge the excellent graphic design provided by Tsunami Graphics, Sacramento, CA.

Much of the Appendix has been reproduced with kind permission from PJD Publications Limited, Westbury, NY 11590, USA, from M. A. Hollinger, *Res. Commun Alc. Sbst. Abuse*, vol. 16, pp. 1–23, 1995. Copyright 1995 by PJD Publications Ltd.

Preface to the first edition

The topic of pharmacology usually escapes the attention of many college students by virtue of the fact that pharmacology itself is rarely taught on the undergraduate level. It generally is reserved for postbaccalaureate students who are enrolled in health curricula associated with medicine, dentistry, nursing, and the veterinary sciences; however, certain upper level undergraduates are interested in the subject. This book is the product of teaching undergraduates the principles of pharmacology over the last 20 years. During that period the author continually searched for an appropriate textbook for students who normally had some background in biochemistry and physiology. Medical school texts were of no use since their coverage is far too extensive. Alternatively, "softer" texts tended to overemphasize certain areas, such as drug abuse, which were often the driving force behind their creation. Although both types of texts were good in their own right, they missed the mark. Students frequently expressed a desire for more "hard" science that would not inundate them with boiler plate text. It is because I agree with this sentiment that this book was created. The goal of this book is not to be a mini-medical school pharmacology text. Rather, it is intended to address a wider audience of advanced undergraduate students who have an interest in learning about the diverse aspects of pharmacology in society—not simply about the curative aspects of drugs. It is hoped that not only students in the biological sciences but also those in the social sciences will find some, if not all, of the book's contents informative and useful.

This book has been organized to provide a logical continuum of information relating to drugs, beginning with the inevitable historical discovery of drugs in food. With this background, important pharmacological principles will be considered relating to drug absorption, distribution, metabolism, and elimination. This material forms the corpus of the chapters that constitute Part 1. In essence, the emphasis is placed upon pharmacokinetic aspects of drug action. Having gained access to the body, how do drugs produce an effect and how can the effect be quantified for comparative purposes? In Part 2, the student is exposed to the concepts of drug–receptor interaction and the transduction of drug binding into pharmacodynamic or toxicodynamic responses. Factors influencing drug toxicity, as well as underlying principles of managing drug overdose, also will be presented as the inevitable "other side of the coin." Part 3 reiterates, in more detail, the concept introduced in Part 1 that drugs can be classified into four broad categories: (1) drugs that replace physiological inadequacies, (2) drugs that cure, (3) drugs that treat symptoms, and (4) drugs that alter mood or behavior. In this regard, hormones, antibiotics, and neuroactive agents provide examples, respectively, in their own chapters. In addition, the pharmacology of substance abuse as well as the evolution of drug abuse laws and the use of drugs in sports are also discussed. In Part 4, the final three chapters deal with the development of drugs by the pharmaceutical industry and the challenges they face in new drug discovery as well as dealing with the FDA. The section concludes with a discussion of the controversial use of experimental animals in research, an area often neglected in the study of pharmacology.

Mannfred A. Hollinger
Davis, California

Preface to the second edition

Since the publication of the first edition I have reevaluated the content of the book as well as its purpose. It became clear over the years that certain important areas that had been omitted in the first edition needed to be included in a revision, if a revision was to be meaningful. Therefore, additional areas added to the second edition include cardiovascular drugs, anticancer drugs, neuroleptics, designer drugs, bioterrorism, placebos, recombinant DNA technology, apoptosis, gaseous anesthetics, local anesthetics, vitamins, and the cigarette industry Master Settlement Agreement. In the intervening period since the publication of the first edition, the issue of alternative medicine has also become very topical, and a new chapter on this subject has been added.

Although identifying areas of omission was relatively straightforward, the question of how to make the book more attractive to my intended audience was more illusive. It has always been my goal to reach upper-level undergraduate students beyond those in the traditional "hard" science paths. Surely there must be students and faculties in the humanities, in fields such as sociology and psychology, for example, who would find certain aspects of the study of drugs interesting and perhaps even provocative? Areas such as animal experimentation, the development of drug laws, drugs in sports, the drug discovery process, and bioterrorism are not typical subjects expanded upon in graduate level texts. These are stand-alone subjects that do not require mastery of pharmacokinetics and pharmacodynamics, which are covered essentially in the introductory chapters in Parts 1 and 2.

In order to assist the student in evaluating his/her progress in dealing with the subject matter, I have included a set of 10 self-assessment questions at the end of each chapter (answers are provided at the back of the book). These questions are intended to emphasize the important facts, principles, and personalities that the student should become familiar with in the field of pharmacology. To further enhance the teaching power of the book the new edition contains 41 new tables and 33 new figures. Finally, in the hope of helping students and faculty, wherever, I encourage constructive input and am willing to try to answer any questions. My email is mahollinger@ucdavis.edu.

Mannfred A. Hollinger
Oro Valley, Arizona

Part I

Fundamentals of pharmacokinetics

Chapter 1

Introduction

HISTORY

Pharmacology is one of the pillars of the drug discovery process. While the medicinal/organic chemist may create the candidate compound (sometimes referred to as a new chemical entity, NCE), it is the pharmacologist who is responsible for testing it for pharmacological activity. An NCE is eventually investigated by several other groups of scientists (toxicologists, microbiologists, and clinicians) if it has demonstrated a potential therapeutic effect.

Pharmacology studies the effects of drugs and how they exert their effects. For example, penicillin cures certain bacterial infections and acetylsalicylic acid (ASA) can reduce inflammation. How do they accomplish these respective effects? Through research we now know that penicillin can disrupt the synthesis of cell walls in susceptible bacterial strains by inhibiting a key enzyme, while ASA can inhibit the action of a human cell membrane enzyme known as cyclooxygenase, which is responsible for the synthesis of a number of inflammatory mediators.

Modern pharmacology owes part of its development to Friedrich Worler, who inaugurated the field of synthetic organic chemistry in 1828 with the synthesis of urea. This achievement catalyzed the formation of an entire industry (the German dye industry), which ultimately led to the synthesis of NCEs, many of which were subsequently introduced as possible therapeutic agents. Prior to this achievement physiological pharmacologists had been restricted to the study of crude preparations of natural substances such as strychnine (Francois Magendie showed that its convulsant action was produced at the spinal cord level) and curare (Claude Bernard demonstrated that it produced paralysis of skeletal muscle by blocking the neuromuscular junction).

Another key figure in the development of pharmacology as a discipline was Oswald Schmiedeberg (1838–1921). He obtained his medical doctorate in 1866 with a thesis on the measurement of chloroform in blood. He worked at the University of Dorpat in Hungary under Rudolph Buchheim (see Chapter 5) in what is generally considered to be the first department of pharmacology, ultimately succeeding him in 1869. Only three years later he was a professor at the University of Strasbourg and head of an institute of pharmacology. In 1878 he published the classic text *Outline of Pharmacology*.

In his 46 years at Strasbourg, Schmiedeberg trained a number of preeminent scientists who populated the great centers of scientific learning throughout many countries. One of these was John Jacob Abel. Abel became the first chairman of pharmacology

Table 1.1 Important figures in the development of pharmacology

Dioscorides (AD 57), Greek, produced one of the first material medica of approximately 500 plants and remedies

Paracelsus (1493–1541), Swiss scholar and alchemist, often considered the "grandfather of pharmacology"

William Withering (1741–1799), English, published *An Account of the Foxglove* in 1785

Frederich Sertürner, German pharmacist's assistant, isolated morphine—the first pure drug—in 1805

Paul Ehrlich, German pathologist and Nobel prize winner, credited with developing the concept of chemotherapy

Gerhard Domagk, German pathologist and Nobel prize winner, observed the antibacterial property of a prototypical sulfonamide (Prontosil) that is considered to be the first selective antimicrobial agent

Horace Wells and *William T. G. Morton*, introduced volatile anesthetics in the 1840s

Henri Bequerel (1896), *Pierre and Marie Curie* (1898), discovery and awareness of radioactive principles

Alexander Fleming, discoverer of penicillin

Rosalyn Yalow (1921–), development of the radioimmunoassay, Nobel prize winner in 1977

Stanley Cohen and *Herbert Boyer*, genetic engineering in the 1980s

in the United States at the University of Michigan. Abel was an excellent scientist and is credited with the isolation of both epinephrine and histamine and with the preparation of crystalline insulin. Additional important individuals in the history of pharmacology are shown in Table 1.1.

Clinical pharmacology owes much of its foundation to the work of William Withering. Born in 1741 in Shropshire, England, Withering was interested in various aspects of science, and graduated with an MD from the University of Edinburgh. Withering became interested in the disorder known as "dropsy" and learned about a herbal treatment for this disorder from an old woman herbalist in Shropshire. However, her herbal recipe contained more than 20 plants. Fortunately, because of his interest and knowledge of botany, he identified the active ingredient as coming from the plant *Digitalis purpurea*. With the publication of his book *An Account of the Foxglove* in 1785, Withering introduced *Digitalis* for the therapy of congestive heart failure, or dropsy, as he knew the condition.

Withering was unaware that dropsy was caused by cardiac insufficiency. In common with his time, he believed that the kidney was responsible for dropsy (peripheral fluid accumulation) and was therefore the site of action of *Digitalis* in the condition. Nevertheless, his clinical observations were precise: "Let the medicine therefore be given in doses, and at the intervals mentioned above; let it be continued until it either acts on the kidneys, the stomach, the pulse or the bowels; let it be stopped upon the first appearance of any one of these effects, and I will maintain that the patient will not suffer from its exhibition, nor the practitioner be disappointed in any reasonable expectation."

In the process of observing the pharmacological effects of *Digitalis*, Withering identified desired endpoints to include increased urine production (now believed to be the result of increased cardiac output and increased blood flow through the kidneys) and a decreased pulse rate. He also noted the toxic central and cardiac effects

Table 1.2 Pharmacologic definitions

Pharmacodynamics is the study of how drugs act, with an emphasis on mechanisms

Pharmacokinetics is the study of how the body absorbs, distributes, metabolizes, and excretes drugs; the calculation of various rates brings a quantitative component to assessing drug action

Pharmacotherapeutics is the use of drugs to treat disorders; the emphasis is on clinical management

Pharmacoepidemiology is the study of the effect of drugs on populations; questions dealing with the influence of genetics are particularly important

Pharmacoeconomics is the study of the cost-effectiveness of drug treatments; the cost of medications is of worldwide concern, particularly among certain groups such as the elderly and AIDS patients

---

of *Digitalis*. Withering's major contribution was not so much a discovery as the construction of a way of rationally approaching a therapeutic problem. He replaced the anecdotal (testimonial) basis of medicine with evidence-based medicine, derived from careful observation uncontaminated with prejudice.

DEFINITIONS

Pharmacology is the science of drugs (Greek *pharmakos*, medicine or drug, and *logos*, study). Pharmacology has been defined as an experimental science that studies changes brought about *in vivo* and *in vitro* by chemically acting substances, whether used for therapeutic purposes or not. In the broadest sense, pharmacology is the science of studying the effect of drugs on living organisms. It attempts to describe the biological responses produced by drugs and to define the underlying mechanisms by which the responses are generated. Because of this, pharmacology is an integrative discipline involving other fields of study such as physiology, biochemistry, microbiology, and immunology. Pharmacology should be distinguished from the profession of pharmacy, whose responsibilities include the identification, verification, standardization, compounding, and dispensing of drugs and dosage forms of drugs. Additional useful definitions relative to pharmacology are shown in Table 1.2.

Associating the word science with pharmacology implies a systematic investigation of observable phenomena that can be quantified and controlled—a state that reflects much of modern pharmacology. However, as we shall see, this has not always been the case. As mentioned earlier, pharmacology involves the study of drugs. However, what is a drug?

The word drug is believed to have been derived from the French word *drogue*, which refers to a dry substance and probably reflects the use of herbs in early therapy. Broadly defined, a drug is a chemical substance that can alter or influence the responsiveness of a biological system. The action of a drug is mediated by a naturally occurring process of the body. A drug either mimics, facilitates, or antagonizes a normally occurring phenomenon. Although people can, and do, argue about what a drug is to them, perhaps it may be helpful at this point to present several "official" views as to what a drug is. To begin with, let us examine how the governmental agency most concerned with drugs defines a drug. According to the Food and Drug Administration (FDA):

A. All drugs are chemicals, BUT, all chemicals are not drugs;

    1. All drugs are poisons, BUT, all poisons are not drugs;

B. Definitions

    1. chemical—a substance composed of a combination of elements (electrons, protons, and neutrons);

    2. drug—a chemical which is utilized for the diagnosis, prevention, cure or amelioration of an unwanted health condition;

        a. Federal Food, Drug, and Cosmetic (FDC) Act Sec. 201. [321] (g)(1)— The term "drug" means (A) articles recognized in the official United States Pharmacopeia, official Homeopathic Pharmacopoeia of the United States, or official National Formulary, or any supplement to any of them; and (B) articles intended for use in the diagnosis, cure, mitigation, treatment or prevention of disease in man or other animals; and (C) articles (other than food) intended to affect the structure or any function of the body of man or other animals; and (D) articles intended for use as a component of any articles specified in clause (A), (B), or (C)....

1) "Food" (201). [321] (a) (f) means (1) articles used for food or drink for man or other animals, (2) chewing gum, and (3) articles used for components of any other such article.

As one can appreciate, deciding what a drug is, or is not, can become an exercise as complicated as one wishes. For example, are salt water, sugar water, synthetic saliva (there is such a product—Salivart®), artificial tears, placebos, or tetrodotoxin drugs? However, with this official orientation behind us, we may now proceed to investigate the world(s) of drugs and their diverse influences on the human experience.

BACKGROUND

The roots of pharmacology extend backward in time to our earliest Pleistocene hominid ancestors on the African savanna, approximately five to ten million years ago. These primitive forebearers grubbed for existence in the brush, where berries, shoots, leaves, tubers, flowers, seeds, nuts, and roots were plentiful. Our predecessors became specialized vegetarians who only later acquired an appetite for meat. It was their vegetarian diet that served to join gastronomic needs with pharmacological discovery.

As our species evolved, we developed the higher reasoning centers of the brain. One of the manifestations of this increased capacity for thought was the ability to recognize cause-and-effect relationships between our environment and us. One specific relationship that our ancestors learned was that the dietary ingestion of certain plants (regardless of which part) produced significant, corresponding physiological changes in their bodies, in addition to providing essential minerals and calories. Thus began our long-standing relationship with plants that continues to the present time.

HISTORY—ROLE OF PLANTS

Since time immemorial, plants have been used for treating diseases in humans and animals, as well as being involved in the spiritual needs in humans. The role of plants in early religion can be seen in friezes (carvings) from the eighth century BC in Mesopotamia. These carvings clearly depict mandrake flowers and poppy heads. Early belief in the curative powers of plants and certain substances rested exclusively upon traditional knowledge, that is, empirical information not subjected to critical examination (i.e., ethnopharmacology).

The question has been asked: "how over time, have we been 'shaped' by the shifting alliances that we have formed and broken with various members of the vegetable world as we have made our way through the maze of history?" The answer, in part, is that plants have always played a significant role in mediating human cultural experiences in the world at large, be that role dietary, medicinal, or to alter consciousness. These are roles that they still play today, whether in the realm of medicine, religion, or jurisprudence.

One of the most provocative theories relating to our relationship with plants is the suggestion that their consumption may have contributed to the relatively rapid organization of the human brain's information-processing capacity. This is a process that occurred over a relatively short anthropological time frame. Specifically, this proposal suggests that hallucinogenic compounds such as psilocybin, dimethyltryptamine, and harmaline were present in the protohuman diet and that their psychopharmacological effects catalyzed the emergence of human self-reflection.

The theory boldly suggests that the tripling of human brain size from *Homo hablis* was facilitated by mutagenic, psychoactive plants that functioned as a chemical "missing link." While this proposal certainly does not represent a mainstream scientific view, it illustrates, nevertheless, the impact that plants, particularly psychoactive ones, continue to have in our attempts to define ourselves.

We can only speculate as to the actual sequence of events in the genesis of our relationship with plants. However, the knowledge of plant effects undoubtedly began with individual experiences. It was only after the epigenetic (i.e., learned rather than genetically based) development of language (i.e., communication) that members of a familial or tribal group could receive "instruction" based upon the experience of senior members. This view is based, of course, upon the premise that language, of any kind, is the primary fulcrum of teaching and/or learning.

Verbal communication does not appear to be an absolute prerequisite, however. For example, mother chimps routinely offer choice tidbits of food to their infants and will snatch unusual, possibly dangerous, foods from their mouths. Primatologists in Tanzania have observed that chimpanzees periodically include leaves of the *Aspilia* plant in their diet. Despite its bitter taste, it is consumed by both sexes of all ages, the healthy as well as the sick. The chimps eat these leaves regularly, but consume very few of them at one time, indicating that their nutritional value is in doubt. In the rainy season, however, when intestinal worms and other illnesses plague apes, ingestion increases dramatically. Analysis of these leaves has shown them to contain the chemical thiarubrine-A, which has antibacterial properties.

Leaves from the same plant are also used by natives of the area to treat wounds and stomachaches. How is "chimpanzee ethnomedicine" possible? Could it be based on some kind of hereditary information? Or, more probably, is this *cultural* information passed on—by emulation or instruction—from generation to generation, and subject to rapid change if the available medicinal plants change, or if new diseases arise, or if new ethnobotanical discoveries are made? With the exception of the lack of professional herbalists, chimpanzee folk medicine does not seem so different from human folk medicine etiology. While the *Aspilia* story is particularly instructive, chimps are also known to eat plants other than *Aspilia* to treat intestinal disorders, as well as soil from particular cliff faces, presumably to provide mineral nutrients such as salt.

It has been said that until experience can be summarized by symbols—whether words or manual gestures—and the symbols grouped, filed, isolated, and selected to perform the thinking process, then experience is no more than a silent film. Symbols allow us to store information outside of the physical brain for retrieval and transmission across space and time. The capacity to relate past experiences to future possibilities and deal in symbols, particularly language, is an inheritance from our Pliocene past that has evolved from warning cries in the Oldavi gorge to Senate filibusters and "rap" music.

In this way, knowledge of the effect of plants on bodily functions probably became part of our collective memory. Before the advent of writing, this collective memory had to be communicated verbally and became the responsibility of certain members of the group—a practice that continued into the Middle Ages in the form of lyrical song or verse in order to make the information easier to remember.

There are many examples of plants that played significant roles in the lives of ancient man. Perhaps one of the more interesting deals with a parasitic shrub that is still used in traditional Christmas celebrations. Mistletoe (*Viscum album*) was celebrated for its mysterious powers by the ancient Celts (fourth century BC). Celtic priests (the Druids) were fascinated by the haphazard growing and blooming of the shrub and considered it the most sacred plant of all. Interestingly, the presence of mistletoe pollen in the peat moss "grave" of the 1500-year-old "Lindow Man," unearthed in 1984 near Manchester, England, contributed to the theory that this individual had in fact been a Druid prince.

Druids harvested the mistletoe berry yearly and used it in their winter celebrations, known as *samain* and *imbolc*, which were centered on the winter solstice. For this celebration, the Druids concocted a strong potion of the berries, which researchers have subsequently discovered contains a female-like steroid that may have stimulated the libido (presumably structurally related to either estrogen or progesterone). Mistletoe has, of course, become a contemporary symbol to Yuletide merrymakers as a license to kiss.

The Celts, and others, also used mistletoe for medical purposes. The Roman historian Pliny the Younger wrote that mistletoe was "deemed a cure for epilepsy; carried about by women it assisted them to conceive, and it healed ulcers most effectually, if only the sufferer chewed a piece of the plant and laid another piece on the sore." Modern herbalists continue to recommend mistletoe for the treatment of epilepsy, hypertension, and hormone imbalances. However, it should be appreciated that homemade brews prepared from the berries and leaves of the North American species (*Phoradendron flavescens*) are poisonous and should be avoided.

In the New World, specialists similar to the Druids existed in "primitive" societies and functioned as shamans. The shaman is a priest-doctor who uses "magic" to cure the sick, to divine the hidden, and to control events that affect the welfare of the people. The shaman seeks to achieve "ecstasy," often by the use of plants containing psychedelic drugs. The central role that drugs played in fourteenth-century life in Columbia, for example, is clearly illustrated by much of their artwork. Sculptures depict the use of coca leaves as well as the veneration of the mushroom. The writings of Carlos Castaneda and others have popularized the shaman and the use of hallucinogenic drugs in contemporary literature.

While shamans were inculcating the role of drugs in the New World, the Middle Ages were not a particularly good time for plants and drugs. For example, the medieval church actively suppressed knowledge of plants suspected of playing a role in the nocturnal activities of the practitioners of witchcraft. Specifically, use of extracts from the thorn apple (*Datura*) was prohibited since the application of ointments containing this substance was believed to confer the gift of flight.

Throughout medieval Europe witches routinely rubbed their bodies with hallucinogenic ointments made from belladonna, mandrake, and henbane—all structurally related to *Datura*. In fact, much of the behavior associated with witches was attributed to these drugs. Their journey was not through space, however, but across the hallucinatory landscape of their minds. A particularly efficient means of self-administering the drug for women was through the moist tissues of the vagina; the witches broomstick or staff was considered a most effective applicator.

Fortunately, a Swiss named Phillippus Theophrastus von Hohenheim (1493–1541) began to question doctrines handed down from antiquity. In 1516 he assumed the name Paracelsus (para meaning beside, beyond; Celsus was a famous Roman physician). He encouraged development of knowledge of the active ingredient(s) in prescribed remedies, while rejecting the irrational concoctions and mixtures of medieval medicine. He discounted the humoral theory of Galen, whose rediscovered works became the foundation of medicine at the time. Galen postulated that there were four humors in the body (blood, phlegm, yellow bile, and black bile); when these were in balance, one enjoyed health, and when there was imbalance, sickness ensued. Paracelsus was a freethinker and an iconoclast. His disenchantment with the teaching of medicine at the University of Basle reached its climax on July 24, 1527, when he publicly burned the standard medical textbooks of the day (e.g., Galen). All of this behavior was deemed heresy, and not acceptable to the medical community of his time.

Paracelsus prescribed chemically defined substances with such success that enemies within the profession had him prosecuted as a poisoner. This was primarily based upon his use of inorganic substances in medicine, because his critics claimed that they were too toxic to be used as therapeutic agents. He defended himself with the thesis that has become axiomatic in pharmacology/toxicology: "If you want to explain any poison properly, what then isn't a poison? All things are poisons, nothing is without poison; the dose alone causes a thing not to be poison."

Plants, and natural products, continue to play a vital role in modern society both as the source of conventional therapeutic agents and as herbal preparations in "health food" stores. In 1994, half of the top 25 drugs on the market in terms of sales were either natural products or based on natural products, now made synthetically or semisynthetically. Examples of active plant compounds with therapeutic uses are shown in Table 1.3.

It is estimated that 80 percent of people in developing countries are almost totally dependent upon traditional healers for their health care, and that plants are the major source of drugs for their traditional medical practitioners. In theory, in as

Table 1.3 Plant compounds and their therapeutic uses

Compound	Therapeutic use
Atropine	Anticholinergic (mydriatic)
Caffeine	CNS stimulant
Cocaine	Local anesthetic
Colchicine	Antigout
Digoxin	Cardiotonic
Ephedrine	Bronchodilator
Morphine	Analgesic
Oubain	Cardiotonic
Physostigmine	Cholinergic
Quinine	Antimalarial
Scopolamine	Anticholinergic
Theophylline	Bronchodilator
D-Tubocurarine	Skeletal muscle relaxant
Vincristine	Antineoplastic

much as 80 percent of the world's population live in developing countries, approximately 64 percent of the world's population depends, therefore, almost entirely on plants for medication.

As indicated earlier, a large proportion of over-the-counter (OTC) drugs, prescription drugs, and "health food" products are still derived from plants and natural sources in Western medicine. A few examples include the use of cardiac glycosides from the purple foxglove (*Digitalis purpurea*), opiates from the opium poppy (*Papaver somniferum*), reserpine from the *Rauwolfia* species, quinine from the *Cinchona* species, and Taxol® from the yew tree. Taxol® is the best selling anticancer drug ever.

The antiovarian cancer compound Taxol (paclitaxel) is a classic case of how supply can be critical for drugs based on natural products. In the late 1980s, the only known source of this drug was the bark of the relatively rare Pacific yew tree *Taxus brevifolia*. Unfortunately, in the Pacific Northwest nearly 90 percent of the yew's native habitat was destroyed in the last century. The decline in yew population had serious implications for patients with ovarian cancer.

It has been estimated that six 6-inch-diameter trees would have to be sacrificed for enough Taxol to treat one woman suffering from ovarian cancer. Considering that the number of potential patients in the late 1980s numbered approximately 12,000, an eventual limitation of Taxol was possible. Fortunately, the problem was solved in the early 1990s by the partial synthesis of Taxol from a precursor produced in needles and twigs from the more renewable *Taxus baccata*.

The approval of Taxol for marketing in December 1992 was the culmination of 35 years of work. During this period of time the National Cancer Institute (NCI) and the U.S. Department of Agriculture (USDA) collaborated to collect, identify, and screen U.S. native plant material for antitumor activity. The year 1992 also marked, co-incidentally, the discovery of the "Ice Man" in the Italian Alps. This Bronze Age man, who died 5300 years ago, was found in possession of a pure copper axe set in a yew wood handle and an unfinished 6-foot yew bow. Obviously, the yew tree has played a number of important roles for humans throughout history.

Taxol is a potent inhibitor of eukaryotic cell replication, blocking cells in the late G2, or mitotic, phase of the cell cycle. Interaction of Taxol with cells results in the formation of discrete bundles of stable microtubules as a consequence of reorganization of the microtubule cytoskeleton. Microtubules are not normally static organelles but are in a state of dynamic equilibrium with their components (i.e., soluble tubulin dimers). Taxol alters this normal equilibrium, shifting it in favor of the stable, nonfunctional microtubule polymer.

In addition to being an essential component of the mitotic spindle, and being required for the maintenance of cell shape, microtubules are involved in a wide variety of cellular activities, such as cell motility and communication between organelles within the cell. Any disruption of the equilibrium within the microtubule system would be expected to disrupt cell division and normal cellular activities in which microtubules are involved.

As indicated earlier, plant products can be useful as starting materials for the semisynthetic preparation of other drugs. An important example in this regard is the Mexican yam, which produces a steroid precursor (diosgenin) vital to the synthesis of steroidal hormones used in oral contraceptives (i.e., progesterone). The availability of diosgenin eliminates numerous expensive steps in the organic synthesis of the basic steroid molecule. It was this discovery that contributed to the development of the pharmaceutical company Syntex (now a subsidiary of Hoffman LaRoche) and the development of the first birth control pill.

CONTEMPORARY ISSUES REGARDING PLANTS

It is our historical relationship with plants that has led contemporary ethnobotanists to attempt to raise our consciousness regarding the disappearance of rainforests and their indigenous richness in discovered and undiscovered drug sources. For example, it has been estimated that between 2000 and 40,000 plant species are lost annually through destruction of tropical rainforests. This is significant since less than 1 percent of the world's flowering plants have been tested for their effectiveness against disease. In an attempt to counteract this scenario, several drug companies have committed financial resources to support increased acquisition and evaluation of remaining plant material. In addition, royalties have been guaranteed to South American tribes whose shamans provide successful drug leads.

There are estimated to be at least 250,000 species of higher plants and 30 million botanical species remaining, most of which have not been tested for biological activity. To this end, a drug company was formed in the early 1990s to specifically deal with this challenge (appropriately named Shaman Pharmaceuticals). By forming consortiums with larger drug companies (e.g., Lilly), the company hopes to accelerate the rate of discovery of new drug entities discovered from botanical sources.

Major technological advances in screening processes (see Chapter 13) have promoted the belief that the drug discovery process may become abbreviated. Pharmacologists have traditionally had to analyze in the approximate neighborhood of 15,000 NCEs before one could qualify for testing in humans. This normally requires many years and hundreds of millions of dollars. Until relatively recently, animal testing was the only way to go. However, initial screening can often be done in a matter of days without using animals. This can be achieved by using isolated enzymes or receptors to determine if the drug has any binding affinity at all (see Chapter 13).

However, not everyone agrees that this renewed drug company enthusiasm for going out in the field to seek plant-based drugs will be particularly widespread or particularly effective in the long term. Nonenthusiasts contend that labor-intensive plant collection methods are being supplanted by newer, laboratory-based chemistry techniques (see Chapter 13) that are more efficient in creating new drug leads. For every proven anticancer drug like Taxol, there are hundreds of plant compounds that demonstrate initial promise in the test-tube, only to prove a disappointment later.

In the final analysis, will rational drug design, chemical synthesis, or combinatorial chemistry prove to be enough? Or will the abundant natural diversity of chemical structures found in nature provide new scaffolds and new chemical space for even greater advancement in NCEs?

In the Western hemisphere there are more than 40 species of plants that are used for hallucinogenic purposes alone. Although the structures of hallucinogenic substances vary significantly, most plants owe their hallucinogenic properties to alkaloids, which are cyclic structures containing nitrogen. At least 5000 higher plants contain alkaloids. Despite their wide distribution among plants, our knowledge of their pharmacology is still largely incomplete.

One of the challenges facing early, as well as contemporary, chemists is how to extract the pharmacologically active principle (such as an alkaloid) from a plant. This is desirable because it allows identification, assessment of pharmacological effects, constant dosage, and the opportunity to create liquid forms of the extract. For example, soaking plants in alcohol (ethanol) creates a *tincture*, which was, undoubtedly, one of the first organic extractions performed by man.

In the process of preparing a tincture, some pharmacologically active constituents of the plant are extracted by the alcohol. Although not all substances are soluble in alcohol, those that are include the alkaloids. In the case of a tincture of raw opium, the soluble alkaloids include morphine, codeine, noscapine, and papavarine. Such tinctures of opium were the infamous laudanum preparations of the late 1800s (see Appendix).

In addition to providing drugs, plants have also been recently utilized for ecological purposes via the process of phytoremediation. Phytoremediation refers to the ability of some plants to remove toxic compounds from the soil, concentrate them in their own tissues, and thus, achieve a certain degree of detoxification. Current interest has specifically focused on removing metals from poisoned sites. Among the poisoned sites are abandoned mines containing zinc and lead; military bases contaminated with lead and cadmium; municipal waste containing copper, mercury, and lead; and sewage sludge, where numerous metals can be a problem. Agricultural applications are also being researched (e.g., selenium removal by the mustard plant). The process of metal scavenging appears to be mediated by phytochelatins, small peptides that bind metals in forms that are less toxic to the plant.

MICROORGANISMS

Plants are not the only natural products used as a source for drugs. Microorganisms have, of course, been extensively screened for antibiotics since Alexander Fleming's discovery of the antibacterial activity of *Penicillin notatum* in the 1920s. Numerous useful antibiotics are also produced by bacteria of the *Streptomyces* genus (including streptomycin, neomycin, tetracycline, and chloramphenical) as well as by fungi (griseofulvin and cyclosporin C). Antibiotics are discussed in more detail in Part 3, Chapter 10.

MARINE SOURCES

Drugs and other products from the sea have been a steadily growing area of research interest for the past 20 years. In 1992, the U.S. government spent approximately $44 million in the area of marine biotechnology research. U.S. industrial investment in marine biotechnology was approximately $60 million in 1994 (both small and large companies are involved). By collecting, growing, or synthesizing natural compounds made by an array of marine creatures (e.g., microbes, sponges, corals, sea slugs, and others), investigators are screening compounds in the hope of adding to the medical armamentarium against cancer, acquired immune deficiency syndrome (AIDS), inflammation, and other conditions.

Marine species comprise approximately one-half of total global diversity (estimates range from 3 million to 500 million different species). Therefore, the marine world would appear to offer significant potential resources for novel pharmacological compounds. Unfortunately, much of the literature on marine natural products is characterized by compounds with demonstrable cytotoxicity rather than pharmacological efficacy.

However, toxicological properties can conceivably be utilized therapeutically. For example, one current therapeutic candidate, based upon its cytotoxicity, is bryostatin 1. Bryostatin, from the bryozoan *Bugula neritina*, is now in phase II trials (see Chapter 14 for discussion of clinical trials). Research is currently under way to develop aquaculture techniques for the harvesting of the bryozoan source. Because of the relatively large number of possible drug candidates from marine sources, pharmaceutical companies are forced to utilize their high-throughput screening technologies with extensive arrays of drug target-specific assays (see Part 4, Chapter 13 for more details) to test marine extracts.

An example of a natural product from a marine organism that has been commercialized is an extract from sea whips (*Pseudopterogoogia elisabethae*). This extract is used in the manufacture of certain cosmetic products. The active ingredient is believed to be a class of diterpine glycosides (pseudopterosins) that apparently has some anti-inflammatory activity.

Another marine product undergoing development is docosahexaenoic acid (DHA), developed via fermentation of a microalgae. DHA is a major component in human gray matter and is important for normal healthy development in infants. Various groups, such as the World Health Organization, have recommended DHA's inclusion in infant formulas at levels similar to those found in human milk. DHA is presently used in Belgium and Holland and is expected to gain approval in the United States.

ANIMAL SOURCES

Today, animal products such as insulin (extracted from the pancreas of cows and pigs) are still being used for the treatment of diabetes mellitus and other disorders.

However, it should be appreciated that less attractive members of the animal world can also provide therapeutic features. For example, maggots, which are the larval form of approximately one-half of the more than 85,000 species of flies, have been and still are occasionally used to treat open wounds—a procedure known as maggot debridement therapy (MDT) or, more commonly, maggot therapy. MDT is practiced in more than 150 hospitals in the United States and in 1000 centers worldwide.

The use of maggots to treat wounds dates from ancient times; in fact, the 2000 Academy Award film *Gladiator* portrayed the hero's shoulder being healed by maggot therapy. The modern father of MDT was William S. Baer, who developed the strategy based on his observation during World War I that wounded soldiers whose wounds harbored living maggots did not develop gangrene. The maggots had the lovely habit of selectively debriding the necrotic tissue in the wounds but leaving the healthy tissue unmolested. This is particularly true for the popular *Lucilia sericata* (greenbottle blowfly larvae) that actually starve on healthy tissue, making them ideal for medicinal use. Another of Baer's contributions to the field involved a method to sterilize the maggots. Today, commercial and research laboratories produce sterile larvae.

The ability of maggots to promote healing of lacerations on skin wounds is the result of their secretion of the chemical allantoin. A less offensive source of allantoin is the synthetic form. Synthetic allantoin is available today to accelerate wound healing and is used in skin ulcer therapy when applied topically (similar uses exist in veterinary medicine). An alternative theory to explain the maggots' "mechanism of action" is that they secrete antimicrobial waste products such as ammonium, calcium, or other bicarbonates that break down only the necrotic tissue in wounds; these secretions also change the alkalinity of the wound to help it to heal.

The soft-bodied, legless larvae were widely used to clean wounds until the 1940s, when antibiotics supplanted them. However, interest in this "biosurgery" using specially bred, germ-free maggots is currently increasing within certain clinical specialties (e.g., plastic surgery), particularly in Britain. Three-day-old maggots from the greenbottle fly have been used in the treatment of open wounds such as ulcers. Apparently, 100 maggots can eat 10 to 15 grams of dead tissue a day, leaving wounds clean and healthy (today, the scientific standard of 10 larvae/cm^2 is used). In one case an 83-year-old man with severe leg ulcers was saved the trauma of an amputation due to successful treatment with maggots.

In a similar context, a recombinant version of a protein from a blood-feeding hookworm is currently being investigated for its use in preventing blood clots. The protein, designated NAP–5, is a member of a family of anticoagulant proteins. The protein acts by inhibiting Factor Xa in the initial step of the blood-clotting cascade leading to fibrin formation. If successful, this protein may replace an entire class of 40-year-old "blood-thinning" drugs, called heparins, which are widely used to protect against clot formation in heart-attack patients.

Another natural anticoagulant is hirudin, derived from the saliva of the leech (*hirudo* is the Latin word for leech). Leeches, in fact, are still occasionally used themselves therapeutically for certain topical applications. Another possible drug to be used for the dissolution of blood clots is derived from bat saliva and acts as a plasminogen activator. It appears that saliva is a good place to look for possible drugs affecting the blood-clotting system since sand fly saliva is also being examined for this property.

Snake venoms have also been found to possess ingredients with important pharmacological properties. Perhaps the best-known example is the drug captopril, which is used in the management of hypertension. This drug is a dipeptide analog of bradykinin-potentiating peptides (BPPs), originally identified in the venom of the pit viper, *Bothrops jararaca*. The drug acts by inhibiting angiotensin-converting enzyme (ACE), whose normal function is to catalyze the formation of a vasoconstrictor peptide (angiotensin II). When the snake injects its venom, the BPPs inhibit ACE, thus ensuring circulation of the venom by inhibiting vasoconstriction in the same manner.

DEVELOPMENT OF FORMULARIES

Archeological evidence confirms our assumption that drug taking is an extremely old human characteristic. Human use of alcohol in the form of fermented grains, fruits, and plants is particularly ancient. For example, fragmentary evidence exists that beer and hackleberry wine were used as early as 6400 BC. However, it was not for several more millennia before organized, written compendia (i.e., brief compilations of whole fields of knowledge) were developed.

The Egyptian Ebers papyrus (*circa* 1550 BC) contains the description of several active medicinal ingredients that are still used today. In India an extensive list of the therapeutic uses of plant material was developed by approximately 1000 BC. To put Western knowledge of drugs into perspective, the modern era of pharmacology did not begin until the work of Francois Magendie (1783–1855), who prepared a medical formulary of "purified drugs." His book contained a list of medicinal substances and formulas for making medicines.

The earliest Chinese records indicate the use of natural products after approximately 500 BC. It was also during this period that the Chinese might have been the first to distill alcohol, thus making it the first drug to be isolated and purified.

The Chinese have one of the most extensive herbal traditions. The earliest known written work on Chinese herbs is *The Herbal Classic of the Divine Plowman*, written anonymously in approximately 100 BC. This treatise recommended the therapeutic use of 365 drugs (252 from plants, 67 from animals, and 46 from minerals). It is claimed that the world's first pharmacopoeia (a book containing an official or standard list of drugs along with recommended procedures for their preparation and use) was written during the Tang dynasty in AD 659. Perhaps the most significant written work on Chinese herbs was the *Ben Cao Kong Mu*, published in 1596 and subsequently translated into English, French, German, Russian, and Japanese.

Following the 1911 revolution, the Ministry of Health of the nationalist government sought to curtail or eliminate traditional Chinese medicine. However, after the communist revolution of 1949, the new government reversed the ban on traditional medicine, establishing a number of traditional medical colleges and institutes whose role is to train physicians and further investigate the uses of herbs. Even in Western hospitals in China, apothecaries are available to dispense herbs upon request.

SOURCES OF DRUG INFORMATION

Today, in the United States, there are numerous sources of drug information, including the *Physicians' Desk Reference* (PDR), which is an industry-supported reference. The PDR contains information identical to that contained in package inserts. No comparative information on efficacy, safety, or cost is included. PDR versions covering both trade name protected and generic preparations are available.

The *United States Pharmacopoeia* (USP), founded in 1820, originally contained "recipes" (formulas) for the preparation of drugs and drug products. The evolution of the USP actually began in 1817 when a New York physician, Lyman Spalding, recognized the need for drug standardization. At that time, medicine names and formulations differed from one region to another.

Spalding organized a meeting with 10 other physicians in January 1820 in the U.S. Capitol's Senate Chamber. Following the week-long meeting, the groundwork was laid for the compilation of the first *Pharmacopoeia of the United States of America*. The book was designed to standardize 217 of the most fully recognized and best understood medicines of that era.

USP standards first became legislatively mandated in 1848 when Congress enacted the Drug Import Act. The USP gained further recognition in the 1906 Food and Drugs Act and the 1938 Federal Food, Drug, and Cosmetic Act (see Appendix), in which its standards of strength, quality, purity, packaging, and labeling are recognized. These acts also recognized the standards of the USP's sister publication, the *National Formulary* (NF).

Today, the USP contains standards of identity, strength, quality, purity, packaging, and labeling for more than 3200 drug substances and products. With the incorporation of the NF in 1980, the standards for approximately 250 excipients (inert additives) were also included.

Manufacturer compliance with the combined USP–NF standards ensures that drug products (dosage forms) and their ingredients are of appropriate strength, quality, and purity, are properly packaged, and that the product labeling includes the names and amounts of active ingredients, expiration dates, and storage conditions.

In addition to the publications dealing with ingredients, there are also publications dealing with nomenclature (e.g., United States Approved Name (USAN) and USP *Dictionary of Drug Names*), information indexing (e.g., Index Medicus, National Library of Medicine), and information retrieval (e.g., computer-based Medical Literature Analysis and Retrieval System; MEDLARS and MEDLINE, National Library of Medicine).

There are also over 1500 medical journals and books published in the United States that comprise the primary (research publications), secondary (review articles), and tertiary (textbooks) literature. The pharmaceutical industry also supplies promotional material, often via "detail" persons. With the development of the Internet, vast amounts of drug-related information have become readily available to the general public. Governmental (e.g., NIH), commercial (e.g., Pharminfo), and individual's websites provide hard data as well as controversial platforms for alternative viewpoints regarding drugs.

Reasons for the proliferation of this resource material include the major role that drugs play in modern therapeutics; the considerable profitability associated with their sale; and problems associated with drug abuse. Millions of prescriptions are written every year for more than 700 active ingredients available in several thousand different pharmaceutical preparations. In addition, there are many thousands of OTC preparations.

CLASSIFICATION

In reading any of the above-described drug information sources you will find that drugs can be classified in many different ways, ranging from their chemical structure to the principal effect they produce, or the disease that they treat. Which method of classification used is usually dependent upon one's point of view. For example, the drug amphetamine could be classified in at least five different ways depending upon who was doing the classifying:

1   Physician: appetite-suppressing agent (anorexigenic)
2   Pharmacologist: sympathomimetic
3   Chemist: 2-amino-1-phenylpropane
4   Lawyer: drug of abuse falling in schedule II of the 1970 federal drug law
5   Psychologist: stimulant.

By analyzing the method of classification imposed upon a drug we can gain some insight into which of its characteristics is being emphasized by the classifier. However, there is an alternative classification system to those just described that can also be instructive. This system seeks to put drugs into four functionally distinct categories that divulge important distinctions about therapeutic and nontherapeutic principles. The four categories are listed below. More in-depth coverage is presented in Part 3.

1 *Drugs used to combat infection*. Drugs in this category are based on the concepts of selective toxicity and chemotherapy developed by Paul Ehrlich in the late nineteenth and early twentieth centuries. Ehrlich made the observation that the dye methylene blue specifically stained neural tissue but not any other. From this specific observation he generalized that some molecular characteristic of neural tissue conferred selectivity on the dye and that a similar situation might exist in foreign organisms, which could form the basis for selective chemotherapy.

Unfortunately, there are few pure examples of true selective toxicity. Perhaps the best is penicillin. The therapeutic specificity of this antibiotic is based upon the *qualitative* difference between bacterial cell wall synthesis and mammalian cell membrane synthesis. Synthesis of the former can be inhibited by penicillin while the latter is unaffected. Thus, penicillin is one of the few examples of a drug that can actually "cure" an illness. A similar example involves the sulfa drugs, which interfere with the synthesis of folic acid, used in nucleic acid formation, in bacteria. While bacteria must synthesize their own folic acid, mammalian cells utilize dietary, preformed folic acid and are not susceptible to interference with its formation.

2 *Drugs used to replace inadequacies of naturally occurring substances*. In an ideal sense this class of drugs represents the "purest" form of drug use in that they are

not "foreign" to the body. Examples include the use of hormones, such as insulin, in replacement therapy. Insulin is obviously an endogenous hormone and, if the human preparation is used, is exactly the same in all of us. The therapeutic goal in treating diabetes mellitus is to replace normal, physiological levels of insulin. The neurogenic chemical L-dopa can also be thought of in a similar manner since it is used to treat inadequate brain levels of dopamine in certain cases of parkinsonism. It must be understood, however, that if hormones are given in supraphysiological amounts they have the capacity to produce undesirable effects just as any xenobiotic does.

3 *Drugs that change regulation*. This group contains the largest total number of drugs used because they deal with the treatment of symptoms. Drugs used in this category do not cure, or replace, but can effectively manage acute or chronic disorders, often involving regulatory changes in the cardiovascular or nervous system, for example. Drugs in this category include antihypertensives, antianginals, diuretics, anticoagulants, analgesic and antipyretics, sedatives, anticonvulsants, and birth control pills.

4 *Drugs to alter mood or behavior*. This class includes relatively widely used licit, as well as illicit, drugs such as tranquilizers, alcohol, and tetrahydrocannabinol (THC, the active ingredient in marijuana). In addition, "hard" drugs such as cocaine, opiates, and hallucinogens are also included. This class of drugs is usually taken to change our perceptions of our environment and ourselves. They are often taken to relieve anxiety or to facilitate our involvement in certain social or "recreational" settings.

In addition to the variety of drug classification systems just described, a similar diversity, and somewhat bewildering array, of systems is used to name drugs during their development. This is because in the course of a drug's development, it usually acquires more than one identifying name. An example is the common drug aspirin:

1 *Chemical name*—A systematized and standardized nomenclature that encodes within the name descriptive information about the molecular constitution of the drug (e.g., 2-acetoxybenzoic acid).
2 *Trivial name*—A coined name in general use. It is a common name by which the drug is identified although it may not be intrinsically descriptive. There may be more than one trivial name (e.g., acetylsalicylic acid).
3 *Generic or established name*—A similar or contrived or coined name in general use. It usually refers to the U.S. name adopted by nomenclature groups known as the USAN and USP Committees. The generic or established names are trivial names but they have a somewhat more official status (e.g., aspirin).
4 *Trade name*—A brand or proprietary name; a legally registered trademark of a drug or dosage form of a drug. This name is the property of the registrant. There may be more than one trade name for a drug (e.g., Empirin™).

Before considering the pharmacology of any particular class of drugs, it is important to understand the basic underlying principles of drug action. The following two chapters in this section will deal with an important subject traditionally covered in the area of pharmacology known as pharmacokinetics (i.e., time-related factors such as absorption, distribution, metabolism, and excretion). Pharmacokinetics is the branch of pharmacology that is concerned with both the rates with which drug uptake and elimination proceed and with those processes that influence the time course of drug movement between one biological compartment and another.

The rates of absorption and distribution govern the time of onset of the drug's action; the rates of metabolism and excretion govern its duration; while the size of the dose, in combination with these effects, governs the intensity.

In addition to these fundamental aspects of drug action, the important area of drug interactions will be considered in Chapter 4. Although this subject does not require exhaustive coverage, it is important to appreciate its ramifications early in the study of pharmacotherapeutics since the coincidental administration of drugs can affect their respective pharmacokinetics. In some cases their interaction can be clinically significant.

THE PLACEBO EFFECT

Before we move on to the first "serious" topic of pharmacology it is necessary for at least a cursory consideration of the placebo. To the average pharmacologist this is really not an issue. However, for those of you who go on to be clinicians or, more specifically, clinical pharmacologists, the issue of a placebo effect will often have to be dealt with.

Briefly defined, a placebo is any treatment (including drugs, psychotherapy, quack therapy, and surgery) that achieves an ameliorative effect on a symptom or disease but that is in fact ineffective or is not specifically effective for the condition being treated. The good news is that this phenomenon can be taken advantage of in relieving the symptoms of certain patients. What types of patients? Many effective antianxiety drugs have been prescribed both knowingly and unknowingly at placebo dosages, for example. But how effective can this effect really be? Hundreds of studies have demonstrated the effectiveness of antidepressant drugs for the treatment of depression in a range of 45 to 80 percent—pretty impressive, until we realize that placebo effectiveness in depression is also high, ranging from 30 to 50 percent.

Placebos are effective for a variety of conditions. Patients with angina pectoris (insufficient blood flow to the heart) responded to placebo surgery in which surgeons made only an incision in the chest. And in a study of the drug propranolol that is used after heart attacks to prevent further damage, investigators noticed that patients who took placebo pills regularly had a lower death rate than patients who took placebos sporadically. Therefore, the placebo effect is not unique to psychiatric illness.

Conversely, what types of patients are not really amenable to a placebo effect? If you are a type I (insulin-dependent) diabetic (Chapter 9) who goes into hypoglycemic shock, a placebo effect will not help you. No matter how much you believe in whatever you are or are not taking, nothing will change the physiological dynamics between your circulating blood glucose level and your brain's extremely high need for this energy substrate.

Ideally, in clinical trials the placebo effect should be controlled for. If not, how can the investigator know if it is his/her company's NCE effectiveness or the patient's belief system? On the surface this seems rather straightforward—simply give a "sugar pill" and your problems are solved. But simply having an inert control is inadequate because it can often be detected. Color, shape, texture, dissolution rate, and taste are but a few of the parameters that can be discerned by humans.

ZOMBIES

Throughout this first chapter I have tried to emphasize the extremely wide diversity of drugs and their impact on the human scene. One of the most dramatic and bizarre examples of drug use is the putative creation of zombies. Article 240 of the Haitian penal code deals with zombie poison and prohibits the use of any substance that induces a lethargic coma "indistinguishable from death." Haitians do not fear zombies, they fear being turned into one.

According to one theory, victims are "converted" into a zombie in a two-step process. Initially, the intended victim is treated with the nerve toxin tetrodotoxin applied surreptitiously to an open wound. As the toxin does its work, the victim presents with all the symptoms of death. Often not realizing this error in diagnosis, the victim is placed in a coffin and buried. A day or two later, a priest (bokor) resurrects the highly traumatized victim, who is then forced to eat a strong dose of a plant called the zombie's cucumber (*Datura stramonium*), which brings on a state of disorientation and amnesia.

Tetrodotoxin is present in the puffer fish and is one of the most potent poisons known. It has been estimated to be more than 500 times more potent than cyanide. This makes the voluntary consumption of puffer fish all the more remarkable. In Japan, for example, puffer fish (fugu) is considered a culinary delicacy that requires preparation by specialized fugu chefs. Their job is to reduce the level of the toxin so that the meal is not fatal but retains enough of the toxin to produce some of its effects. These include a mild numbing or tingling of the tongue and lips, sensations of warmth, a flushing of the skin, and a general feeling of euphoria. If the dose is too high, difficulty in breathing occurs and a coma-like state develops. In some cases, people have seemed to have died, and been declared clinically dead, only to rise from the examining table.

SELECTED BIBLIOGRAPHY

Bowman, W. C. (1979) Drugs ancient and modern. *Scot. Med. J.* 24: 131–140.
Brown, W. A. (1998) The placebo effect. *Sci. Am.* 90: 90–95.
Davis, W. (1997) *The Serpent and the Rainbow*. Carmichael: Touchstone Books.
Harvey, A. L. (ed.) (1993) *Drugs from Natural Products*. Chichester: Ellis Horwood Ltd.
Huang, K. C. (1993) *The Pharmacology of Chinese Herbs*. Boca Raton, FL: CRC Press.
Mann, J. (1992) *Murder, Magic, and Medicine*. New York: Oxford University Press.
McKenna, T. (1992) *Food of the Gods*. New York: Bantam Books.
Midgley, J. M. (1988) Drug development: from sorcery to science. *Pharm. J.* 241: 358–365.
Moore, M. (1979) *Medicinal Plants of the Moutain West*. Santa Fe: The Museum of New Mexico Press.
Ross, A. and Robins, D. (1989) *The Life and Death of a Druid Prince*. New York: Touchstone.

Rouhi, A. M. (1997) Seeking drugs in natural products. *Chem. Eng. News* 75: 14–30.

Shapiro, A. K. and Shapiro, E. (1997) *The Powerful Placebo*. Baltimore: The Johns Hopkins University Press.

Suffness, M. (ed.) (1995) *Taxol® Science and Applications*. Boca Raton, FL: CRC Press.

QUESTIONS

1 Which of the following individuals is credited with the first synthesis of an organic compound (urea)?
   a John Jacob Abel
   b Oswald Schmiedeberg
   c Friedrich Worler
   d Francois Magendie
   e Claude Bernard.

2 Which of the following is credited with isolating the first pure drug (morphine)?
   a Friedrich Worler
   b Sertürner
   c Paul Ehrlich
   d Paracelsus
   e William Withering.

3 Man's first experience with pharmacology was the result of which of the following?
   a dreams
   b word of mouth
   c ancient material medica
   d food
   e observing animals.

4 Which of the following statements are true regarding pharmacology?
   a it is an integrative discipline
   b pharmacological effects can be studied *in vitro* and *in vivo*
   c the word pharmacology is believed to be derived from the French word drogue
   d drug effects are mediated by naturally occurring processes in the body
   e all of the above.

5 Drugs play a role in which of the following?
   a sports
   b religion
   c politics
   d the judicial system
   e all of the above.

6 Which of the following apply to a shaman?
   a a fraud
   b a priest-doctor

   c   can employ hallucinogenic drugs
   d   generally works for Western drug companies
   e   both b and c above.

7 The first department of pharmacology in the world is generally associated with which of the following universities?
   a   University of Michigan
   b   Cambridge University
   c   Montpelier University
   d   University of Dorpat
   e   Oxford University.

8 Which of the following is concerned with the study of drug absorption, distribution, metabolism, and excretion?
   a   pharmacodynamics
   b   pharmacokinetics
   c   pharmacotherapeutics
   d   pharmacoepidemiology
   e   pharmacoeconomics.

9 Extracts from which of the following were believed to confer the gift of flight?
   a   mistletoe
   b   tobacco
   c   tomatoes
   d   thorn apple
   e   cannabis.

10 Which of the following produces a steroid precursor that was used in the synthesis of progesterone?
   a   mistletoe
   b   coca plant
   c   North American potatoes
   d   Southwestern mushrooms
   e   Mexican yam.

Chapter 2

Absorption and distribution

BACKGROUND

As mentioned in Chapter 1, our species' earliest experience with "drug effects" occurred unintentionally, as a result of intentionally eating plants for nourishment. Obviously, these effects would have to be classified as "side effects," of sorts, since obtaining nutritive value was, of course, the real goal. Nevertheless, this paradigm illustrates an important principle in pharmacology—that drugs are usually substances that are chemically foreign to the body (i.e., xenobiotics). Therefore, because they are produced in plants (be they botanical or pharmaceutical), they usually have to gain entrance *into* the body in order to produce an effect, the exception being those that produce a topical (skin) effect.

Today, there are a number of methods that can be used to introduce a drug into the body. Because of its convenience, the most common delivery system is the oral route. However, sometimes the oral route is not the most appropriate. In addition to the oral route, some of the alternative routes of drug administration with the oldest history include, not surprisingly, inhalation, and, surprisingly, rectal and vaginal, as illustrated by the following examples.

Upon landing in the New World, members of Columbus's crew described natives on the island of present-day Cuba who inserted burning roles of leaves (called tobaccos) into their nostrils and "drank the smoke." The crew quickly took up this practice and the custom was subsequently introduced into Europe upon their return. Nicotine was a runaway success in Europe for many reasons, not the least of which was the belief that it would increase libido. Nicotine was not the first drug taken for this reason and will not be the last. Inhalation proved to be an extremely efficient method for conveying nicotine into the human body in order to obtain its alleged aphrodisiac effect.

Today, the advantage of inhalation as a therapeutic route of drug administration is utilized for the concentrated localization of certain drugs within the tracheobronchiolar region of the airway. For example, ipratropium and cromolyn are drugs used in the treatment of asthma. However, they are poorly absorbed from the intestine when they are taken orally. Therefore, they are essentially devoid of therapeutic effectiveness when taken by this route. Fortunately, when these drugs are given by inhalers for the treatment of asthma, they are effective in many patients. The large surface area of the terminal alveoli also permits rapid absorption of drugs other than antiasthmatics, such as "crack" cocaine and gaseous anesthetics.

Drug companies around the world are now exploring the possibility of having patients inhale their medicines. Their hope is that tiny particles inhaled deeply into the lung will cross through the thin epithelial cells lining the alveoli into the bloodstream and then make their way to their intended destination. Clinical trials are already under way with inhaled formulations of currently marketed drugs including insulin, morphine, and drugs to fight osteoporosis. As mentioned earlier, asthmatics have long used inhalers to deliver bronchodilators such as albuterol. In 1994, Genentech began marketing the first aerosol-delivered protein, a recombinant form of the natural human enzyme deoxyribonuclease that degrades excess DNA that accumulates in the lungs of patients suffering from cystic fibrosis.

Unfortunately, the current devices for delivering drugs to the lungs, used primarily for asthma medications, are too inefficient at delivering their cargo to make them economically viable for more than a handful of products. These devices, called nebulizers (which deliver drugs in a water-based mist) and metered-dose inhalers (in which the drug is suspended in a propellant), only manage to get approximately 5–10 percent of the drug from the inhaler into the lungs. The nature of the propellent system and the particle size of the drug are prime determinants. For example, particles less than 1 μm in diameter favor coalescence while those of diameter greater than 5 μm tend to be physically trapped due to the architecture of the airway.

The utility of alternate routes for drug administration is not a new phenomenon. The ancient Maya and Peruvians (AD 600–800), for example, employed enemas for drug delivery. The exact nature of the drugs used is unknown, but may have included tobacco, a fermented beverage called *balche*, and morning glory seeds. In Europe, the Danish physician Thomas Bartholin recommended, in 1661, the use of tobacco-juice and tobacco-smoke enemas as purgatives (i.e., to induce vomiting). Delivery of smoke was via pipes specifically designed for this purpose.

Ancient Egyptians used vaginal inserts containing honey mixed with lint as contraceptive devices, while an eighteenth-century French physician named Buc'hoz advocated the use of intravaginal insufflation of tobacco smoke to cure hysteria. These examples illustrate the degree to which our species will go to introduce drugs into the body. In this regard, nicotine has probably been delivered into the body by more routes than any other drug (e.g., oral, nasal, inhalation, vaginal, rectal, and topical).

Because the oral route is basically passive and relatively time-consuming, more direct routes now allow us to inject directly (i.e., intravenously) or indirectly (i.e., intramuscularly or subcutaneously) into the circulatory system. Administration via these routes was facilitated by the invention of the hypodermic syringe, credited to the Scotsman Alexander Wood in 1853, althoug archeological research during the eighteenth century has uncovered medical items that look remarkably similar to the syringe. Before this invention, physicians had used creative devices such as the hollow stems of the lilac plant to introduce drugs into the body. Today, more subtle technologies have been developed for facilitating the movement of drugs across the skin (e.g., transdermal patches and iontophoresis). Traditionally, the principal routes of administration have been divided into two major classes: *enteral*, which refers to the gastrointestinal tract, and *parenteral*, which indicates other than the gastrointestinal tract.

Considerable research in recent years has successfully yielded drug preparations that can also be given intranasally (e.g., calcitonin for osteoporosis) or by inhalation (e.g., bronchodilators for asthmatics). A more complete list of possible routes of drug

Table 2.1 Possible routes of drug administration

Oral	Sublingual
Intravenous	Rectal
Intramuscular	Topical
Subcutaneous	Intravaginal
Inhalation	Intranasal
Intra-arterial	Subarachnoid

administration is presented in Table 2.1. However, we will concern ourselves only with the principal routes of administration. An important point to remember is that all these routes vary in terms of influencing a drug's onset of action.

THE ORAL ROUTE

The human body can be basically thought of as a container of water (a polar medium) within which various aqueous compartments are separated by lipid membranes that contain both polar and nonpolar components. The oral route is, for most drugs, the most desirable route for administration into the body because of the ease of self-administration. However, oral agents must be able to withstand the acidic environment of the stomach and must permeate the gut lining (a mucousal membrane) before entering the bloodstream.

In general, drugs must traverse biological membranes in order to gain access to the circulatory system and, hence, distribution throughout the body. The facility with which a chemical crosses these membranes is a major determinant in estimating rates of absorption and subsequent distribution, and in the eventual pharmacological effect of the drug. This is particularly important for drugs that must cross the mucosal lining of the gastrointestinal (GI) tract. In order to gain some insight into the factors that affect the passage of xenobiotics, such as drugs, across biological membranes in the body, we should have some appreciation of important membrane characteristics that can influence drug absorption, particularly in the GI tract.

The conventional model developed to explain cell membrane characteristics influencing drug permeability is routinely referred to as the fluid-mosaic model (Figures 2.1 and 2.2). In this model the main components, for our purposes, are a phospholipid (e.g., sphingomyelin and phosphatidylcholine) bilayer (8 nm), with polar moieties at both the external and internal surfaces, and with proteins periodically traversing the phospholipid plane perpendicularly.

The bilayer forms because of the physicochemical properties of the phospholipid constituents and their interaction with water. The round "head" regions depicted in the figure are polar because they contain charged phosphate, choline, and ethanolamine groups. However, the tail regions are the predominant component and consist of nonpolar fatty acyl chains. Because orientation of polar groups is favored toward other polar groups, such as water, the bilayer is oriented both inward and outward toward extracellular and intracellular water, respectively. This architecture forms a diffusion barrier that is almost impermeable to charged (polar) molecules and ions attempting to move in either direction.

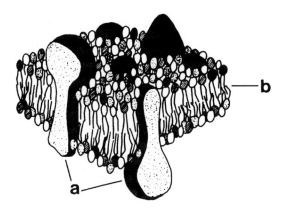

Figure 2.1 The three-dimensional structure of the animal cell membrane. Proteins (a) are interspersed in the phospholipid bilayer (b).

Source: J. A. Timbrell (1995), *Introduction to Toxicology*, 2nd ed. London: Taylor & Francis.

Figure 2.2 The molecular arrangement of the cell membrane: a, integral proteins; b, glycoprotein; c, pore formed from integral protein; d, various phospholipids with saturated fatty acid chains; e, phospholipid with unsaturated fatty acid chains; f, network proteins; g, cholesterol; h, glycolipid; i, peripheral protein. There are four different phospholipids: phosphatidyl serine; phosphatidyl choline; phosphatidyl ethanolamine; sphingomyelin represented respectively as $\bigcirc$; $\circledcirc$; $\oslash$; $\bullet$. The stippled area of the protein represents the hydrophobic portion.

Source: J. A. Timbrell (1995), *Introduction to Toxicology*, 2nd ed. London: Taylor & Francis.

The lipid layer favors uptake of nonpolar compounds (lipophilic; having an affinity for fat), while certain globular proteins embedded in the membrane form aqueous pores or channels, which allow penetration of small polar substances (hydrophilic; having an affinity for water) such as ethanol or ions such as those of sodium chloride.

However, the ordered structure of the phospholipid membrane is not highly conducive to the presence of numerous pores. Therefore, high lipid solubility is a predominant characteristic that favors membrane absorption of a chemical. It is an important feature for oral absorption into the body as well as for distribution within the body, since the body is basically a series of polar, aqueous media chambers separated by phospholipid barriers containing polar groups.

Molecules that do not contain electrical charges (uncharged) or whose electron distribution is not distorted (nonpolar) are compatible with the nonpolar region of cell membranes. For charged or polar molecules, the aqueous pores that exist within the protein channels can provide an alternate route. These pores allow the passage of some poorly lipid-soluble nonelectrolytes, as well as some charged molecules. However, they must be low in molecular weight.

Transmission of extracellular signals to the cell interior is based on receptor-induced recruitment and assembly of proteins into signaling complexes at the inner leaflet of the plasma membrane. Protein–protein and protein–lipid interactions play a crucial role in the process in which molecular proximity in specially formed membrane subdomains provides the special and temporal constraints that are required for proper signaling. The phospholipid bilayer is not merely a passive hydrophobic medium for this assembly process, but is also a site where the lipid and the protein components are enriched by a dynamic process (see Chapter 5).

TRANSMEMBRANE PROCESSES

Transmembrane movement of a chemical can occur by several processes including: (1) *passive diffusion* through the membrane phospholipid according to Fick's law (rate of passage is directly proportional to the concentration gradient, the surface area of the membrane, and the partition coefficient of the chemical, and inversely proportional to membrane thickness). Therefore, a concentration gradient must exist and the xenobiotic must be lipid soluble and nonionized; (2) *filtration* of small molecules through pores in the membrane protein, also down a concentration gradient; (3) *active transport* of a select group of molecules—requires a specific membrane carrier and the expenditure of metabolic energy. Because of these requirements, the process can be inhibited by metabolic poisons, is saturable, and the carrier sites subject to competition from other chemicals. However, active transport can occur against a concentration gradient; (4) *facilitated diffusion*—also utilizes a specific membrane carrier (saturable) and requires a concentration gradient but no energy expenditure is required; (5) *phagocytosis* and *pinocytosis*—involve the invagination of part of the membrane to enclose a particle or droplet, respectively, that might contain a drug.

PARTITION COEFFICIENT

Because lipid solubility is so important for transmembrane movement of a drug, attempts have been made over the years to assess this characteristic as a predictor of drug activity. Perhaps the most useful method employs a simple relationship referred

Table 2.2 Relationship of oil/water partition coefficient to drug absorption

Drug	Partition coefficient	Percent absorbed
Barbital	0.7	12
Aprobarbital	4.9	17
Phenobarbital	4.8	20
Cyclobarbital	11.7	24
Pentobarbital	28.0	30
Secobarbital	50.7	40

to as the oil/water partition coefficient. The coefficient may be obtained relatively easily by adding the drug to a mixture of equal volumes of a nonpolar medium (e.g., an organic aliphatic alcohol such as octanol) and a polar medium (water). The mixture is then agitated (usually with a mechanical shaking device) until equilibrium is reached, whereupon the phases are separated and assayed for the drug. The greater the partition coefficient of a drug (i.e., the greater the concentration in the organic phase), the more lipid soluble the drug. This principle is illustrated in Table 2.2 for a number of structurally related barbiturates.

Comparing the lipophilicity of the barbiturates in Table 2.2 with their uptake across the GI tract (colon) demonstrates that the membrane permeability of each member of the series is proportional to its partition coefficient. Apparently, there can be some differential effect on partitioning depending upon which organic solvent is used in making the determination. For example, the GI membrane is believed to behave more like an octanol/water pairing, while drug uptake into the brain is more closely mimicked by a heptane/water combination.

ADDITIONAL MAJOR FACTORS AFFECTING ABSORPTION

Within the GI tract, the major anatomical absorption site is the upper small intestine because of its huge surface area (e.g., 500–1000 times that of the stomach; Figure 2.3 and Table 2.3). In addition to surface area, other important factors include drug solubility (drugs must dissolve before absorption), particle size, contact time with the absorption surface, membrane integrity, and hydrogen ion concentration (pH). Materials that are insoluble or only slightly soluble in both polar and nonpolar media are pharmacologically inert. For example, barium sulfate is a highly toxic material if absorbed into the body. However, because of its poor solubility in the GI tract, it can be swallowed and used as a contrast medium for radiography in this region without toxicological hazard.

THE EFFECT OF pH

Hydrogen ion concentration (pH) has particular relevance to drug absorption since approximately 75 percent of all clinically utilized drugs can behave as either weak

Figure 2.3 The mammalian gastrointestinal tract showing important features of the small intestine, the major site of absorption for orally administered compounds: a, liver; b, stomach; c, duodenum; d, ileum; e, colon; f, longitudinal section of the ileum showing folding which increases surface area; g, detail of fold showing villi with circular and longitudinal muscles, h and i respectively, bounded by the serosal membrane, j; k, detail of villi showing network of capillaries, m, lacteals, n, and epithelial cells, l; o, detail of epithelial cells showing brush border or microvilli, p. The folding, vascularization, and microvilli all facilitate absorption of substances from the lumen.

Source: J. A. Timbrell (1995), *Introduction to Toxicology*, 2nd ed. London: Taylor & Francis.

Table 2.3 Relative size of the absorptive surface of various parts of the gastrointestinal tract

Oral cavity	0.02
Stomach	0.1–0.2
Small intestine	100
Large intestine	0.5–1.0
Rectum	0.04–0.07

acids or weak bases (i.e., they can take up or release a hydrogen ion and become charged, polar entities). As mentioned earlier, uncharged molecules are compatible with the lipid environment of cellular membranes. Therefore, acidic and basic drugs are preferentially absorbed in their nonionized form, the proportion of which exists at any moment being pH dependent.

Calculations regarding the influence of pH upon the ionization of weak acids and bases may be solved by applying the Henderson–Hasselbalch equation ($pH - pK_a = \log[base/acid]$), which may be familiar to you from taking a class in biochemistry.

This equation essentially describes the relationship between pH and the degree of ionization of weak acids and bases. When applied to drugs, the equation tells us that when pH equals the apparent equilibrium dissociation constant of the drug (pK_a), 50 percent of the drug will be in the unionized form and 50 percent will be in the ionized form (i.e., log[base/acid] = 0 and antilog of 0 = 1, or unity). Application of the Henderson–Hasselbalch equation can, therefore, allow one to mathematically determine the exact proportion of ionized and nonionized species of a drug in a particular body compartment if the pK_a of the drug and the pH of the local environment are known.

The general effect of pH on the degree of ionization of a drug can be determined in a straightforward manner by applying Le Chatelier's principle. This principle states that if the conditions of a system, originally in equilibrium, are changed, the new equilibrium shifts in such a direction as to restore the original conditions. When applying this principle to the effect of pH on drug ionization, the following relationships occur. For a weak acid, the dissociation equilibrium can be expressed as follows:

$$AH \leftrightarrow A^- + H^+$$

In this situation, if the hydrogen ion concentration increases (pH becomes lower), the reaction will be driven to the left by mass action (to the original condition), and the proportion of the drug in the nonionized form will increase and, hence, the number of lipid-soluble molecules. For example, if the pK_a of a weak acid is 5.0 and it is placed in a medium of pH 4.0, 90 percent will be in the unionized form. Therefore, weak acids are preferentially absorbed in a relatively acidic environment. For a weak base, the equilibrium dissociation constant can be expressed as follows:

$$BH^+ \leftrightarrow B + H^+$$

In this situation, if the hydrogen ion concentration increases, the proportion of drug in the ionized form (the original condition) increases. Therefore, consequences of a shift in pH away from equilibrium conditions are opposite for weak acids and weak bases. For example, a solution of the weak base dextromethorphan (a drug present in cough preparations with a pK_a of 9.2) in the stomach (pH 1) will have approximately 1 of every 160,000,000 molecules in the unionized form. Obviously, gastric absorption will be significantly curtailed.

As important as this pH effect is, it can be subordinated by other factors. For example, as indicated earlier, the absorptive area that a drug is exposed to can be a predominating factor. In this context, even though the acidic environment of the stomach favors the absorption of weak acids (e.g., acetylsalicylic acid), aspirin is still absorbed to a greater extent, in totality, in the small intestine. A partial list of the pH of several body compartments is shown in Table 2.4. The fact that there are some variations suggests that the disposition of some drugs may be differentially affected.

The oral route is, of course, the principal enteral route of drug administration. However, two other examples are worthy of note. First, the sublingual route (beneath the tongue) provides relatively good absorption because of its rich capillary bed; it is routinely used for the administration of nitroglycerin tablets in the treatment of

Table 2.4 Comparison of pH values in some human body compartments

Blood	7.35–7.45
Oral cavity	6.2–7.2
Stomach (at rest)	1.0–3.0
Duodenum	4.8–8.2
Jejunum	6.3–7.3
Ileum	7.6
Colon	7.8–8.0
Rectum	7.8
Cerebral fluid	7.3–7.4
Vagina	3.4–4.2
Urine	4.8–7.5
Sweat	4.0–6.8
Milk	6.6–7.0

angina pectoris. Because the stomach is bypassed, acid lability and gut permeability need not be considered. Second, the rectal route can be useful for unconscious or vomiting patients or small children.

Although the oral route is certainly the most convenient mode of drug delivery, it is not appropriate for all drugs or all situations. For example, administration of insulin by the oral route results in destruction of the hormone's physiological activity. This is because the proteinaceous nature of insulin renders it susceptible to degradation within the stomach due to the acidic environment as well as the presence of proteases. Therefore, insulin must be given by injection (note, however, that attempts are being made to develop new insulin preparations that can be given by other routes, e.g., intranasally, thus avoiding the necessity of repeated injections). Absorption from the GI tract is also relatively slow and may not be appropriate for an emergency situation. For these and other reasons, alternative routes of drug administration are often utilized.

INJECTION

As indicated in Table 2.1, drugs may be injected into veins, muscles, subcutaneous tissue, arteries, or into the subarachnoid space of the spinal canal (intrathecal). For obvious reasons, intraarterial and intrathecal injections are reserved for specialized drug administration requirements, such as regional perfusion of a tumor with a toxic drug or induction of spinal anesthesia, respectively. Therefore, the more routine injection routes are intravenous (IV), intramuscular (IM), and subcutaneous (SC). Because these three modalities involve skin puncture, they carry the risks of infection, pain, and local irritation.

Intravenous administration of a drug achieves rapid onset of drug action. For this reason IV lines are routinely established in many emergency rooms and inpatient situations (e.g., unconsciousness) in order to establish a "permanent" portal for drug injection. While IV injection achieves rapid action it also must be used with discretion for several reasons: (1) administration is irreversible; (2) if the rate of injection is too rapid the drug is delivered in more of a bolus form, thus presenting the heart and vascular system with a more concentrated "hit"; (3) severe allergic reactions may be particularly severe for the same reason; (4) accidental injection of air can form air emboli in the circulatory system; and (5) mixing certain drugs may cause a chemical interaction between them, such as precipitation (e.g., precipitation of sulfonamides by tetracyclines).

In addition to the factors listed above, IV drugs must also be delivered in a sterile medium and be free of insoluble material. Failure to respect these requirements can produce serious consequences. For example, it is well recognized that IV drug abusers are a population at particular risk for bacterial endocarditis, viral hepatitis, and AIDS. Fortunately, free-needle programs can significantly reduce the likelihood of cross-infections when implemented.

Drug abuse often involves attempts to "solubilize" oral medication for IV injection. This practice, with drugs such as amphetamine or cocaine, for example, can result in severe pulmonary injury. This is due to the inadvertent coadministration of insoluble talc (hydrous magnesium silicate) that is routinely present as a filler material in the original preparation manufactured for oral use. Because of their size, the insoluble talc particles (particularly in the 10–17 μm range) can become trapped in small blood vessels in the lung and serve as "foreign body" loci for connective tissue accumulation. Depending upon the quantity of talc deposited, patients will experience varying degrees of compromised lung function ranging from dyspnea (difficulty in breathing) to death.

Fortunately, not all drugs need to be injected intravenously. Common alternatives include IM and SC injections, which can provide depot sites for more prolonged entrance of drugs into the circulatory system. If a drug is given by either IM (directly into muscle) or SC (beneath the skin) injection, it passes through capillary walls to enter the bloodstream. The rate of absorption is influenced by several factors including the drug's formulation (oil-based preparations are absorbed slowly, aqueous preparations are absorbed rapidly) and regional blood flow.

For drugs deposited in the proximity of the peripheral capillary beds of muscle and subcutaneous tissue, lipid solubility is considerably less important than the oral route since even ionized forms of drugs are absorbed with relative ease. The capillary wall in these areas is of sufficient porosity that even drugs with molecular weights as great as 60,000 daltons may be absorbed by passive diffusion. This explains why a protein, such as insulin (5808 daltons), can be given subcutaneously and is absorbed into the bloodstream.

The rate and efficiency of drug absorption following IM or SC injection may be greater than, equal to, or less than that following oral administration, depending upon the drug under consideration. In addition, blood flow in the area of drug injection is a major determinant in the rate of drug absorption from both IM and SC sites. This fact can be utilized in altering the absorption of certain drugs. For example, local anesthetics are usually injected in combination with a vasoconstricting agent such as epinephrine. Epinephrine serves to elicit contraction of the vascular smooth muscle, achieving a reduction in both the absorptive surface area of the vessel and the blood flow through the area. The cumulative effect is that the local anesthetic remains in the proximity of the injection site (sensory nerve) for a longer period of time.

BIOAVAILABILITY

An important consequence of administering drugs by different routes is that there can be a difference in their bioavailability. Bioavailability refers to that fraction of a drug administered that gains access to the systemic circulation in an unchanged form. The standard of comparison in determining bioavailability, against which all other routes are compared, is the IV dose. In practice, drug serum or plasma levels are monitored at different time points following various routes of administration, such as oral, and the respective ratios of the area under the curve (AUC) are calculated:

$$\text{Bioavailability} = \text{AUC}_{oral}/\text{AUC}_{iv}$$

In Figure 2.4 the serum concentrations of three tablet forms of a drug are compared with its IV form. As you can see, tablets A and B have approximately the same bioavailability (AUC). Tablet C, on the other hand, has significantly less. Poor oral bioavailability can obviously influence a drug's ideal mode of delivery. It is because of poor oral bioavailability (approximately 25 percent) of heavily charged weak bases, such as the opiates (pK_a values in the range of 8.0–9.0), that heroin and morphine abusers resort to injection of the drugs to maximize their effects.

If drugs have the same bioavailability (i.e., the same AUC) they are said to be bioequivalent. This is a particularly important aspect in the development of generic drugs (discussed later). However, it should be appreciated that bioavailability refers ultimately to plasma concentration per se. It does not tell us anything about therapeutic

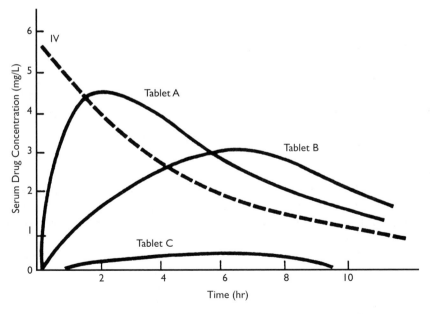

Figure 2.4 Comparative bioavailability of three oral forms of a drug. Reference is serum level of the drug administered in its intravenous (IV) form.

Source: Pharmacia and Upjohn, *Pharmacokinetics Applied to the Treatment of Asthma.* Reprinted with permission.

equivalence, which deals with comparable efficacy and safety (issues to be addressed in subsequent chapters).

Generic products tested by the FDA and determined to be therapeutic equivalents are listed by the FDA in their publication *Approved Drug Products with Therapeutic Equivalence Evaluations*. These products contain the same active ingredients as their brand-name counterparts and also meet bioequivalence standards. The FDA recommends substitution only among products listed as therapeutically equivalent.

Factors that can affect bioavailability include metabolism (to be discussed in more detail in Chapter 3), lipid solubility of the drug, chemical stability of the drug (e.g., penicillin G is unstable at gastric pH), and the nature of the drug formulation (i.e., particle size, salt form, presence of inert binders, etc.).

GENE THERAPY

After nearly 30 years of speculation, one of the most provocative avenues of "drug" administration currently receiving substantial interest and financial resources is the area of gene therapy. There are at least two different kinds of gene therapy—the choice of which to use depends on an assessment of the disease and the needs of the patient. In "traditional" replacement-gene therapy, a functional copy of the gene in question is administered to replace the faulty activity of the defective gene in question. Pharmacological-gene therapy transmits a gene not for replacement but for the production of a novel therapeutic product, essentially turning the patient's own cells into pharmaceutical manufacturing plants. To date, clinical research has focused on gene-replacement therapy.

One of the first patients to be treated with gene replacement was a 4-year-old girl in 1990. She was born with a defective gene for making the essential enzyme adenosine deaminase (ADA), which is vital for the function of the immune system. Since that time, hundreds of clinical trials (mostly phase I safety trials—see Part 4) have been started, dealing with single gene disorders such as cystic fibrosis, as well as acquired disorders such as cancer and AIDS. Clinical progress with acquired disorders seems to be occurring at a faster rate using gene addition as a greater diversity of approaches is possible.

This diversity of approaches in treating acquired illnesses is illustrated in the gene therapy strategies that have been proposed for treating AIDS and various cancers. Treatment of human immunodeficiency virus (HIV) infection could conceivably be based on the interruption of viral processes that contribute directly to the pathogenesis of AIDS. This could be achieved by several potential mechanisms, including inserting a gene that produces antisense mRNA or ribozymes (see Chapter 13 for more information), or a dominant negative mutant protein.

There are many reasons why gene therapy has not proven to be straightforward. Challenges to be dealt with include: Is it the right form of the gene to solve the specific disease problem? Is the gene product stable enough to act as a replacement for the missing or aberrant "natural product"? What is the most effective promoter to get the new gene to express properly (in time, space, and amount)? Finally, how does one get the introduced gene to breach the numerous membrane barriers and other defense mechanisms that have evolved to keep out foreign genetic material?

Vectors

Although all of the notoriety of gene therapy rests in finding prospective genetic solutions to various diseases, the pedestrian issue of safe and effective transport and delivery of genetic "magic bullets" can make or break a therapeutic protocol. Therefore, creating an efficacious gene or gene product depends on the development of a corresponding carrier, i.e., the appropriate vector.

A major challenge in gene therapy is to find safe vectors capable of transporting genes efficiently into target cells and getting these target cells to express the genes once inserted. The most commonly used retrovirus vectors are based on Moloney murine leukemia virus (MMLV), which can infect mouse and human cells. Inactivated versions of this retrovirus have been loaded with genes and used in approximately 40 percent of human trials to date.

Although this murine retrovirus is relatively easy to make and use, retroviruses insert genes only into cells that are actively dividing and growing and possess, therefore, some theoretical danger of eliciting tumor formation. For these reasons, retroviruses have been used in ex vivo procedures such as ADA deficiency. For example, in the case of the 4-year-old girl mentioned earlier, a sample of her blood was removed, T lymphocytes were isolated from it, the gene for ADA was inserted into the cells via a retrovirus, and the cells reinfused into her body.

Attempts to obviate the limitations of retrovirus vectors include the use of alternative virus vectors such as adeno-associated viruses (now used in approximately 20 percent of clinical trials) and lentiviruses, as well as nonviral vectors such as plasmid-based vectors, either alone, in combination with liposomes, or linked to a ligand. Other, more theoretical, strategies proposed involve the creation of a "human artificial chromosome." In this case, a 25th chromosome containing "suites" of genes would, it is hoped, be introduced into the nucleus of a target cell.

In the final analysis, it is likely that no universal vector will be found to be appropriate for all situations.

The future

Although the potential therapeutic benefits of gene therapy appear to be great, it remains to be seen how successful attempts will be to overcome present problems. These problems include the need to develop improved gene transfer methodology and reduced vector antigenicity as well as the appreciation of new pharmacokinetic paradigms. For example, with in vivo gene transfer, it will be necessary to account for the fate of the DNA vector itself (e.g., volume of distribution, clearance rate, etc.), as well as determining the consequences of altered gene expression and protein function.

In addition to the challenges of gene transfer and expression, there are also potential adverse consequences that could occur as a result of gene transfer. These include immunological responses to both the newly transcribed protein and to the vector itself. The death in 1999 of an 18-year-old boy (the first reported death from gene therapy) being treated for a deficiency of ornithine transcarbamylase has been ascribed to an immunological response to the massive doses of an adenovirus vector that are needed in clinical trials. Furthermore, a state of replication defectiveness must be maintained in the vector to protect against the potential inherent pathogenicity of the carrier.

To date, clinical trials of gene therapy have shown little evidence of positive therapeutic effects. An NIH report in 1995 indicated that all the "vectors" used so far to transfer genes into target cells were inefficient with a "very low" rate of gene transfer. In addition, the same report concluded that gene therapists and their sponsors were "overselling" the technology and that there should have been less hype and more emphasis on good biology.

Despite these disappointing results and the increasing awareness of the limitations of gene therapy, pharmaceutical companies have invested nearly $1 billion in gene biotechnology companies since the summer of 1995. Research firms have estimated that the market for gene therapy treatments will generate between $2 billion and $3 billion in worldwide revenues early in the new millennium. In addition, current NIH funding for gene therapy will remain at approximately $200 million per year.

Perhaps the most significant cause for renewed enthusiasm for gene therapy lies in the results of two phase I studies reported in 2000. In a phase I gene transfer trial for hemophilia B, "significant reduction in whole blood clotting times was observed in patients for several months after receiving intramuscular administration of the lowest dose of a recombinant adeno-associated virus expressing the human coagulation factor IX gene." In another study, patients who received autologous transplants of bone marrow stem cells transformed *in vitro* using an MMLV-derived vector containing the complement to the normal gene for X-linked SCID (bubble-boy syndrome) have "reconstituted their immune systems for up to one year and the children are now living normally with their families."

DISTRIBUTION

After a drug is administered to the body it goes through various phases of distribution. If we were to make periodic plasma measurements of a drug following its administration, its plasma profile would be a composite of various dynamic processes serving to increase or decrease its concentration. The processes of distribution can be considered in terms of *compartments*.

Absorption of a drug into the theoretical central or main compartment may be followed by distribution into one or more peripheral compartments, or the drug may undergo excretion or metabolism from the central compartment. While compartmental analysis of drug distribution can be informative, it is beyond the scope of this book. For more details on the effect of multicompartmental distribution of a drug on pharmacokinetics, see references in the Bibliography.

With the exception of the more complicated aspects of gene delivery methodologies described earlier, after a drug is absorbed into the systemic circulation via a conventional route of administration it is basically transported throughout the body either free or bound to plasma proteins. In order for a drug to reach its site of action, it must leave the bloodstream. Drug permeability occurs largely in the capillary bed, where both surface area and contact time are maximal due to extensive vascular branching and low velocity of flow. However, capillary beds in different organs vary in their penetrability (i.e., pore size between adjacent endothelial cells). For example, the liver capillary bed is "leaky" while brain is not.

Before steady state is reached (when the concentrations of drug in all body compartments are constant), distribution is principally dependent upon blood flow.

Table 2.5 Tissue perfusion (percent of cardiac output in the human)

Brain	14.0
Heart	3.3
Kidney	22.0
Liver	26.5
Viscera	30.0
Adipose tissue	4.7

Source: Data derived from U.S. Environmental Protection Agency, Reference Physiological Parameters in Pharmacokinetic Modeling, A. D. Arms and C. C. Travis, Office of Risk Analysis, EPA No. 600/6-88/004, 1988.

In fact, the fraction of drug that can diffuse into a specific organ is proportional to the blood flow into that organ. A comparison of organ perfusion is shown in Table 2.5. Tissues that are highly perfused, such as kidneys, liver, heart, and brain, are therefore promptly exposed to a drug. A useful concept in drug distribution is referred to as the apparent volume of distribution (V_d) of a drug. It is defined as:

V_d = total drug dose (mg)/plasma concentration at equilibrium (mg/ml)

Therefore, V_d is the apparent fluid volume, usually expressed in milliliters or liters, in which the drug is dissolved. Values of V_d compatible with the known volume of a body compartment may suggest that the drug is confined to that compartment. Values of V_d greater than the total body volume of water indicate that the drug is concentrated in a tissue compartment.

Many lipid-soluble drugs are stored in body fat, for example, which can range from 10 to 50 percent of body weight. Therefore, fat can serve as an important reservoir for highly lipid-soluble drugs. This can have important implications for the distribution and time course of drug action. It has been shown, for example, that 3 hours after the intravenous administration of the short-acting barbiturate thiopental, 70 percent of the dose can be found in the fatty tissues, thus contributing to the rapid termination of its action.

Another example of the effect of fat storage on a drug is provided by THC, the psychoactive component in *Cannabis sativa*. THC is quite lipid soluble (hence its ability to affect the brain and be stored in adipose tissue). It is released very slowly from fat cells, which explains why it can have a lingering effect and can be detected in the urine many days following a single exposure. The potential liability of this pharmacokinetic fact is obvious in this era of workplace drug testing. A person could test positive for urinary THC, as it slowly equilibrates out of adipose tissue, without being under its influence. Conversely, rapid weight loss (i.e., fat reduction) could also result in accelerated release of THC.

Some relevant volumes of body compartments are (in liters): plasma water (3), erythrocyte water (3), extracellular water excluding blood (11), and intracellular water (24). The total body water is approximately 41 L. A comparison of selected drugs with apparent volumes of distribution (in liters) approximating various body compartments is shown in Table 2.6.

Table 2.6 Comparison of apparent volumes of distribution (liters)

Acetylsalicylic acid	11
Amoxicillin	29
Captopril	40
Chloroquine	13,000

It should be noted that percent body water varies between infants and adults. Infants possess approximately 77 percent body water and adults approximately 58 percent. Conversely, the elderly have a lower percent body water. This can have significant implications in terms of drug clearance (see Chapter 3).

In certain cases of drug distribution there can be advantageous cellular selectivity. For example, tetracyclines, organic arsenicals, griseofulvin, and cyanocobalamin (vitamin B_{12}) concentrate in bacteria, trypanosomes, fungi, and bone marrow, respectively. The antimalarial drug chloroquine also concentrates outside of the plasma, localizing in parasitic protozoans. This aspect of chloroquine's pharmacokinetics explains its therapeutic usefulness as well as an apparent volume of distribution in excess of 10,000 L. This value is obviously a physiological impossibility and therefore represents only a mathematical concept. Many drugs have very large distribution volumes because they are highly bound to tissue proteins. However, the site of concentration within the body is not necessarily a drug's target organ.

If a drug passes through cell membranes but is not taken up into any particular cells, it will be evenly distributed throughout the total body water when equilibrium is reached. It will therefore have a volume of distribution of about 41 L. A prime example of such a drug is ethanol.

After arriving at a particular organ, the free, unbound form of the drug is able to cross first the endothelial cells of the capillaries into the interstitial space, and subsequently the cellular membrane of the tissue. Capillary permeability is largely determined by (1) capillary structure and (2) the chemical nature of the drug. The membrane-related factors influencing distribution of drugs between blood plasma and tissues are essentially the same as those described previously between the GI tract and blood plasma.

CHIRALITY

To this point, various physicochemical properties of drugs such as lipophilicity, ionization, and partition coefficient have been discussed. While these are certainly major factors, there is an additional factor that can influence drug distribution, namely chirality. Chirality is a relatively unique structural characteristic of certain molecules that can exist in two asymmetric, nonsuperimposable isomers (enantiomers) due to the presence of a chiral center (a carbon atom that is attached to four different functional groups (see Chapters 5 and 13).

Chirality does not really become a significant factor unless enantioselectivity exists in processes such as active transport. The distribution of a drug can be markedly affected by its ability to bind to plasma proteins since only a free drug is able to cross cell membranes and the blood–brain barrier. The plasma proteins to which drugs bind are enantioselective and the fraction of the free, active drug can be widely different between the enantiomers of highly protein-bound drugs such as ibuprofen and warfarin (50 percent) in each case.

BLOOD–BRAIN BARRIER

In the periphery, capillary walls are generally quite porous depending upon the area (e.g., liver > kidney > muscle > brain). Most drugs, whether ionized or not, are able to pass through gaps (fenestrations) between endothelial cells and within the basement membrane. An important exception to this, however, is the central nervous system (CNS; brain and spinal cord), where capillary endothelial cells are tightly packed adjacent to each other, precluding the existence of gaps, and are closely associated with astrocytes. Therefore, in the CNS, as in the GI tract, drug absorption is also significantly influenced by its lipophilicity (i.e., its state of ionization and polarity).

The result of this anatomical characteristic of endothelial cells in the CNS is an increased resistance to water-soluble and ionized drugs entering the brain, and cerebrospinal fluid (CSF), from capillary blood. However, in a few areas of the brain the barrier is absent. These areas include the lateral nuclei of the hypothalamus, the area postrema of the fourth ventricle, the pineal body, and the posterior lobe of the hypophysis. Highly lipophilic compounds can cross the barrier. Tranquilizers such as diazepam and its analogs are known to gain access rapidly to the CSF with a half-life ($t^{1/2}$) entry time of less than 1 minute.

In addition to the more tightly packed endothelial cells in CNS capillaries, the capillaries are also surrounded by glial cells (astrocytes), which form an additional sheath surrounding the capillary network. The CNS, therefore, has two protective barriers between free drug and brain tissue. This membrane complex is referred to as the blood–brain barrier or the blood–CSF barrier. Under normal circumstances it is quite effective. However, if the barrier membranes become inflamed, a wider range of substances can pass through because of the development of "leaky" pores. In addition, this barrier is incompletely developed at birth, so neonates are less protected against drugs gaining access to the CNS.

PLACENTAL TRANSFER

A relatively unique but particularly significant aspect of drug distribution is the placental transfer of drugs from the maternal circulation into that of the fetus. Any xenobiotic that gains access to the maternal circulation should be considered capable of crossing the placenta unless demonstrated to the contrary. In general, lipophilic, unionized, low-molecular-weight drugs in their unbound form tend to cross the placenta. Although the human placenta contains some detoxification enzymes (see Chapter 3) responsible for oxidation, reduction, hydrolysis, and conjugation, their capacity is extremely limited and they do not contribute significantly to drug clearance.

A number of drugs are known to have adverse or teratogenic effects on the developing fetus. The most infamous, of course, is thalidomide (a sedative used during the early 1960s). Thalidomide was manufactured in the former West Germany and was used by millions of people in 46 nations before it was discovered that it caused birth defects during the first trimester of pregnancy. This is the period of gestation when the developing fetus is most susceptible to teratogenic effects and a single dose of thalidomide at the right/wrong time was sufficient to produce its effect.

Specifically, thalidomide produced a characteristic stunting of limb bud tissue, apparently due to interference with normal vascularization. The result was the development of a relatively unique syndrome known as phocomelia. At least 10,000 children, most of them German, were born with "flippers" instead of arms or legs. Unfortunately, some thalidomide babies are still being born in South America where the drug continues to be manufactured and many people are unaware of its proper uses (it is used fairly extensively for treating certain skin lesions in leprosy patients).

Despite thalidomide's embryotoxicity it is relatively nontoxic in other contexts. Therefore, research projects are currently under way, or proposed, to investigate thalidomide's possible use in cancer patients because of its presumed antiangiogenesis and immune-modulating effects. In addition, some AIDS patients have also reported that thalidomide seems to provide some relief for their rapid weight loss and possibly provides relief for mouth ulcers.

ETHANOL

At the present time there are several contemporary drugs that pose particular dangers to the developing fetus because of the relative prevalence of their use and their distribution across the placenta. These include alcohol, tobacco, and cocaine.

As mentioned earlier, ethanol distributes within total body water. This includes the body water of a developing fetus. Maternal consumption of ethanol is, therefore, a major cause of birth defects today, with its maximal expression being the fetal alcohol syndrome (FAS). FAS is characterized by (1) growth retardation, (2) CNS abnormalities, and (3) a particular pattern of craniofacial abnormalities. The minimal amount of maternally consumed ethanol needed to elicit the syndrome is controversial. However, consumption of at least 165 grams per week or 1 ounce per day is generally accepted as sufficient to generate abnormalities. Not surprisingly, the fetus is particularly sensitive to binge drinking, where blood levels can reach devastating amounts and exceed the mother's capacity to inactivate it (see Chapter 3). The fetotoxic effects of ethanol are probably mutifactorial. However, restricted placental blood supply is a possible cause mediated by the release of prostaglandins resulting in fetal hypoxia.

TOBACCO

Concern regarding the exposure of pregnant women to tobacco dust and smoke has existed since at least the middle of the nineteenth century. During the subsequent years many studies have reported the association of cigarette smoking with numerous problems of pregnancy. One of the most important observations in experimental animals was reported in 1940. In this study it was found that the young of nicotine-treated as well as tobacco-smoke-exposed rats were underweight compared to those of control rats. This observation was confirmed in 1957. In general, babies of pregnant women who smoke are 200 grams lighter than babies born to comparable pregnant women who are nonsmokers. In addition to lower birthweight, smoking increases prematurity, spontaneous abortion, and prenatal mortality.

The fetotoxic causative agent(s) in tobacco is(are) not known with certainty. One of the reasons for this is that a lit cigarette generates more than 2000 known compounds. These can be divided into five groups: (1) tobacco alkaloids and their metabolites; (2) nitrosamines; (3) tobacco gases; (4) metals; and (5) toxic hydrocarbons. The three components in the highest concentration per cigarette are carbon dioxide (68.1 mg), carbon monoxide (16.2 mg), and nicotine (0.1–2.5 mg). Proposed mechanisms for tobacco fetotoxicity include decreased utilization of amino acids (negative nitrogen balance) and hypoxia due to the displacement of oxygen from hemoglobin (e.g., the affinity of hemoglobin for carbon monoxide is approximately 300 times that for oxygen).

COCAINE

One of the most significant contemporary pediatric problems is cocaine abuse in pregnant women ("crack" cocaine being a particularly prevalent form; see Part 3). Surveys indicate that women of childbearing age (18–34 years) constitute 15 percent of all regular users of cocaine. It is estimated that 2–3 percent of pregnant women use cocaine in the United States. The use of cocaine by pregnant women has caught the attention of the courts. In some U.S. jurisdictions, mothers have been sentenced for causing the addiction of their baby.

The hazards of cocaine specific for pregnant women include premature rupture of placental membranes, spontaneous abortion, abnormal labor, and several general medical risks (e.g., hypertension). Their babies typically have growth retardation with consequent lowered birthweight. Cocaine use is also related to sudden infant death syndrome, characterized by abnormal respiratory control, particularly during sleep.

It is not clearly understood to what extent cocaine and/or its metabolites contribute to fetotoxicity. However, the end result appears to be a reduction in uterine blood flow, possibly via blockade of neuronal amine reuptake (see CNS section for more details). Cocaine may also decrease placental transport of amino acids.

SELECTED BIBLIOGRAPHY

Albert, A. (1979) *Selective Toxicity*. London: Chapman & Hall.

Brody, T. M., Larner, J., Minneman, K. P. and Neu, H. C. (eds) (1994) *Human Pharmacology: Molecular to Clinical*, 2nd ed. St Louis, MO: Mosby.

Goldstein, A., Aronow, L. and Kalman, S. (1974) *Principles of Drug Action: The Basis of Pharmacology*, 2nd ed. New York: John Wiley & Sons.

Hardman, J. G., Limbird, L. E. and Gilman, A. G. (eds) (2001) *Goodman and Gilman's The Pharmacological Basis of Therapeutics*, 10th ed. New York: McGraw-Hill.

Mutschler, E. and Derendorf, H. (eds) (1995) *Drug Actions: Basic Principles and Therapeutic Aspects*. Boca Raton, FL: CRC Press.

Niesink, R. J. M., de Vries, J. and Hollinger, M. (eds) (1995) *Toxicology: Principles and Applications*. Boca Raton, FL: CRC Press.

Rama Sastry, B. V. (1995) *Placental Toxicology*. Boca Raton, FL: CRC Press.

Smith, C. M. and Reynard, A. M. (eds) (1995) *Essentials of Pharmacology*. Philadelphia: W. B. Saunders.

Timbrell, J. A. (1995) *Introduction to Toxicology*, 2nd ed. London: Taylor & Francis.

QUESTIONS

1 Following oral administration of a drug, the first major organ the drug would reach would be which of the following?
   a   heart
   b   lung
   c   brain
   d   liver
   e   kidney.

2 Following intravenous administration of a drug, the first major organ the drug would reach would be which of the following?
   a   heart
   b   lung
   c   brain
   d   liver
   e   kidney.

3 A drug, which is highly lipid soluble:
   a   is absorbed slowly from the GI tract
   b   is rapidly excreted by the kidneys
   c   is probably active in the CNS
   d   requires an active transport system
   e   is none of the above.

4 Administering a drug by way of inhalation:
   a   can be a slow way to get the drug in the bloodstream
   b   can be an ideal route for certain drugs
   c   is a good route to ensure a long duration of drug action
   d   is the fastest way to get a drug into the bloodstream
   e   is the ideal route for all drugs.

5 You have overheard a physician talking about the parenteral administration of a drug. Which route would he/she *not* have been referring to?
   a   sublingual
   b   topical
   c   intradermal
   d   inhalation
   e   intramuscular.

6 Advantage(s) of the intravenous (IV) route is/are which of the following?
  a   once injected intravenously the drug can be easily removed
  b   rapid injections can be made free of acute toxic effects
  c   large volumes of drug solution can be introduced over a long period of time
  d   ideal route to deliver drugs to the liver
  e   both b and c above.

7 The blood–brain barrier is believed to be:
  a   fully developed at birth
  b   impermeable to lipid-soluble drugs
  c   a specialized lining of blood vessels in the brain and adjacent astrocytes
  d   a means of keeping drugs out of the peripheral nervous system
  e   all of the above.

8 Which of the following is/are *not* true regarding Fick's law?
  a   rate of passage directly proportional to concentration gradient
  b   rate of passage directly proportional to surface area of membrane
  c   rate of passage directly proportional to partition coefficient
  d   rate of passage directly proportional to membrane thickness
  e   none of the above.

9 Which of the following is/are true regarding the effect of pH on drug absorption?
  a   weak acids are preferentially absorbed in relatively acidic environments
  b   weak bases are preferentially absorbed in relatively acidic environments
  c   weak acids are preferentially absorbed in relatively basic environments
  d   both b and c above
  e   none of the above.

10 The fetus is most susceptible to teratogenic effects of drugs during which period(s) of gestation?
  a   first trimester
  b   second trimester
  c   third trimester
  d   fourth trimester
  e   equally throughout.

Chapter 3

Metabolism and elimination

GENERAL PRINCIPLES

After a drug or any xenobiotic gains access to the body and distributes within it, there must be some mechanism(s) whereby the molecule has its bioactivity terminated. Otherwise, drug effects could last the lifetime of the recipient. For most drugs, their duration of action is inversely proportional to the rate at which they are metabolically inactivated. For example, if hexobarbital (a sedative/hypnotic drug that can produce sleep) is given to mice and dogs, dogs will sleep, on average, 26 times longer than mice even if they receive half the dose on a per weight basis. This increased sleeping time in dogs correlates reasonably well with the elevated half-life (time required for the blood level to decrease by one-half) of hexobarbital in that species.

In view of the fact that we have evolved in a manner in which we obtain our energy primarily by way of the gastrointestinal (GI) system, this route also became the most likely portal for the inadvertent introduction of toxic substances. Therefore, as a survival necessity, the body had to evolve a strategy for the early interception and processing of potentially lethal xenobiotic substances. Anatomically, this is accomplished by the hepatic–portal venous system, which delivers substrates absorbed from the gut directly to a succession of chemical-transforming enzyme systems located in the liver.

An important consequence of the hepatic–portal system is that before a drug can reach the heart and from there the rest of the body, it has to pass through the liver. This is referred to as the first-pass effect and can result in nearly complete metabolism (> 90 percent) of certain substances. It is for this reason that some drugs are not given orally (e.g., nitroglycerin) but by an alternative route (e.g., transdermally across the skin or sublingually across the mucous membrane beneath the tongue) because they are so completely inactivated. Xenobiotics introduced into the body via alternative routes will, of course, ultimately find their way to the liver via the general circulation (i.e., hepatic artery).

The chemical modification of xenobiotics in the body is called biotransformation, metabolism, or metabolic clearance. Enzymes involved in metabolism are either membrane bound (e.g., endoplasmic reticulum and mitochondria) or freely soluble within the cytosol. Because these metabolic enzymes are not particularly substrate specific, they can metabolize compounds with fairly diverse chemical structures, including some endogenous compounds such as steroids, bile acids, and heme (endobiotics).

In general, all biotransformation reactions can be assigned to one of two major categories called phase I and phase II reactions (Table 3.1). Phase I reactions are

Table 3.1 Examples of metabolic phase I and phase II reactions

Phase I	Phase II
Oxidation	Glucuronidation
Reduction	Methylation
Hydrolysis	Acetylation
	Amino acid conjugation
	Glutathione conjugation

Table 3.2 Tissue localization of xenobiotic-metabolizing enzymes

Relative amount	Tissue
High	Liver
Medium	Lung, kidney, intestine
Low	Skin, testes, placenta, adrenals
Very low	Nervous system tissues

nonsynthetic biotransformation reactions that modify the drug molecule by oxidation, reduction, or hydrolysis. Phase II reactions are synthetic reactions and involve conjugation of the drug with a new moiety. Often, a drug may undergo sequential biotransformation through both phase I and phase II pathways. The usual net effect of these reactions is to produce metabolites that are more polar (i.e., more water soluble and less lipophilic). Therefore, the metabolites are partitioned into the aqueous media and are less likely to cross subsequent cellular membranes than the parent molecule and, conversely, more likely to be excreted by the kidneys.

PHASE I REACTIONS

Enzymatic oxidation in the liver is one of the most important processes in the disposition of xenobiotics in many species, including humans. This process is often the rate-limiting step in the elimination of a compound from the body. Large differences can exist between different species, as illustrated earlier by hexobarbital sleeping time in the mouse and dog, as well as between different individuals within a species in their capacity to metabolize xenobiotics. The reason that mice sleep significantly less following administration of two times as much hexobarbital as dogs is that mice have a liver hydroxylase (the enzyme that inactivates hexobarbital) activity nearly 17 times higher than dogs. Although the liver is the most important xenobiotic-metabolizing organ, other tissues can have varying activity (Table 3.2).

Interspecies and interindividual variability in drug metabolism is influenced by both genetic and environmental factors. The basal rate of drug metabolism in a particular individual is determined primarily by genetic constitution, but also varies with age, gender, and environmental factors such as diet, disease states, and concurrent use of other drugs.

For most drugs, oxidative biotransformation is performed primarily by the mixed-function oxidase enzyme system, which is present predominantly in the smooth endoplasmic reticulum of the liver. This system comprises (1) the enzyme NADPH cytochrome P450 reductase; (2) cytochrome P450, a family of heme-containing proteins that catalyze a variety of oxidative and reductive reactions; and (3) a phospholipid bilayer that facilitates interaction between the two proteins. Important exceptions to this rule are ethyl alcohol and caffeine, which are oxidatively metabolized by enzymes primarily present in the soluble, cytosolic fraction of the liver.

Cytochromes P450 (named for their absorption of light at 450 nm when complexed with carbon monoxide) are a superfamily of heme-containing enzymes found throughout the animal and plant kingdoms and in yeast and bacteria. These proteins are classified into families and subfamilies on the basis of their amino acid similarities. The mammalian P450s involved in the oxidation of foreign compounds are designated CYP1, CYP2, CYP3, and CYP4. More than 20 different human CYP isoforms have been characterized. It has been estimated that over 50 percent of the most commonly used prescribed drugs are metabolically cleared primarily by CYPs. The mechanism of oxidation by CYPs within the mixed-function oxidase enzyme system has been determined in some detail but is beyond the scope of this book. The interested reader may consult any major medical pharmacology text for in-depth coverage; the mini-review by Snyder cited at the end of this chapter is also a good start. However, the mechanism can be summarized as:

$$Drug + NADPH + H^+ + O_2 \rightarrow Drug\text{-}O + NADP^+ + H_2O$$

Examples of oxidative reactions are shown in Table 3.3. Generally, reduction and hydrolysis reactions play subordinate roles in xenobiotic metabolism compared to oxidation reactions. Examples of reduction and hydrolysis reactions are shown in Tables 3.4 and 3.5, respectively. To reiterate: the net result of phase I reactions is the

Table 3.3 Examples of oxidative reactions

Reaction class	Structural change		Drug example
Hydroxylation	RCH_2CH_3	$\rightarrow RCH_2CH_2OH$	Phenobarbital
Dealkylation	$RNHCH_3$	$\rightarrow RNH_2 + CH_2O$	Morphine
Desulfuration	R_1CSR_2	$\rightarrow R_1COR_2$	Thiopental
Deamination	$RC(NH_2)HCH_3 \rightarrow RCOCH_3 + NH_3$		Amphetamine
Sulfoxide formation	R_1SR_2	$\rightarrow R_1SOR_2$	Cimetidine

Table 3.4 Examples of reduction reactions

Reaction class	Structural change		Drug example
Aldehyde reduction	$RCHO$	$\rightarrow RCH_2OH$	Chloral hydrate
Azo reduction	$R_1N = NR_2 \rightarrow R_1NH_2 + R_2NH_2$		Azo gantrisin
Nitro reduction	O_2NR	$\rightarrow H_2NR$	Chloramphenicol

Note
Tend to occur when oxygen tension is low.

Table 3.5 Examples of hydrolysis reactions

Reaction class	Structural change	Drug example
Ester hydrolysis	$R_1COOR_2 \rightarrow R_1COOH + HOR_2$	Acetylsalicylic acid
Amide hydrolysis	$R_1CONHR_2 \rightarrow R_1COOH + H_2NR_2$	Procaineamide

Note
Esters and amides are hydrolyzed by the same enzymes, but esters are hydrolyzed much faster.

formation of more polar, less lipid-soluble metabolites that will have a greater tendency to remain within the circulatory system until they are eliminated via the kidneys.

PHASE II REACTIONS

Phase II reactions involve a different type of mechanism whereby either the parent drug or the oxidized metabolite becomes conjugated to a new moiety. The resulting conjugate is, once again, more polar and less lipid soluble. Conjugation of weak acids is particularly important because they tend to be unionized at the relatively low pH of urine and are therefore subject to reabsorption (remember Le Chatelier's principle). There are a number of drugs that are primarily cleared metabolically by phase II reactions, including tricyclic antidepressants, β_2-agonists, and some anti-AIDS drugs.

There are a variety of phase II conjugating enzyme systems that react with functional groups such as –OH, –COOH, –NH_2, and –SH, which are either present originally on the target xenobiotic or have been generated by phase I reactions.

Glucuronide conjugation and sulfate conjugation are the major phase II conjugation pathways and are enzymatically mediated by uridine diphosphoglucuronosyltransferase and sulfotransferase, respectively. In addition to the transferase enzymes, these two conjugation reactions require coenzymes and adenosine 5′-triphosphate (ATP). In both cases, the conjugated moiety is provided by an activated donor source (e.g., uridine diphosphate-glucuronic acid [UDPGA] and 3′-phosphoadenosine 5′-phosphosulfate, respectively). Other important conjugating substances include glutathione and amino acids such as glycine.

An example of glucuronide conjugation is shown in Figure 3.1. In general, both glucuronide and sulfate conjugation result in the formation of a biologically inert metabolite that is more readily excreted. In relatively rare situations, however, exceptions can occur. For example, morphine 6-glucuronide is more active than the parent molecule (see section on bioactivation for a broader discussion).

Glutathione is one of the most important molecules in the body's defense against toxic compounds, including drugs. This protective function is largely due to its ability to undergo conjugation reactions with electrophiles catalyzed by *S*-transferases. Reduced glutathione (its active form) is a tripeptide composed of glutamic acid, cysteine, and glycine. It is found in most cells but is particularly abundant in mammalian liver, where it reaches a concentration of 5 mM. The presence of cysteine is the key component of glutathione since its sulfhydryl group is nucleophilic and will tend to attract highly reactive, toxic electrophiles (see Chapter 7).

Figure 3.1 Conjugation of a phenol and a carboxylic acid with glucuronic acid.
Source: J. A. Timbrell (1991), *Principles of Biochemical Toxicology*. London: Taylor & Francis.

Electrophiles may be chemically reactive products of phase I reactions or they may be somewhat more stable xenobiotics that have been ingested. Therefore, reduced glutathione can protect cells by removing reactive metabolites (discussed later) via conjugation. Unlike glucuronic acid conjugation, however, reduced glutathione is not part of an activated donor source utilizing ATP. Instead it provides a direct target for electron-seeking electrophiles.

BIOACTIVATION AND BIOTOXIFICATION

While the term biotransformation generally implies inactivation and detoxification, there are exceptional cases where a metabolite is more chemically active or more toxic than the parent compound. In these situations, the processes of bioactivation and biotoxification are said to have occurred, respectively. An example of bioactivation is the formation of the commonly used drug acetaminophen from phenacetin in the liver (see Figure 3.2). The latter drug was once widely used as an analgesic agent but because of kidney toxicity has been replaced by other more potent, less toxic substitutes including, of course, acetaminophen itself. In this particular bioactivation pathway the process occurs via normal oxidative dealkylation.

In this context, phenacetin can be thought of as a prodrug, that is, an inactive or less active precursor of a more active drug form. The classic example of a prodrug is prontosil, which was the first antibacterial sulfonamide, introduced in 1935 by Gerhard Domagk. However, within a year it was discovered that prontosil itself was inactive. The actual active substance was found to be sulfanilamide, which was formed from prontosil by bacterially mediated fission of the parent compound in the gut (see Chapter 10 for additional coverage).

Aspirin, one of the most widely used drugs in the United States (estimated annual consumption of 10–20 thousand tons), also has a prodrug background. The antifebrile

Figure 3.2 Comparison of metabolic bioactivation and biotoxification processes.

property of willow bark (*Salix alba*) has been known by many cultures for centuries and is due to the presence of a glucoside called salicin. In the human, salicin is hydrolyzed in the gastrointestinal (GI) tract to glucose and salicyl alcohol. The latter substance subsequently undergoes cytoplasmic oxidation to salicylic acid, the true active ingredient. However, because of the irritating effect of sodium salicylate when administered orally, the molecule was subsequently modified to acetylsalicylic acid and became commercially available in 1899. Today, considerable research is being devoted to the development of prodrugs that can be activated in target tissues other than the liver or gut.

An example of biotoxification is the formation of paraoxon from the insecticide parathion via sulfoxidation. The simple substitution of an oxygen atom for a sulfur atom in the molecule results in a cholinesterase inhibitor with several times more potency. Similarly, the toxic action of methanol in producing blindness is the result of its metabolism to formaldehyde. Examples of bioactivation and biotoxification reactions are shown in Figure 3.2.

It should also be pointed out that there are reports in the literature relating to the paradoxical toxicity of glutathione conjugates. Glutathione conjugates of drugs such as menadione and *p*-aminophenol have been reported to produce nephrotoxicity in rodents. Therefore, although thiols such as reduced glutathione are generally considered to be antioxidants, the redox cycling (see Chapter 7) of thiols may lead to the formation of reactive oxygen species.

ENZYME INDUCTION

One of the more interesting and clinically relevant aspects of the drug-metabolizing capacity of the liver is that it is subject to fluctuations in activity. As mentioned previously, the basal rate of many liver enzymes can be modified by a number of factors

Table 3.6 Examples of phenobarbital-like enzyme inducers

Drug group	Example	Strength of induction
Antibiotic	Rifampin	4
Anticonvulsant	Diphenylhydantoin	3
Antihistamine	Chlorcyclizine	2
Antipsychotic	Chlorpromazine	2
Muscle relaxant	Carisoprodol	1
Nonsteroidal anti-inflammatory	Phenylbutazone	3
Oral hypoglycemic	Tolbutamide	3
Sedative	Phenobarbital	4

including xenobiotics (e.g., drugs, environmental pollutants, natural products, and pesticides). Enzyme activity can be either increased or decreased. When enzyme activity is increased the process is referred to as hepatic enzyme induction.

The induction of liver enzymes has been demonstrated in many species, including humans, and probably represents a homeostatic, defense mechanism. Induction usually requires multiple exposures to the inducing agent over a period of several days, the time required for the synthesis of new protein. Enzymes induced include the cytochrome P450 monooxygenase system; glucuronyltransferase; the microsomal ethanol oxidative system; and the steroid-metabolizing system.

There are basically three types of cytochrome P450 inducers: (1) phenobarbital-like (the major class); (2) methylcholanthrene-like (which actually increases a P448 isozyme); and (3) anabolic steroids. The former two have been the most frequently studied. Research over the past 40–50 years indicates that their mechanism of action involves genetic interaction, possibly via derepression of a "repressor" gene, and the subsequent synthesis of mRNA for the specific enzyme proteins. Examples of phenobarbital-like enzyme inducers, the most common, are shown in Table 3.6.

There are a number of clinical consequences of liver drug-metabolizing enzyme induction by phenobarbital-like drugs. For example, a drug can increase its own rate of metabolism. If the nonsteroidal anti-inflammatory drug phenylbutazone is administered for 5 days to a dog, the dog's blood level will decrease by 85 percent even though the dose remains constant. The decline in blood level is the result of enzyme self-induction. Similarly, phenobarbital can increase its rate of metabolism by inducing cytochrome P450, thus requiring the need for a higher dose. This type of tolerance is referred to as pharmacokinetic tolerance.

In addition to self-induction, the metabolism of other drugs and endogenous compounds can also be increased (i.e., cross-induction). In one classic case, a hospitalized heart patient was treated with an anticlotting drug (warfarin) to prevent additional heart attacks. In order to assist the patient in sleeping, the sedative/hypnotic phenobarbital was administered. After several days, the effectiveness of warfarin began to wane and its dose was increased. Following release from the hospital, the use of phenobarbital was discontinued but the elevated dose of warfarin was continued. The result was a severe bleeding episode because the inducing effect of phenobarbital is reversible, and the higher, compensatory dose of warfarin was being metabolized at a reduced rate.

A similar type of situation has been reported in female epilepsy patients who were participants in a program studying the effectiveness of birth control pills. In this case, users of the antiepilepsy medication diphenylhydantoin (see Table 3.6) were found to have a higher incidence of pregnancy. This was subsequently shown to be due to the induction of liver enzymes metabolizing the steroids in their birth control pills. Obviously, the simultaneous use of enzyme-inducing drugs in women taking birth control pills has potentially significant complications and must be monitored carefully.

Rifampin, a semisynthetic antibiotic effective in the treatment of tuberculosis, is a well-characterized inducer of the CYP3A4 isoform in man and is known to result in significant drug interactions with a relatively diverse range of drugs. The capacity for metabolic clearance of drugs by CYP3A4 can increase between five- and eightfold following treatment with rifampin, which translates into a 20- to 40-fold reduction in plasma concentration of subsequently administered drugs such as oral contraceptives, cyclosporin, verapamil, and nifedipine.

ENZYME INHIBITION

Drug metabolism in the liver can also be inhibited by certain xenobiotics. Enzyme inhibition can occur by decreased synthesis of drug-metabolizing enzymes, increased degradation of the enzyme, or competition of two or more drugs for the same binding site. In general, inhibition of the capacity of the liver for detoxification is the result of pathological changes in the organ. For example, cirrhosis of the liver has been reported to diminish the glucuronidation of several drugs, including morphine and acetaminophen. In addition, hepatotoxicants such as carbon tetrachloride and toluene can also produce an inhibitory effect.

Relatively innocuous factors can also sometimes influence liver enzyme activity. For example, the metabolic elimination of the bronchodilator theophylline has been reported to be prolonged in patients with influenza A or adenovirus infections. In 1990, an influenza epidemic in Seattle resulted in the admission of 11 children with high serum levels of theophylline and confirmed drug toxicity. These effects appear to be confined to cytochrome P450-based drug biotransformation. They may be related to the generation of interferons as a result of these infections, which, presumably, are causally related to the inhibitory effect on hydroxylases and demethylases.

In addition, something as innocuous as grapefruit juice has been shown to inhibit the metabolism of certain calcium channel blockers (e.g., nifedipine, taken to treat hypertension; see Chapters 4 and 12). This effect is caused by the presence of relatively high concentrations of specific flavenoids in grapefruit juice. Patients taking calcium channel blockers should be warned of the food–drug interaction since blood levels of the drug can increase by 100–150 percent, resulting in rapid decrease in blood pressure.

RENAL ELIMINATION

In order for a drug or its metabolite(s) to be completely eliminated from the body it must undergo excretion as well as metabolism. Excretion represents the final common

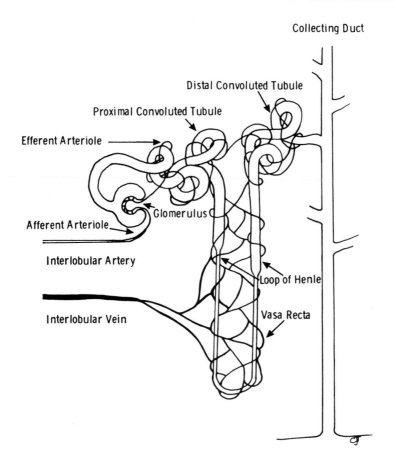

Figure 3.3 Structure of the mammalian kidney.
Source: J. A. Timbrell (1991), *Principles of Biochemical Toxicology*. London: Taylor & Francis.

pathway for the elimination of drugs. The kidneys are the most significant of the excretory sites. Extrarenal sites include biliary, pulmonary, sweat, salivary, and mammary glands, in order of decreasing importance. For the purposes of our discussion the renal pathway will be emphasized. The renal processes operating to modify the blood level of a drug include (1) glomerular filtration; (2) tubular secretion; and (3) tubular reabsorption.

The fundamental functional unit of the kidney is the nephron, of which approximately 1.2 million are present in each human being (Figure 3.3). If placed end to end, one person's nephrons would stretch approximately 50 miles. Structurally, each nephron consists of a porous tube within a nonporous tube and is U-shaped. At the beginning of each nephron is a small tuft of blood capillaries called the glomerulus. Blood flows unidirectionally into this tuft, which has a porous membrane that retains large blood components (e.g., erythrocytes) and most of the plasma protein (e.g., albumin; the presence of excess protein in the urine is suggestive of kidney damage) but allows passage of low-molecular-weight compounds (< 500 daltons). Therefore, drugs that are bound to plasma proteins will not be filtered and their clearance will be directly related to the free fraction.

After traversing the proximal and distal regions of the nephron, the filtrate eventually exits into the ureter, which leads to the urinary bladder. Molecules and ions that the body needs are reabsorbed back across the epithelial layer of the tubules into the blood. The human kidneys produce approximately 180 liters of glomerular filtrate per day, with the tubules reabsorbing all but 1.5 liters of water and many dissolved endogenous and exogenous substances.

Glomerular filtration

The kidneys receive approximately one-fifth of the cardiac output (i.e., 1200 ml/min of blood). Therefore, each minute they are exposed to approximately 650 ml of plasma. However, the normal rate of plasma filtration in the specific region of the glomeruli is 125 ml/min (i.e., the glomerular filtration rate). The volume of plasma filtered by the glomeruli per unit time is independent of the plasma concentration of the drug. In individuals, the actual glomerular filtration capacity of the kidneys can be quantified. This is accomplished by measuring the urinary excretion of a substance that is unbound and does not undergo appreciable tubular secretion or reabsorption (e.g., creatinine, which is only processed by glomerular filtration).

At the early stage of the elimination process in the glomerulus, lipophilic drugs are filtered just as readily as hydrophilic. If a drug is excreted solely by glomerular filtration, its excretion rate (mg/min) will be the product of its glomerular filtration rate (ml/min) and its plasma concentration (mg/ml). However, if drug disappearance studies show that the renal clearance is either significantly greater or lower than 125 ml/min, some other factor(s) must be involved.

Tubular secretion

In the case of certain drugs, such as the penicillin class, there are energy-dependent active secretory processes that take place in the proximal tubule cells. These secretory processes selectively facilitate the excretion of certain acids (anions) and bases (cations) from the plasma over and above that provided by glomerular filtration. Therefore, in these cases renal clearance is the sum of glomerular filtration and tubular secretion.

Because carrier systems are involved, the secretory process has a limited carrying capacity and can be saturated. Therefore, in distinction from glomerular filtration, tubular secretion is dependent upon the plasma concentration of the drug. Like all active transport processes, secretion of a drug into the tubular fluid can be competitively inhibited by other drugs that are transported by the same carrier.

For example, coadministration of the drug probenecid reduces the tubular secretion of penicillin G because both are organic acids that are transported by a common carrier. The oral administration of probenecid in conjunction with penicillin G results in higher and more prolonged concentrations of the antibiotic in plasma than with penicillin alone. The elevation in plasma penicillin level can be at least twofold and sometimes much greater. The ability to reduce the dose of the antibiotic required is particularly important in the treatment of resistant infections.

Reabsorption

The renal clearance of many drugs is low because they are significantly reabsorbed passively from the distal portion of the tubules due to the large concentration gradient that exists between the free drug in the tubular lumen and that in plasma. Reabsorption depends on two separate routes: a transcellular pathway (through cell cytoplasm via selective pumps and cotransporters on epithelial cell plasma membranes) and a paracellular pathway (through the intercellular space between cells). For most drugs reabsorption is a passive process that is influenced by the lipid solubility of the drug, the pK_a of the drug, and the pH of the urine. Lipophilic drugs, which are well absorbed in the GI tract, are also generally reabsorbed across the tubule epithelium. Conversely, hydrophilic drugs, which are poorly absorbed orally, are also reabsorbed poorly and are therefore more readily excreted in the urine.

If urine flow increases, the time that a drug is exposed to the reabsorptive surface of the kidney is decreased. This principle forms the basis for the treatment of certain extreme cases of acute drug overdose. In these situations patients undergo forced diuresis with large volumes of fluid in order to accelerate drug clearance (e.g., meprobamate poisoning).

The effect of urinary pH on drug ionization also has toxicological implications. For example, in cases of phenobarbital (a weak acid barbiturate) overdose the urine can be alkalinized (the pH elevated) by administering sodium bicarbonate to the patient. The resultant increase in pH shifts the dissociation equilibrium for this weak acid to the right, producing an increase in the proportion of the ionized form, less reabsorption in the kidneys, and more rapid elimination. Conversely, acidifying the urine with ammonium chloride will increase the excretion rate of drugs that are weak bases since they will be more protonated (ionized) and less reabsorbed (more polar, less lipophilic).

CLEARANCE, ELIMINATION RATE CONSTANT, AND HALF-LIFE

In this chapter we have seen that drugs are distributed in the body and subsequently metabolized and eliminated. All of these factors contribute to regulating the ultimate duration of the drug's presence in the body. In concluding this section, there are some basic kinetic relationships between volume of distribution of a drug (discussed in Chapter 2), circulating drug concentration, and duration of drug in the body that the introductory student should be familiar with. These relationships allow us to quantify important drug parameters that have significant pharmacological and toxicological implications.

An important concept relating to the ability of the body to eliminate a drug is total body clearance (CL_t), a term that indicates the rate at which a drug is cleared from the body. It is defined as the volume of plasma from which all drug is removed in a given time (i.e., ml/min) by all routes as expressed in the following equation:

CL_t = rate of drug removal (mg/min)/plasma concentration of drug (mg/ml)

Since drug elimination mechanisms in humans generally follow first-order kinetics (nonsaturated), an elimination rate constant (K_e) can be determined according to the following formula (assuming a one-compartment model):

$$K_e = \text{total body clearance (ml/min)}/V_d \text{ (ml)}$$

The important feature of first-order kinetics in this context is that they are not saturated. In other words, the reactions are not operating maximally. This has important toxicological implications.

For example, if a drug has a total body clearance rate of 100 ml/min and its V_d is 2000 ml, the corresponding K_e would be 0.05 min^{-1}. This value indicates that approximately 5 percent of the remaining drug is eliminated per minute. In a first-order process, the concentration of the remaining chemical is rate limiting.

It should be understood that the total body elimination rate constant is a composite parameter. It encompasses all rate constants for all routes of elimination including excretion in the urine and feces, biotransformation, and sequestration in tissues.

Determination of clearance rate (for first-order reactions) also allows us to calculate another very important drug characteristic, namely its half-life ($t^{1/2}$), according to the following formula:

$$t^{1/2} = 0.693/K_e$$

Therefore

$$t^{1/2} = 0.693 \times V_d \text{ (ml)}/\text{clearance (ml/min)}$$

In this equation, 0.693 is a constant obtained during the derivation of the formula (log 0.5). If we substitute our hypothetical values as used above, we would obtain a $t^{1/2}$ of approximately 14 minutes. This is an important value to know since the time required to reach a steady-state plateau, and maintain it, depends only on the half-life of the drug. In our case, therefore, it would take approximately 70 minutes (i.e., 5 half-lives) to reach approximately 97 percent of steady state. In first-order reactions $t^{1/2}$ is independent of dose, since, under normal circumstances, i.e., therapeutic, the system is not saturated since dosage is in the subgram amount.

In the example given, the drug has a very short half-life. In fact, this would not be practical for a therapeutic agent, particularly if given orally. While this relationship between half-life and duration holds true for most drugs, there are exceptions. Adrenal glucocorticosteroids, for example, produce many of their anti-inflammatory effects after gaining access to intracellular receptors that transport the steroid into the nucleus. The steroid then induces gene expression of a specific protein. As with all protein synthesis this process takes time (i.e., a latent period). It continues after blood levels of the steroid have become diminished but the effect lingers on.

When possible, a "once a day oral dose" represents an ideal regimen for drug administration. Since approximately 90 percent of a dose is eliminated within three plasma half-lives of a compound, this would indicate that a half-life of approximately 8 hours would be ideal. Compounds that have half-lives in humans in excess of

12 hours are likely to demonstrate systemic accumulation with daily dosing, in that all of the previous days' dose will not be 100 percent eliminated before the successive dose is administered. Obviously, this has significant toxicological implications.

It should be pointed out at this point that although most drug elimination is via first-order kinetics, there can be some important exceptions. Drugs that saturate routes of elimination will disappear from plasma in a nonconcentration-dependent manner, which is zero-order kinetics. The most common example of a drug that has zero-order kinetics is ethanol. The reason that ethanol displays zero-order kinetics is that it is usually consumed in 5–10 gram quantities that overwhelm (saturate) alcohol dehydrogenase in the liver.

Important characteristics of zero-order reactions are that (1) a constant amount of drug is eliminated per unit time since the system is saturated (maximized); and (2) the half-life is not constant for zero-order reactions but depends on the concentration. The higher the concentration, the longer the half-life. Therefore, the term zero-order half-life has little practical significance since it can change; and (3) zero-order kinetics is also known as nonlinear or dose-dependent. For example, if the body can metabolize ethanol at a rate of 10 ml per hour, then if one consumes 60 ml, it will take 3 hours to metabolize half of it (the half-life under these circumstances). However, if 80 ml is consumed the half-life will now become 4 hours. This is particularly significant regarding ethanol toxicity.

BLOOD ALCOHOL LEVEL

The amount of alcohol (ethanol) in your bloodstream is referred to as the blood alcohol level (BAL). It is recorded in milligrams of alcohol per 100 milliliters of blood, or milligrams percent. For example, a BAL of 0.10 means that one-tenth of 1 percent (or one-thousandth) of your total blood content is alcohol. When you drink alcohol it goes directly from the stomach into the bloodstream and distributes evenly throughout the body. BAL is primarily influenced by weight, gender, genetic factors, and rate of consumption. On average, it takes the liver approximately an hour to metabolize the amount of alcohol found in 12 ounces of beer, 4 ounces of wine or 1 ounce of 50 proof (25 percent) hard liquor.

The National Highway Traffic Safety Administration in the United States estimates that it takes a 170-pound male 4–5 drinks (5 ounce glasses of 11 percent wine) within an hour on an empty stomach to reach a BAL of 0.08 percent. Conversely, it is estimated that a 137-pound female requires only three drinks over the same time frame to reach the same BAL. Therefore, the difference between 0.08 and 0.10 percent could be one drink in an hour for a large man, or half a drink for a small woman. The significance of BAL in terms of behavior and toxicity is shown in Table 3.7.

The reason for the significant increase in severity of effects from an elevated BAL is that, basically, from the first drink liver enzymes are saturated and continued drinking will only elevate BAL. This fact is little appreciated by binge drinkers—defined as four drinks within an hour for females and five for males. Binge drinking has become an unfortunate aspect of college life. Surveys indicate that college students are not dissuaded by drink-related deaths: deaths include one student who died celebrating his twenty-first birthday by consuming 20 shots within 10 minutes and another

Table 3.7 Relationship of BAL (mg percent) to human behavior and toxicity

0.02	Mellow feeling, slight body warmth, less inhibited
0.05	Noticeable relaxation, less alert, less self-focused, impairment of coordination begins
0.08	Drunk driving limit in many states, definite impairment in coordination and judgment
0.10	Noisy, possible embarrassing behavior, mood swings, reduction in reaction time
0.15	Impaired balance and movement, clearly drunk
0.30	Many lose consciousness
0.40	Most lose consciousness, some die
0.50	Breathing stops, many die

15 shots within 15 minutes. One student died with a BAL of 0.588—a level that would require 20–25 drinks in an hour. This is equivalent to unintentional suicide. Each new school year brings the inevitable addition of new names to this death list. Binge drinking can no longer be viewed as a rite of passage; it is a major health threat.

Those dying from alcohol poisoning experience no pain because the central nervous system is severely compromised. Initially, blood glucose begins to drop, signaling hypoglycemia. This is critical because blood glucose is the principal metabolic substrate for the brain to function. Following hypoglycemia, hypothermia sets in. The body's temperature drops, and because the mechanism that regulates the body's temperature is impaired, natural responses to a cold environment, such as shivering, do not occur. Veins dilate and allow heat to escape at the skin level, causing the body's exterior to feel hot even as its core temperature is dropping.

The next phase involves the development of acidosis, in which the body's pH level begins to fall. In an acid environment, the body's many vital systems go awry and start trying to compensate for the imbalance. Breathing may speed up and then slow down. The kidneys may attempt to excrete more acids. Blood pressure rises. All of these conditions—hypoglycemia, hypothermia, and acidosis—begin in most people when BAL reaches 0.15 to 0.20 percent and higher.

EXTRARENAL CLEARANCE OF DRUGS

In addition to metabolism, the liver contributes to clearance by secreting approximately 0.5–1.0 liters of bile daily (Figure 3.4). Important constituents of bile include conjugated bile salts, cholesterol, phospholipid, bilirubin diglucuronide, electrolytes, and drugs. Biliary excretion is primarily important for compounds with a molecular weight greater than 500 while compounds with a molecular weight less than 300 are preferentially excreted into the urine.

Bile is initially concentrated in the gall bladder and subsequently transported to the small intestine (duodenum) via the bile ducts. Drugs entering the duodenum may be eliminated in the feces or recycled back into the general circulation (i.e., enterohepatic circulation). Therefore, biliary excretion is truly a route of elimination only to the extent that the excreted drug fails to be reabsorbed. A mechanism facilitating the reabsorption of certain drugs is the hydrolysis of glucuronide conjugates via β-glucuronidase present in intestinal flora.

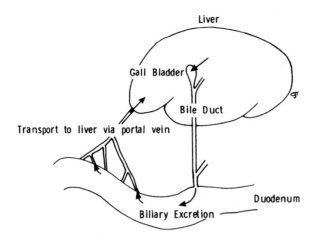

Figure 3.4 Biliary excretion route for foreign compounds.
Source: J. A. Timbrell (1991), *Principles of Biochemical Toxicology*. London: Taylor & Francis.

The lungs are the primary site of elimination for gaseous anesthetics and any other compounds that are volatile. For example, certain aromatic hydrocarbons are largely eliminated in the expired air. The major pathway for the elimination of ethanol, of course, is metabolism by the liver. However, approximately 2 percent is eliminated via the lungs. The equilibrium partition coefficient for ethanol between blood and alveolar air in humans is approximately 2100 : 1. Therefore, the ethanol concentration in end-expiratory air can be measured and multiplied by 2100 (e.g., by the Breathalyzer machine) to provide a fairly accurate estimate of ethanol concentration in the blood.

A number of drugs are eliminated partially by transport into milk during lactation. For most drugs, their concentration in milk is similar to that in the mother's circulation. The usual maternal dose transferred to the infant is in the range of 0.05 to 2 percent. In some cases, a significant pharmacological effect can be produced in babies who are breast-feeding. Among the drugs that are specifically contraindicated during breast-feeding are cocaine, lithium, and methotrexate. In addition, a number of drugs should be used with caution, including aspirin and phenobarbital.

SELECTED BIBLIOGRAPHY

Albert, A. (1979) *Selective Toxicity*. London: Chapman & Hall.
Brody, T. M., Larner, J., Minneman, K. P. and Neu, H. C. (eds) (1994) *Human Pharmacology: Molecular to Clinical*, 2nd ed. St Louis, MO: Mosby.
Goldstein, A., Aronow, L. and Kalman, S. (eds) (1974) *Principles of Drug Action: The Basis of Pharmacology*, 2nd ed. New York: John Wiley & Sons.
Hardman, J. G., Limbird, L. E. and Gilman, A. G. (eds) (2001) *Goodman and Gilman's The Pharmacological Basis of Therapeutics*, 10th ed. New York: McGraw-Hill.

Mutschler, E. and Derendorf, H. (eds) (1995) *Drug Actions: Basic Principles and Therapeutic Aspects.* Boca Raton, FL: CRC Press.

Rowland, M. and Tozer, T. N. (1980) *Clinical Pharmacokinetics: Concepts and Applications.* Philadelphia: Lea & Febiger.

Smith, C. M. and Reynard, A. M. (eds) (1995) *Essentials of Pharmacology.* Philadelphia: W. B. Saunders.

Snyder, R. (2000) Profiles in toxicology: microsomal enzyme induction. *Toxicol. Sci.* 55: 233–234.

Timbrell, J. A. (1995) *Introduction to Toxicology*, 2nd ed. London: Taylor & Francis.

QUESTIONS

1 In the process of drug action, the primary function of the liver is:
  a to initiate the deactivation process
  b to aid in the transportation of the drug to the site of action
  c to excrete the drug
  d to speed up the absorption of the drug into the bloodstream
  e to initiate the activation process.

2 During the metabolism of a drug, most chemical changes of the drug's molecular structure result in products that are:
  a less ionized
  b less rapidly excreted by the kidneys
  c more lipid soluble
  d more active pharmacologically
  e more water soluble.

3 Mechanisms for metabolizing certain drugs in the body may be impaired by:
  a illness or damage to the liver
  b inadequate diet
  c advanced age
  d grapefruit juice
  e all of the above.

4 A drug may be excreted through the:
  a lungs
  b urine
  c skin
  d kidneys
  e all of the above.

5 The primary enzymes responsible for the oxidation of drugs are located in the:
  a cytoplasm
  b mitochondria
  c smooth endoplasmic reticulum
  d nucleus
  e cell membrane.

6 Which of the following is a phase II reaction?
  a   reduction
  b   oxidation
  c   hydrolysis
  d   conjugation
  e   a, b, and c above.

7 The consequences of stimulation of the smooth endoplasmic reticulum are more likely with regard to which of the following?
  a   acute administration of a drug
  b   chronic administration of a drug
  c   phenobarbital
  d   rifampin
  e   b, c, and d above.

8 The mixed-function oxidase system is composed of which of the following?
  a   a superfamily of heme-containing proteins
  b   cytochrome P450s
  c   cytochrome P450 reductase
  d   b and c above
  e   a, b, and c above.

9 Which of the following is/are true regarding "prodrugs"?
  a   they are an inactive or a less active precursor of a more active metabolite
  b   they have only been developed during the past 10 years
  c   their "activation" occurs primarily in the gastric mucosa
  d   they are far more potent than drugs considered "amateurs"
  e   a and b above.

10 Which of the following drugs is/are most likely to be eliminated by zero-order kinetics?
  a   birth control pills
  b   penicillin
  c   digoxin
  d   alcohol (ethanol)
  e   b and d above.

Chapter 4

Drug interactions

There are currently approximately 13,000 prescription drugs available in the United States and 3000 in the United Kingdom. A new entity is approved for human use approximately every 2–3 weeks and two-thirds of all physician visits culminate in a drug being prescribed. No other risk factor compares with polypharmacy as a cause of adverse drug reactions and interactions, particularly in the geriatric population. A number of British and American studies have indicated that persons over 65 years of age living independently take an average of 2.8 drugs per day. In skilled nursing homes the number increases to an average of 3.4, while approximately 9 drugs per day are prescribed for the hospitalized elderly.

It has been reported that there is a ninefold increased risk of having an adverse drug reaction when four or more drugs are taken simultaneously. In addition, 3–5 percent of all hospital admissions are related to adverse drug reactions, and of all the admissions for the elderly, 15–25 percent are complicated by an adverse drug reaction. Some of these reactions are life-threatening, and it is estimated that fatal adverse drug reactions in the United States may run in the thousands each year.

Results obtained by counting the number of interactions of major clinical significance indicate substantial variation among different drug classes. For example, oral anticoagulants appear to have the greatest tendency, followed by oral antidiabetics, monoamine oxidase inhibitors, phenothiazines, and anticonvulsants. The former two are not surprising since they are among the most frequently prescribed in the elderly.

When it comes to drug interactions, there is a spectrum of pharmacological issues that should be considered. For example, some drug interactions are very common, such as the lipid-elevating effect of combining thiazide diuretics and beta blockers, but the clinical consequences are usually not life-threatening, produce few symptoms, are easily managed, transient, and well tolerated. However, in other situations, the statistical risk of incurring a drug interaction may be very low but the drug-related consequences may be life-threatening (e.g., cardiac arrhythmias produced by the combination of erythromycin and terfenadine—the latter subsequently withdrawn from the market). To minimize an inadvertent drug interaction, numerous pharmacies maintain records of prescription drugs currently used by individuals. Compendia of possible drug interactions are also available in both written and computer-based formats.

As the number of drugs continues to proliferate and the population ages, the likelihood of drug interactions will undoubtedly continue to increase. Of all prescription drugs, 25 percent are taken by people over 65 years of age, although this group presently comprises approximately 12 percent of the population. The average older person fills more than twice as many prescriptions as those under age 65. Polypharmacy, variable compliance, and multiple diseases, combined with altered physiological response, make the elderly especially prone to adverse drug reactions.

In addition to the elderly, patients with AIDS have a higher incidence of toxic reactions to medications than other subgroups treated with similar drugs. These individuals frequently consume 5–10 different medications daily, including anti-retroviral drugs, as well as a number of antibiotic or antifungal agents that are used for prophylaxis against opportunistic infections. Often, nonapproved drugs are also used. Although the exact reasons for this increased sensitivity to drug-related side effects are not fully understood, it is possible that HIV-infected individuals tend to take multiple medications for long periods and also have multiorgan system compromise.

INTERACTIONS DURING DISTRIBUTION AND METABOLISM

As mentioned previously, it is the free, unbound form of a drug that is able to be absorbed across cellular membranes. However, many drugs are reversibly bound to red blood cells and plasma proteins (particularly albumin which represents 50–65 percent of the total). In humans, the blood concentration of albumin is normally 4 percent and each molecule possesses 109 cationic and 120 anionic groups at physiological pH. Albumin is referred to as "high capacity, low affinity." Acidic drugs tend to bind to albumin while basic drugs tend to bind to α1-acid glycoprotein (AAG), which is present in plasma at approximately 1 percent of the concentration of albumin. Plasma levels of AAG are more subject to change than albumins. AAG is often referred to as "low capacity, high affinity" in terms of binding sites.

The drug fraction bound to plasma protein cannot diffuse, cannot be metabolized, and cannot be excreted because the molecular weight of the drug–protein complex exceeds 65,000 daltons. The bound fraction represents, therefore, a storage form that is released when the concentration of free drug decreases. The normal therapeutic dose of a drug is determined taking this into account.

One of the potentially significant ramifications of plasma protein binding of drugs is in the area of drug interactions. The binding sites that exist on albumin, the principal plasma protein for drug binding, are designated as two forms, type I (warfarin site) and type II (benzodiazepine site). They are nonspecific and finite in number. Therefore, whenever two different drugs (which are normally significantly albumin bound, i.e., > 80 percent) are in the bloodstream together, competition for binding sites can occur. Binding is usually expressed in percentage terms, which describes the fraction of the concentration of drug in plasma that is bound to plasma proteins.

The drug with the higher affinity constant will successfully displace the drug with the lower. The result is an increase in the free drug concentration of the latter. For example, tolbutamide (an oral hypoglycemic agent used in maturity-onset *diabetes mellitus*) is approximately 95 percent bound and 5 percent free (see Table 4.1). In the presence of the anti-inflammatory drug phenylbutazone (which is nearly 100 percent

Table 4.1 Comparison of drug plasma protein binding

Drug	Percent bound
Caffeine	0
Alcohol	0
Procainamide	10–20
Digoxin	30–40
Gentamicin	40–50
Penicillin G	50–60
Theophylline	60
Phenobarbital	70
Carbamazepine	70–80
Quinidine	85
Phenytoin	90
Tolbutamide	92–95
Propranolol	92–95
Diazepam	92–95
Digitoxin	97
Warfarin	99.5
Phenylbutazone	99.5
Dicumarol	99.9

bound), essentially all of the bound tolbutamide can be displaced (i.e., a 20-fold increase from 5 to 100 percent), leading to potential toxicity (e.g., severe lowering of blood sugar).

Whether or not a drug interaction of this type is clinically significant depends on the distribution and elimination properties of the drug affected. Competition between two drugs for the same plasma protein binding site is fairly common. However, it is only clinically relevant if the drugs have high protein binding, a low therapeutic index (see Part 2), and a relatively small volume of distribution.

In the case of tolbutamide, second-generation derivatives (e.g., gliburide) have been developed with less protein binding affinity and, hence, less probability for this type of interaction. It should also be remembered that even if the unbound fraction of a drug becomes elevated vis-à-vis a receptor site, it is also presented to the eliminating organs, resulting in more rapid clearance. Consequently, with the exception of the criteria mentioned above, the principal effects of a protein binding displacement are to decrease total concentration and increase percent unbound. Therefore, a new equilibrium between drug effect and drug elimination is achieved, which tends to dampen any consequences of this type of interaction.

In addition to displacement of plasma protein-bound drug, another major example of drug interactions includes acceleration or inhibition of drug metabolism (discussed previously in Chapter 3). Among the drugs that are known to increase the metabolism of selected drugs are ethanol, antihistamines, phenytoin, barbiturates, and glutethimide. For more specific examples the reader is referred to more advanced medical pharmacology texts. Similarly, drugs such as phenylbutazone, chloramphenical, allopurinal, cimetidine, desipramine, and methylphenidate inhibit the metabolism of certain drugs.

Table 4.2 Mechanisms by which nutrients and drugs can influence each other

Process	Mechanism
Ingestion	Both drugs and disease can cause changes in appetite and nutrient intake; resultant malnutrition can impact on drug efficacy
Absorption	Drugs and foods can have mechanical effect, via binding or adsorption, that can influence the absorptive processes, resulting in ↑ or ↓ drug and nutrient absorption. Some drugs can affect GI motility, thereby ↑ or ↓ absorption of nutrients. Chemical factors, in particular pH of the stomach contents and the influence of foods therein, can affect the subsequent absorption of drugs
Transluminal transport	The ability of drugs and nutrients to be transported can depend on such factors as lipid solubility and competition for amino acid transport systems
Metabolism	The effectiveness of the mixed function oxidase (MFO) and conjugase systems in the liver and elsewhere for converting drugs and nutrients into their active and, ultimately, excretory forms is dependent on the availability of specific nutrient cofactors. In addition, certain drugs can increase the activity of the MFO systems required to convent nutrient precursors into their active forms. Nonnutritive components in foods can induce MFO activity, thereby affecting drug metabolism
Distribution	The utilization of both drugs and nutrients depends on body composition, the availability and functional integrity of transport proteins, receptor integrity, and intracellular metabolic machinery
Elimination	Drugs and nutrients can synergistically and competitively interact to cause increased or decreased excretion. Systemic factors such as pH and physiological state (e.g., sweating) can dictate whether a drug or nutrient is excreted or reabsorbed

Source: E. J. Massaro (ed.) (1997), *Handbook of Human Toxicology*. Boca Raton, FL: CRC Press. Reprinted with permission.

There are also other types of drug interactions, including impaired uptake of drugs from the GI tract and altered renal clearance, for example. A summary of mechanisms by which nutrients and drugs can influence each other is shown in Table 4.2.

INTERACTION IN THE GASTROINTESTINAL TRACT

Because drugs are often taken orally at the same time, the GI tract is a relatively common site for drug interactions to occur. Possible interactions during absorption include changes in local pH (e.g., antacids), altered gastric emptying and intestinal motility, and the formation of complexes.

With regard to complex formation, tetracyclines and cholestyramine are common examples—although their mechanisms are different. In the case of tetracyclines, complexes of the antibiotic can be formed with a number of positive, polyvalent mineral ions such as Al^{3+}, Ca^{2+}, and Mg^{2+}. Such minerals are commonly present in antacids and milk. The result of such complex formation is diminished absorption of tetracycline. This is the reason why patients taking tetracyclines are directed to avoid taking milk with their medication.

Complexes can also be formed with compounds that act as ion-exchange resins. The cholesterol-lowering drug cholestyramine acts in this manner and can complex with acidic (anionic) compounds such as the oral anticoagulant drug coumadin. Similar interactions have been reported for thyroid hormone, tetracyclines, bile acids, and iron compounds. In each case, the result is interference with absorption.

INTERACTIONS DURING EXCRETION

A number of drugs are known to inhibit the renal secretion of certain other drugs, resulting in decreased clearance of the latter. Examples of drugs decreasing the renal clearance of other drugs include probenecid, salicylates, sulfinpyrazone, phenylbutazone, and thiazide diuretics. As mentioned previously, the inhibition of penicillin secretion by probenecid due to competition between the two for renal tubule "carriers" is used therapeutically to increase penicillin blood levels.

DRUG–FOOD INTERACTIONS

For many drugs it is not known how food intake affects their pharmacokinetic profile (other than the obvious physical effect). However, as a generalization, it can be said that such interactions do occur and that they can be clinically significant. A selected list of some drug–food interactions is shown in Table 4.3. In addition, although there can be disagreement regarding classifying alcoholic beverages as food or drug, alcohol consumption can potentially have a number of important interactions with drugs (Table 4.4).

An important example of a food–drug interaction involves a drug used in the treatment of AIDS. Saquinavir®, a protease inhibitor, has very low bioavailability—only about 4 percent of the drug taken orally reaches the general circulation. This is partly because the drug is poorly absorbed, and partly because it is rapidly destroyed by the cytochrome P450 system (cytochrome P450 3A4, also called CYP3A4) that is present in the liver and also the intestinal wall. Some foods inhibit this enzyme, thus increasing the AUC of Saquinavir. One such food is grapefruit juice. Human studies indicate that when a 150-ml glass of ordinary reconstituted frozen grapefruit juice is taken with the Saquinavir followed by another equal volume 1 hour later, the AUC is increased by 50 percent.

In published studies with other drugs (triazolam, midazolam, cyclosporin, coumarin, nisoldipine, and felodipine), grapefruit juice had comparable effects. Orange juice, however, had no effect. When the bioflavinoid naringin—the component of grapefruit juice, which was suspected to be the active ingredient in increasing the bioavailability of these drugs—was tried instead of grapefruit juice, it had much less effect than the juice itself. A summary of grapefruit juice–drug interactions is shown in Table 4.5.

SUMMATION AND POTENTIATION

When the effect of two drugs given concurrently is additive, this is referred to as summation. However, if the effect of two drugs exceeds the sum of their individual effects, this is referred to as potentiation or synergism. Potentiation requires that the

Table 4.3 Some selected drug–food interactions

Drug	Food	Adverse interaction
Calcium antagonists (felodipine, nifedipine, nitrendipine); terfenadine; caffeine	Grapefruit juice	Increased bioavailability; inhibition of first-pass metabolism; increased toxicity
Monoamine oxidase (MAO) inhibitors	Foods containing tyramine (liver, pickled herring, cheese, bananas, avocados, soup, beer, wine, yogurt, sour cream, yeast, nuts)	Palpitations, headache, hypertensive crises
Digitalis	Licorice	Digitalis toxicity
Griseofulvin	Fatty foods	Increased blood levels of griseofulvin
Timed-release drug preparations	Alcoholic beverages	Increased rate of release for some
Lithium	Decreased sodium intake	Lithium toxicity
Quinidine	Antacids and alkaline diet (alkaline urine)	Quinidine toxicity
Thiazide diuretics	Carbohydrates	Elevated blood sugar
Tetracyclines	Dairy products high in calcium; ferrous sulfate: or antacids	Impaired absorption of tetracycline
Vitamin B_{12} (cyanocobalamin)	Vitamin C—large doses	Precipitate B_{12} deficiency
Fenfluramine	Vitamin C addition	Antagonism of antiobesity effect of fenfluramine
Thiamine	Blueberries, fish	Foods containing thiaminases
	Alcohol	Decreased intake, absorption, utilization
Benzodiazepines	Caffeine	Antagonism of antianxiety action

Source: C. M. Smith and A. M. Reynard (eds) (1995). Essentials of Pharmacology. Philadelphia: W. B. Saunders. Reprinted with permission.

Table 4.4 Summary of adverse interactions of drugs with alcoholic beverages

Drug	Adverse effect with alcohol
Anesthetics, antihistamines, barbiturates, benzodiazepines, chloral hydrate, meprobamate, narcotics, phenothiazines, tricyclic antidepressants	1 Increased central nervous system depression due to additive effects 2 Decreased sedative or anesthetic effects with chronic use due to tolerance
Phenothiazines	Increased extrapyramidal effects, drug-induced Parkinsonism
Diazepam	Increased diazepam blood levels, varying with beverage
Amphetamines and cocaine	Increased cardiac work; possible increase in probability of cerebrovascular accident
Calcium channel antagonists—felodipine, verapamil, nifedipine	Increased bioavailability; possible toxicity
Acetaminophen	Hepatotoxicity
Anticoagulants	Chronic—decreased anticoagulant effect Acute—increased anticoagulant effect
Bromocriptine	Nausea, abdominal pain (due to increased dopamine-receptor sensitivity?)
Disulfiram, chloramphenical, oral hypoglycemics, cephalosporins, metronidazole, quinacrine, moxalactam	Disulfiram–alcohol syndrome reactions
Cycloserine	Increased seizures with chronic use
Imipramine (see also above)	Lower blood level with chronic alcohol consumption
Isoniazid	Increased hepatitis incidence, decreased isoniazid effects in chronic alcohol use due to increased metabolism
Propranolol	Decreased tremor of alcohol withdrawal; decreased propranolol blood levels
Sotalol	Increased sotalol blood levels
Phenytoin	Decreased metabolism with acute combination with alcohol; but increased metabolism with chronic alcohol consumption; increased risk of folate deficiency
Nonsteroidal anti-inflammatory agents (aspirin and related)	Increased gastrointestinal bleeding

Source: C. M. Smith and A. M. Reynard (eds) (1995), Essentials of Pharmacology. Philadelphia: W. B. Saunders. Reprinted with permission.

Table 4.5 Drugs that interact with grapefruit juice

Calcium channel blockers (felodipine, nifedipine, amlodipine, diltiazem, verapamil, and pranidipine)
Tranquilizers (benzodiazapam)
Antihistamines (Hismanal®)
AIDS drugs (protease inhibitors Crixivan® and Saquinavir®)
Antifungal (Sporanox®)

Table 4.6 Factors complicating assessment of drug interactions with herbal products

Failure to inform physician or pharmacist of concomitant use of herbal products
Incomplete and inaccurate product information (FDA analysis of 125 products containing ephedra
    alkaloids revealed a range of 0 to 110 mg/dose)
Lack of standardization of product purity or potency (the fungal hepatotoxin aflatoxin often
    found as a natural contaminant)
Multiple ingredients in product (the presence of a cardiac glycoside has been found in Chinese
    herbal preparation)
Product adulteration (up to seven adulterants have been found in a single product)
Product dosage not standardized
Product misidentification
Variations between labeled and actual product content
Variations in crop conditions and yield (batch-to-batch variability)

Source: *Drug Facts and Comparisons*. (1999) St Louis, MO: Facts and Comparisons, a Wolters Kluwer Company.
Reprinted with permission.

two drugs act at different receptors or effector systems. An example of potentiation involves the multiple uses of drugs in the treatment of AIDS. Significant improvement in virtually all criteria relating to the disease has been achieved with the combination of AZT and 3TC (nucleoside analogs that can inhibit the HIV reverse transcriptase) as well as a protease inhibitor (a protease plays a vital role in the virus's replication in T cells). It has been estimated that for HIV to develop resistance to a protease inhibitor alone, one mutation could suffice; for AZT and 3TC the virus would have to produce progeny with four mutations. However, in order to survive against all three drugs, eight mutations appear to be necessary.

DRUG INTERACTIONS WITH NATURAL (HERBAL) PRODUCTS

Because as many as 70 percent of patients may not be informing their physician or pharmacist of complementary medicine use, including herbal products, the real potential for interactions is not adequately monitored. Making informed decisions regarding drug interactions with herbal products requires accurate and complete information. Because the contents of herbal products are not standardized, the information needed to determine the potential for drug interaction is often not readily available. Table 4.6 presents some of the factors complicating assessment of drug interactions with herbal products.

Table 4.7 Interaction of popular OTC drugs with other OTC products and prescription drugs

Ibuprofen–anticoagulants and aspirin-containing drugs	Abnormal bleeding and gastric irritation
Naproxen–anticoagulants; any drug containing aspirin	Abnormal bleeding and stomach irritation
Aspirin–anticoagulants; any drug containing ibuprofen	Abnormal bleeding and stomach irritation
Diphenhydramine–antihistamines, sedating drugs, muscle relaxants	Oversedation
Famotidine–OTC antacids and antifungal drugs (ketoconazole, itraconazole)	Antacids can reduce the effectiveness of famotidine, while famotidine itself can reduce the effectiveness of these antifungals
Dextromethorphan–monoamine oxidase inhibitors	Elevated blood pressure and tremors as well as more severe responses possible
Calcium carbonate–tetracycline	Reduces absorption

It should be kept in mind that there exist numerous opportunities for interaction between herbal preparations and prescription drugs. The most potentially serious of these involve drugs with narrow therapeutic indexes (i.e., low margin of safety; see Chapters 6 and 7) and those drugs used in life-threatening situations. For example, it has been reported that the concomitant use of St John's Wort with a protease inhibitor (indinavir) results in a significant reduction in plasma concentration of the anti-AIDS drug. Apparently, some component in the St John's Wort is capable of inducing the cytochrome P450 that degrades indinavir. Obviously, a consequence of this interaction could be a curtailment of indinavir's efficacy.

OVER-THE-COUNTER (OTC) DRUG INTERACTIONS WITH PRESCRIPTION DRUGS

There are hundreds of drugs available as OTC preparations that are used for self-medication. Obviously, these drugs also lend themselves to interacting with not only prescription medications but also herbal preparations. Table 4.7 lists the generic name of some of the most popular OTC medications, followed by the prescription drug they are most likely to interact with, followed by the effect(s).

SELECTED BIBLIOGRAPHY

Brody, T. M., Larner, J., Minneman, K. P. and Neu, H. C. (eds) (1994) *Human Pharmacology: Molecular to Clinical*, 2nd ed. St Louis, MO: Mosby.

Drug Interactions and Side effects Index. (1994) Oradell, NJ: Medical Economics Co.

Goldstein, A., Aronow, L. and Kalman, S. (1974) *Principles of Drug Action: The Basis of Pharmacology*, 2nd ed. New York: John Wiley & Sons.

Mutschler, E. and Derendorf, H. (eds) (1995) *Drug Actions: Basic Principles and Therapeutic Aspects*. Boca Raton, FL: CRC Press.

Smith, C. M. and Reynard, A. M. (eds) (1995) *Essentials of Pharmacology*. Philadelphia: W. B. Saunders.

QUESTIONS

1 Which of the following population groups are most likely to experience a drug reaction?
   a neonates
   b teenagers
   c geriatric
   d the indigent
   e all are equal.

2 Competition for albumin binding sites by two drugs is really only clinically significant if which of the following is/are true?
   a they are both of the same pharmacological class
   b they are both highly bound
   c they have a low margin of safety
   d they have a relatively small volume of distribution
   e all but a above.

3 Which of the following are possible types of drug interactions?
   a displacement from albumin binding sites
   b alteration of drug metabolism
   c complex formation in the GI tract
   d interaction with food
   e all of the above.

4 When the pharmacological effect of drug A and drug B given concurrently is greater than the sum of each given alone, this process is referred to as:
   a induction
   b additive
   c activation
   d potentiation
   e none of the above.

5 Which of the following are factors contributing to the difficulty in assessing drug interactions with herbal products?
   a physician may not be aware of concurrent use
   b product labeling may not be consistent with actual contents of main ingredient
   c product purity may vary from batch to batch
   d product may contain adulterants
   e all of the above.

6 Which of the following effect(s) is/are most commonly produced by aspirin- and ibuprofen-containing drugs when interacting with prescription drugs?
   a tremors
   b incontinence
   c skin discoloration
   d abnormal bleeding and gastric irritation
   e constipation.

7 An example of potentiation involves which of the following drug/herb pairs?
   a   diphenhydramine–phenobarbital
   b   St John's Wort–indinavir
   c   AZT (reverse transcriptase inhibitor)–3TC (protease inhibitor)
   d   grapefruit juice–aspirin
   e   phenobarbital–phenobarbital.

8 Which of the following foods can interact with a tetracycline to reduce its effectiveness?
   a   licorice
   b   dairy products containing calcium
   c   caffeine
   d   grapefruit juice
   e   none of the above.

9 Which of the following has the least percentage bound to plasma protein?
   a   ethanol
   b   phenobarbital
   c   penicillin G
   d   warfarin
   e   phenylbutazone

10 Which of the following has the highest percentage bound to plasma protein?
   a   ethanol
   b   phenobarbital
   c   penicillin G
   d   procainamide
   e   warfarin.

Part 2

Fundamentals of pharmacodynamics and toxicodynamics

Chapter 5

Drug receptors

INTRODUCTION

Part 1 began by stating that the science of pharmacology involves the measurement of drug effects (i.e., pharmacodynamics). The beginning of pharmacodynamics as a component of pharmacology is attributed to the efforts of Rudolf Buchheim (1820–1879). Buchheim is believed to have established the world's first pharmacological laboratory at the University of Dorpat in Hungary during the mid-nineteenth century.

Buchheim believed that the mode of action of drugs should be investigated by scientific means in order to quantify their effects and introduce a more rational basis for therapy. The second section of this book deals with drug–receptor interactions within the body and the quantitation of these resulting effects. In addition, toxicological aspects of drug–receptor interactions and the treatment of toxicological problems are discussed.

HISTORY

The development of the concept that receptors mediated the effect of drugs was based primarily upon a series of observations made during the late nineteenth and early twentieth centuries. These observations correlated chemical structure with biological activity, and demonstrated the fact that relatively small amounts of drug can elicit an effect. One of the earliest proposals associating chemical structure with function was that of J. Blake in 1848. Blake suggested that the biological activity of certain metallic salts was due to their metallic component, rather than the complex in its entirety (e.g., the lead moiety in lead acetate or lead nitrate). This important concept received theoretical support in 1884 when Arrhenius introduced his theory of electrolytic dissociation, whereby salts dissolved in water become dissociated into oppositely charged ions.

The effect of ionization on the pharmacological action of drugs was also recognized in the latter half of the nineteenth century. In Scotland, Crum Brown and Fraser demonstrated that quarternization (i.e., the addition of a fourth alkyl group) of several alkaloids resulted in their transition from muscle contractors to muscle relaxants. These researchers concluded that "a relation exists between the physiological action of a substance and its chemical composition and constitution, understanding by the latter term the mutual relations of the atoms in the substance."

It was at the turn of the twentieth century that the importance of lipid solubility in drug action was also independently described by Meyer and Overton (the significance of the oil/water partition coefficient was discussed in Chapter 2). The importance of lipid solubility in drug action subsequently became manifested in the "lipoid theory of cellular depression." In essence, this theory correlated a pharmacological effect (e.g., CNS depression) with a physical property (i.e., lipid solubility) rather than a structure–activity relationship. In the process, the theory was attempting to explain the diverse chemical structures that exist within the hypnotic and general anesthetic classes of drugs (see Chapter 11). Today, we realize the limitations of the "lipoid theory" and appreciate that the distinction between physical and chemical factors is illusory, since chemical structure is a determinant of physical properties.

Despite the undeniable importance of Meyer and Overton's observations, a number of experimental reports of drug action were emerging that clearly indicated that drug molecules must be concentrating on small, specific areas of cells in order to produce their effects. These characteristics included (1) the fact that some drugs can express an effect despite significant dilution (e.g., 10^{-9} M); (2) drugs can be effective despite interacting with only a small fraction of tissue (e.g., acetylcholine decreases frog heart rate when only a six-thousandth of the surface is covered); (3) high chemical specificity (e.g., discrimination between drug stereoisomers); and (4) high physiological specificity (e.g., opiates have a significantly greater effect on smooth muscle than on skeletal muscle).

The concept of drugs acting upon receptors is generally credited to John Langley, who alluded to their existence in 1878. While studying the antagonistic effect of atropine against pilocarpine-induced salivation, Langley wrote "that there is some substance or substances in the nerve endings or gland cells with which *both* [emphasis mine] atropine and pilocarpine are capable of forming compounds." In 1905 Langley subsequently referred to this factor as "receptive substance." Despite this observation, the specific word "receptor" was not introduced into the medical literature until the turn of the century by Paul Ehrlich.

Ehrlich based his hypothesis upon his experiences with immunochemistry (i.e., the selective neutralization of toxin by antitoxin) and chemotherapy (e.g., the treatment of infectious diseases with drugs derived from the German dye industry; see Chapter 10). Ehrlich believed that a drug could have a therapeutic effect only if it has "the right sort of affinity." He specifically wrote "that combining group of the protoplasmic molecule to which the introduced group is anchored will hereafter be termed *receptor*." (It might be appropriate at this point to give credit to the Italian Amedo Avogadro (1776–1856) who coined the term molecules, from the Latin for "little masses".) At that time Ehrlich conceived of receptors as being part of "side-chains" in mammalian cells. As we shall see later in this chapter, Ehrlich was not far off in his visualization.

Today, we realize that drug binding/receptor sites that produce pharmacological effects may be part of any cellular constituent: for example, nuclear DNA, mitochondrial enzymes, ribosomal RNA, cytosolic components, and cell membranes and wall, to name the most obvious. Nevertheless, in contemporary pharmacology, some authors and researchers apply a more restricted use of the term receptor, reserving it for protein complexes embedded in, and spanning, cellular membranes. However, exceptions to this classification system clearly exist. For example, steroids are known to interact with cytosolic receptors that transport them into the nucleus (their site of action), certain anticancer drugs bind to nucleic acids to produce their effects, and bile acids interact with nuclear receptors to modulate cholesterol synthesis. Regardless of how rigid one's definition of receptor is, receptor theory provides a unifying concept for the explanation of the effect of endogenous or xenobiotic chemicals on biological systems.

Although the great preponderance of drugs interact with membrane receptors or some intracellular site, there are a few exceptions. Examples of non-receptor-mediated drug action include: antacids such as sodium bicarbonate, which act to buffer excess hydrogen ions; chelating agents such as ethylenediaminetetraacetic acid, which form inactive complexes with inorganic ions; and osmotic cathartics such as magnesium sulfate, which produce their pharmacological response by attracting water.

THE NATURE OF RECEPTORS

Proteins, glycoproteins, proteolipids, and associated proteinaceous species appear to be particularly suited to act as receptors because they can assume three-dimensional configurations, the three-dimensional shape being the net result of primary, secondary, and tertiary structures. Three dimensionality requires that drugs, or any binding ligand, achieve binding specificity, referred to as "induced fit." If the drug is an active one, the result of this binding is believed to be a conformational change in the receptor, with subsequent modification of membrane permeability or activation of intracellular enzymes.

The concept of a "lock and key" relationship between drug and receptor is based upon the analogous hypothesis of the German chemist and enzymologist Emil Fischer, who originally developed the theory in relation to the interaction between enzymes and substrates. In 1895 Fischer wrote that an enzyme's specific effect might be explained "by assuming that the intimate contact between the molecules necessary for the release of the chemical reaction is possible only with similar geometrical configurations. To use a picture, I would say that the enzyme and the substrate must fit together like lock and key." This lock and key relationship implies extreme precision in the interaction, since extra or improperly placed atoms in the drug, like an additional tooth on a key, can exclude its binding. Failure to achieve "induced fit," therefore, precludes optimal conformational change in the receptor.

The specificity inherent in achieving appropriate geometrical configurations between ligand (i.e., drug) and receptor can extend to stereoisomerism. For example, there are many drugs whose chemical structure contains an asymmetric carbon atom and can thus exist as mirror-image isomers; asymmetry is possible only if all four valences of carbon are utilized by different groups. These asymmetric carbon atoms are often referred to as chiral centers or, conversely, centers of chirality. An example of an optical isomer is the antitussive drug dextromethorphan (found in many OTC cough and cold preparations), which is the *d* isomer of the codeine analog levorphanol. However, unlike the *l* isomer levorphanol, dextromethorphan has no analgesic or addictive properties and does not act through opioid receptors.

Although most drug preparations exist as a racemic mixture (i.e., an equimolar mixture of optical isomers), often only one of the isomers produces the desired pharmacological effect. Therefore, although racemic mixtures are commonly regarded as

Table 5.1 General characteristics of membrane receptors

Protein: generally lipoprotein or glycoprotein in nature
Typical molecular weight in the range of 45–200 kDa
Can be composed of subunits
Frequently glycosylated
K_d of drug binding to receptor (1–100 nM); binding reversible and stereoselective
Receptors saturable because of finite number
Specific binding of receptor results in change in ion flow signal transduction to intracellular site
Specificity of binding not absolute, leading to drug binding to several receptor types
May require more than one drug molecule to bind to receptor to generate signal
Magnitude of signal depends on number of receptors occupied or on receptor occupancy rate;
　　signal can be amplified by intracellular mechanisms
By acting on receptor, drugs can enhance, diminish, or block generation or transmission of signal
Drugs are receptor modulators and *do not* confer new properties on cells or tissues
Receptors must have properties of recognition *and* transduction
Receptor populations can be upregulated, downregulated, or sequestered

single drugs, this may not be technically correct. The two racemic components may have similar or quite different receptor specificities and exert independent pharmacological effects. Considerable research is presently being carried out in this area and is discussed in more detail in Chapter 13.

Chemists have long appreciated that a protein's primary amino acid sequence determines its three-dimensional structure. It has also been known for some time that proteins are able to carry out their diversified functions only when they have folded up into compact three-dimensional structures. The protein-folding problem first gained prominence in the 1950s and 1960s, when Christian Anfinsen demonstrated that ribonuclease could be denatured (unfolded) and renatured reversibly.

During the 1960s and 1970s, receptor proteins, primarily membranous in nature, were isolated and the amino acid sequences of various receptor subunits were determined. In the past two decades complete amino acid sequences of receptors have been determined, and also been successfully cloned. Today we recognize that various types of receptors exist, which can be further divided into different subtypes that, if acted upon by the same ligand (e.g., acetylcholine), can produce either ion channel changes or the generation of secondary messengers (see later discussion). Some general features of receptors are listed in Table 5.1. A pictorial summary of the development of our conceptual understanding of receptors from Ehrlich's time to the present is shown in Figure 5.1.

CHEMICAL BONDS

If most drugs achieve their effects via interaction with a receptor, then by what chemical binding force is this achieved? Ehrlich recognized very early that the combining forces must be very loose. He wrote in 1900: "If alkaloids, aromatic amines, antipyretics or aniline dyes be introduced into the animal body, it is a very easy matter, by means of water, alcohol or acetone, to remove all of these substances quickly and easily from the tissues." This is the reason why isolated organ tissue

Figure 5.1 Comparison of receptor models beginning with (A) Ehrlich's first pictorial representation of his "side-chain" theory in 1898, (B) scheme of drug–receptor interaction in 1971, (C) acetylcholine ion-channel in 1982, and (D) G-protein-coupled receptor system in 1989.

baths containing smooth muscle preparations, such as the guinea pig ileum, can be used experimentally for the sequential assessment of drug activity, since "wash-out" phases can restore the tissue essentially to its original condition.

Based upon the development of knowledge relating to chemical bonds during the first half of the twentieth century, we can now identify the principal binding forces involved in drug–receptor interaction. Of particular importance to this field was some of the research carried out by Linus Pauling in the 1930s. Pauling described (1) a scale of electronegativity that could be used to determine the ionic and covalent character of chemical bonds; (2) the concept of bond–orbital hybridization (the organization of electron clouds of atoms in molecules in configurations that favor bonding); and (3) the theory of resonance (distribution of electrons between two or more possible positions in a bond network).

Simple organic compounds such as hydrocarbons, which by definition only contain carbon and hydrogen atoms, are electrically neutral since the valence electrons comprising the bond are shared equally between the carbon and hydrogen atoms. In contrast, more sophisticated molecules comprising pharmacological receptors in cellular membranes, for example, contain atoms such as oxygen, nitrogen, sulfur, or phosphorus in addition to carbon and hydrogen.

The presence of these additional atoms produces an unequal sharing of electrons due to the differing electronegativities of the elements involved (as Pauling described). Such bonds have the overall effect of shifting the distribution of electrons within the molecule such that areas of positive and negative charge are created (thereby introducing polarity and reactivity into the molecule). Drugs also require the presence of similar atoms in their structure in order to possess areas of positivity and negativity.

The binding of a ligand to a membrane-bound receptor in the aqueous environment of the body is an exchange process, whereby ligand and receptor, both solvated by water molecules, bind together releasing some of the water molecules. Therefore, both the ligand and the receptor lose their interactions with water in favor of interaction with one another. This exchange process includes both favorable and unfavorable free energy changes.

The four most favorable forces in chemical bond formation between ligand and receptor in pharmacology are (1) ionic bonds (i.e., electrostatic); (2) hydrogen bonds; (3) van der Waals forces; and (4) covalent bonds. The first three bond types are easily reversible by energy levels normally present in biological tissue at temperatures between 20 and 40°C (i.e., approximately 5 kcal/mol). Therefore, they are the principal bond forces involved in normal drug action. Covalent bonds are an exception, however, since they require approximately 50–100 kcal/mol to break. This can have significant implications for both the duration of a drug's effect and its toxicity, as described later.

Ionic bonds

These are the principal electrostatic bonds that are formed between two ions of opposite charge (e.g., Na^+ and Cl^-) in which the atom lacks or has surplus electrons. The extent to which ionic bonds may be formed depends on the degree of ionization of groups that form cations (e.g., amino groups) and groups that form anions (e.g., carboxyl groups), and this in turn depends, of course, on the pH of the medium and the pK_a value of the ionizable groups.

Ligands that bind to catecholamine receptors, for example, all contain an amino group that has a dissociation constant greater than 7 so that the ligand will be partly or fully positively charged at neutral pH. It has been assumed, therefore, that the binding of these ligands to their receptors will involve an electrostatic interaction with a negatively charged group on the receptor. A leading candidate to fulfill this role is the carboxyl group of an aspartic acid residue within the binding domain.

Because the intermolecular binding force of the ionic bond decreases only with the square of the interatomic distance (r^2), it is the most effective bond type in attracting a drug molecule from the medium toward the receptor site. In a biological environment, the duration of an ionic bond at a receptor might be only 10^{-5} seconds due to the presence of inorganic salts in the medium that can compete for binding sites. However, when an ionic bond is reinforced by the presence of bonds that act over shorter ranges, the union can become stronger, and last for longer.

Hydrogen bonds

The hydrogen nucleus is strongly electropositive, being essentially a bare proton. This high concentration of electropositivity enables the hydrogen atom to act as a bond between two electronegative atoms (e.g., O, N, and F), assuming the interatomic distance is appropriate. Extensive structure–activity studies using dopamine receptors have shown that at least one hydroxyl group on the benzene ring of an agonist is desirable for activity. It is assumed that the hydroxyl groups are involved in hydrogen bonds with amino acid side chains on the receptor (most likely through O or N).

Hydrogen bonds are expressed over a short distance with the binding force decreasing by the fourth power of the interatomic distance (r^4). For this reason, hydrogen bonds are considered to be important at the more intimate levels of drug–receptor interactions and can act in support of ionic bonds. Individually, hydrogen bonds are weak, but collectively they can significantly stabilize the association of a drug with its receptor.

van der Waals forces

These are the most common of all attractions between atoms. van der Waals forces are the result of the formation of "induced dipoles" when atoms of different electronegativity are bonded together. The intermolecular attraction arises from the fluctuations of charge in two atoms or molecules that are close together. Since the electrons are moving, each molecule has an instantaneous dipole moment that is not zero. If the electron density fluctuations in the two atoms or molecules were unrelated there would be no net attraction. However, an instantaneous dipole in one atom or molecule induces an oppositely oriented dipole in the neighboring atom or molecule, and these instantaneous dipoles attract each other. van der Waals forces are significant only over very short distances since their power varies inversely with the seventh power of the interatomic distance (r^7). However, when a number of atoms become closely juxtaposed, significant attraction can occur and confer stability to a drug–receptor association.

Table 5.2 Examples of drugs forming covalent bonds

Drug	Example
Nitrogen mustards	Cyclophosphamide
Anticholinesterase	Malathion
Hepatotoxic drugs	Acetaminophen
α-Adrenoreceptor antagonist	Phenoxybenzamine

Covalent bonds

The covalent bond, as mentioned earlier, is the most tenacious type of chemical bond since it involves the mutual sharing of orbital electrons. It is the type of bond that holds organic compounds such as proteins, carbohydrates, and lipids together. Fortunately, for these important biochemical entities, it normally does not lend itself to easy reversibility. However, it is not the typical drug–receptor bond type. If it were the typical bond formed between drugs and their receptors, all pharmacological effects would have an inordinately long duration of action.

The strongest bond that can be broken nonenzymatically at body temperature requires approximately 10 kcal/mol. Therefore, covalent bonds (50–100 kcal/mol) are not examples of reversible drug–receptor interactions. We have seen that conjugation reactions occurring in type II biotransformation reactions can involve the formation of covalent linkage (e.g., glucuronidation). This is an example of a "good" type of covalent bond virtually assuring that the conjugate will be successfully excreted. However, certain bioactivated metabolites can form "bad" covalent bonds with normal macromolecular complexes and produce tissue injury. This is a focus in Chapter 7 dealing with drug toxicity. Table 5.2 presents examples of drugs forming covalent bonds with biological molecules.

RECEPTOR CLASSES

Table 5.3 presents a representative list of major receptor classes with their respective subtypes and endogenous transmitters. The receptors are further divided into either ion channel or second-messenger categories.

Ligand-gated ion channel receptors

The nicotinic acetylcholine (ACh) receptor is a well-characterized receptor of this type consisting of five subunits. It is present on the skeletal muscle cell end-plate in the neuromuscular junction, at all autonomic ganglia, and in the central nervous system (CNS). The function of this receptor is to convert ACh binding into an electrical signal via increased Na^+ or K^+ permeability across the cell membrane (i.e., membrane depolarization). When two molecules of ACh bind to the α subunit of the receptor, a conformational change in the receptor induces opening of the channel to at least 0.65 nm for approximately 1–2 ms.

Table 5.3 Examples of classical receptors

Type	Subtype[a]	Endogenous transmitter	Ion channel	Secondary messenger
Acetylcholine	Nicotinic	Acetylcholine	X	—
	Muscarinic: M_1, M_2, M_3, M_4, M_5	Acetylcholine		X
Adrenergic	α_1, α_2	Epinephrine and norepinephrine	—	X
	$\beta_1, \beta_2, \beta_3$	Epinephrine and norepinephrine		X
GABA	A	GABA	X	—
	B	GABA	?	X
Acidic amino acids	NMDA, kainate, quisqualate	Glutamate or aspartate	X	?
Opiate	$\mu, \mu_1, \kappa, \delta, \varepsilon$	Enkephalins	X[b]	X
Serotonin	$5\text{-}HT_1, 5\text{-}HT_2, 5\text{-}HT_3$	5-HT	—	X
Dopamine	D_1, D_2, D_3, D_4, D_5	Dopamine	—	X
Adenosine	A_1, A_2	Adenosine	—	X
Glycine	—	Glycine	X	—
Histamine	H_1, H_2, H_3	Histamine	—	X
Insulin	—	Insulin	—	X
Glucagon	—	Glucagon	—	X
ACTH	—	ACTH	—	X
Steroids	—	Several	—	Special

Source: Brody et al. (1994), *Human Pharmacology: Molecular to Clinical*. 2nd ed. St Louis, MO: Mosby. Reprinted with permission.

Notes
a Other subtypes in various stages of documentation have been proposed, especially where no endogenous transmitter is defined yet.
b Results not clear.

Another important ligand-gated ion channel receptor is the type A gamma-aminobutyric acid (GABA) receptor. The GABA receptor is extremely important because it is the primary endogenous inhibitory transmitter in the CNS. The inhibitory action of the GABA receptor system is enhanced by drugs such as the benzodiazepine class (e.g., minor tranquilizers), which are believed to augment opening of a chloride-ion channel via interaction at an allosteric site.

Voltage-dependent ion channel receptors

These types of receptors are typically present in the membranes of excitable nerve, cardiac, and skeletal muscle cells and are subject to voltage-mediated channel opening. In this situation, membrane depolarization induces conformational opening of channels and allows a transient influx of ions such as Na^+ and Ca^{2+}. Blockade of these respective ion channels is believed to explain the mechanism of action of local anesthetics and certain antihypertensive agents (calcium channel blockers, for example). In certain situations, prolonged opening of a channel can result in hyperpolarization of a cell (e.g., Cl^- influx), resulting in resistance of the cell to subsequent depolarization. Human disorders associated with known mutations of genes encoding for K^+ channels now total 14 and include episodic ataxia, certain forms of epilepsy, and hyperinsulinemia hypoglycemia of infancy.

G-protein-coupled second-messenger receptors

Ligand binding to cell-surface receptors initiates a series of events known collectively as signal transduction. In this process, receptors alter the status of other proteins, which in turn leads to a cascade of changes inside the cell. The cell uses this cascade of information to describe what is occurring in the cellular environment and then make the necessary alterations. Without the ability to transduce the initial receptor signal, the cell would be unresponsive to many environmental changes, making homeostasis more difficult to maintain. Understanding signal transduction is critical to gaining insight into how cells communicate with each other as well as how we can influence cell activity pharmacologically.

A very important class of membrane receptors transmits their signal by coupling with guanine nucleotide-binding proteins (G proteins). In fact, G-protein-coupled receptors (GPCRs) are the largest family of cell-surface molecules involved in signal transmission. These receptors are activated by a wide variety of ligands, including peptide and nonpeptide neurotransmitters, hormones, growth factors, odorant molecules, and light. GPCRs are the target of approximately 60 percent of the current therapeutic agents on the market, including more than a quarter of the 100 top-selling drugs, with sales in the range of several billion dollars per year. Additional examples of GPCR systems include the β-adrenergic receptor (involved in regulating cardiac contractility), the opioid and dopamine receptors (involved in brain function), and the N-formyl peptide receptor (involved in the immune response). Abnormalities in GPCR signaling are involved in numerous diseases and disorders and are therefore a major target for future therapeutic intervention.

G proteins consist of three subunits (α, β, and γ) in one of two states: an inactive form in which guanosine on the α subunit is in the diphosphate form (GDP), or an active state in which GDP is displaced by guanosine triphosphate (GTP). Activation results in dissociation of the α subunit and interaction of its C-terminal region with the appropriate enzyme. Because G proteins have intrinsic GTPase activity they are capable of rapid transformation from active to inactive status.

GPCRs are known to generate second messengers as the method of transducing their transmembrane signaling mechanism. The principal messengers formed are cyclic adenosine monophosphate (cAMP), inositol triphosphate (IP_3), and 1,2-diacylglycerol (DAG). G proteins provide the link between ligand interaction with the receptor and formation of the second messenger generally via enzyme activation of adenylate cyclase and phospholipase C. However, an inhibitory G protein for adenylate cyclase does exist.

The generation of all three second messengers (cAMP, IP_3, and DAG) leads to the activation of protein kinases and the subsequent phosphorylation of important cellular enzymes. [Note: nine amino acids have the potential for adding phosphate, but in biological systems phosphorylation has been described primarily on three of these —serine, threonine, and tyrosine.) The phosphorylation of these key enzymes, in turn, produces activation or inactivation of significant cellular biochemical pathways. In summary, the process is a cascade resulting in amplification of the original receptor signal through a series of four steps: (1) binding of the ligand to the membrane-bound receptor; (2) activation of the membrane-bound G protein; (3) activation of the membrane-bound enzyme; and (4) activation of intracellular kinases.

Receptors with tyrosine kinase activity

A group of receptors exists that responds to so-called growth factors such as insulin, epidermal growth factor, platelet-derived growth factor, etc. These receptors have an extracellular domain that binds the growth factor and an intracellular domain that possesses latent kinase activity. The interaction of insulin, for example, results in autophosphorylation of the intracellular domain and subsequent internalization of the insulin–receptor complex. The internalized complex now possesses the properties of a tyrosine kinase and can phosphorylate cell substrates that produce the appropriate intracellular effect. However, these kinases differ from the usual protein kinases in that they phosphorylate proteins exclusively on tyrosine hydroxyl residues. The ensemble of proteins phosphorylated by the insulin receptor has not yet been identified, but there is supportive evidence that tyrosine kinase activity is required for the major actions of insulin. For example, it is possible that a membrane-linked glucose transport system becomes activated following insulin-stimulated phosphorylation.

RECEPTOR DYNAMISM

An important concept to appreciate regarding receptors is that they are not static, stand-alone components of a cell. On the contrary, they are an integral part of the overall homeostatic balance of the body. For example, receptors can become desensitized upon continuous exposure to an agonist. When desensitization involves a specific class of agonists it is referred to as *homologous desensitization*. If response is reduced by disparate classes of drugs, the term *heterologous desensitization* is applied.

GPCR-mediated signal transduction can be attenuated with relatively fast kinetics (within seconds to minutes after agonist-induced activation) by a process called *rapid desensitization*. Rapid desensitization is characterized by functional uncoupling of receptors from the heterotrimeric G proteins, which occurs without any detectable change in the total number of receptors present in cells or tissues. Rapid desensitization of certain GPCRs is associated with a process called *sequestration*, which involves a physical redistribution of receptors from the plasma membrane to intracellular membranes via endocytosis. The process of internalization is thought to promote dephosphorylation by an endosome-associated phosphatase. Dephosphorylation and subsequent recycling of receptors back to the plasma membrane contribute to a reversal of the desensitized state (resensitization), which is required for full recovery of cellular signaling potential following agonist withdrawal.

GPCRs are also regulated by mechanisms that operate over a much longer time scale. A process called *downregulation* refers to an actual decrease in the total number of receptors in cells or a tissue, which is typically induced over a period of hours to days after prolonged or repeated exposure to an agonist ligand. Downregulation of GPCRs can be differentiated in at least three ways from the process of sequestration: (1) downregulation typically occurs much more slowly than rapid internalization; (2) downregulation is characterized by a reduction in the total number of receptors present in cells or tissues; and (3) internalization is characterized by a physical redistribution of receptor status (uncoupling) without a detectable change in total receptor number.

In addition to the possibility of decreases in receptor number, a corresponding condition of *upregulation* can take place. In this case sensitization can occur by an increase in receptor number. For example, chronic exposure to high levels of thyroid hormone (i.e., thyroxin) can lead to an increase in myocardial β receptors with corresponding increased sensitivity to β agonists. A corresponding result could be elevated heart rate, which is often present in hyperthroidism.

The question of how receptor numbers can be modified is an intriguing one. Because transmembrane receptor proteins are amphipathic in nature (i.e., they possess both extracellular and intracellular polar groups), they are prevented from moving into or out of the membrane lipid bilayer or changing their orientation. However, they can freely diffuse laterally in the plane of the membrane. One theory proposes that upon binding, drug–receptor complexes rapidly migrate to specialized membrane areas called "coated pits." Here they hypothetically undergo a sequence of internalization and recycling. Presumably, there is some feedback mechanism that either accelerates or decelerates the process and hence affects the number of regenerated free receptors available.

Disease states can also influence normal receptor function. For example, modified receptor function occurs in certain autoimmune diseases. Myasthenia gravis is a neuromuscular disease characterized by weakness and marked fatigability of skeletal muscles. The defect in myasthenia gravis is in synaptic transmission at the neuromuscular junction. Initial responses in the myasthenic patient may be normal, but they diminish rapidly, which explains the difficulty in maintaining voluntary muscle activity for more than brief periods.

Animal studies performed during the 1970s indicated that the disease represented an autoimmune response directed toward the acetylcholine receptor. Antireceptor antibody was soon identified in patients with the disorder. In fact, receptor-binding antibodies are detectable in sera of 90 percent of patients with the disease. The result of the autoimmune reaction is receptor degradation with loss of function at the motor end-plate.

Treatment of the disorder usually involves the administration of acetylcholinesterase inhibitors (see Chapter 11). Drugs such as neostigmine increase the response of myasthenic muscle to nerve impulses primarily by preserving endogenously released acetylcholine from enzymatic inactivation. With release of acetylcholine, receptors over a greater surface of the motor end-plate are exposed to the transmitter. Grave's disease (hyperthyroidism) is another receptor-mediated autoimmune disease. However, in this case the antibodies developed against thyrotropin receptors in the thyroid behave like agonists rather than antagonists. The result is enhanced thyroid hormone production by the gland, producing elevated levels of circulating thyroid hormone, i.e., hyperthyroidism.

OPIATE AND TETRAHYDROCANNABINOL RECEPTORS

One of the more interesting chapters in the history of receptors has been their impact on the discovery of endogenous substances. The fact that substances of plant origin such as curare, nicotine, and muscarine could produce neuropharmacological effects suggested that there might exist corresponding endogenous substances. Eventually, this led to a deliberate search for unknown neurotransmitters as a counterpart of neuroactive plant products. One of these is the classic study of Otto Lowi and the discovery of "vagusstoff" (see Chapter 11).

It was only a matter of time, several decades later, when neuropharmacologists began to think that if endogenous mediators existed, and they had their own receptors, then it seemed reasonable to propose that neuroactive drugs, such as morphine for example, might be interacting with receptors that normally accommodate endogenous ligands. One of the first compounds studied in this way was, in fact, morphine. Intensive research on both sides of the Atlantic did establish the existence of opioid receptors in the brain. The question then became: "Is it sensible to suppose that such highly specific receptors developed, over the long course of evolution, only to combine with morphine, which is a product of the opium poppy? Was it not more likely that there were natural morphine-like neurotransmitters in the brain, and that these receptors had evolved to accommodate them?"

In 1975, Hans Kosterlitz and John Hughes in Scotland were able to isolate from thousands of pig brains two endogenous active substances that acted just like morphine. Surprisingly, the chemical composition of these substances was peptide in nature, being only five amino acids in length. They were given the name enkephalins. A database analysis of all known amino acid sequences revealed the presence of this 5-amino-acid sequence in a larger 31-amino-acid peptide found in the pituitary and designated beta-endorphin. Another 17-amino-acid opioid peptide was subsequently isolated several years later and named dynorphin. These endogenous opioid peptides play important physiological and pharmacological roles in analgesia, behavior, emotion, learning, neurotransmission, and neuromodulation by interacting with a number of opioid receptor subsets (e.g., μ, κ, and δ).

A similar situation has occurred with tetrahydrocannabinol (THC). THC acts on a seven-helix receptor that has been identified in those parts of the brain that could reasonably mediate changes in mood and perception caused by marijuana. The receptor has been isolated and its amino acid sequence determined. As was the case with the opiates, the question of an endogenous THC-like material was raised. At the present time, the most likely candidate for an endogenous ligand for the THC receptor is known as anandamide (the ethanolamide of arachidonic acid). Interestingly, anandamide has been found to be present in chocolate and cocoa powder. This discovery may be relevant to the well-known phenomenon of "chocolate craving." Can people become dependent on this confection? Do they periodically need an anandamide fix?

SELECTED BIBLIOGRAPHY

Albert, A. (1979) *Selective Toxicity, The Physico-Chemical Basis of Therapy*, 6th ed. London: Chapman & Hall.
Brody, T. M., Larner, J., Minneman, K. P. and Neu, H. C. (eds) (1994) *Human Pharmacology: Molecular to Clinical*, 2nd ed. St Louis, MO: Mosby.
Kenakin, T. P., Bond, R. A. and Bonner, T. I. (1992) *Definition of pharmacological receptors*. *Pharmacol. Rev.* 44: 351–362.
Woolf, P. J. and Lindeman, J. J. (2001) *From the static to the dynamic: three models of signal transduction in G protein-coupled receptors*. In *Biomedical Applications of Computer Modeling* (ed. A. Christopoulos). Boca Raton, FL: CRC Press.
Wyman, J. and Gill, S. J. (1990) *Binding and Linkage. Functional Chemistry of Biological Macromolecules*. Mill Valley, CA: University Science Books.

QUESTIONS

1 Which of the following individuals first referred to drugs acting on a "receptive substance"?
   a   Crum Brown
   b   John Priestley
   c   John Langley
   d   Paul Ehrlich
   e   c and d.

2 The concept of a "lock and key" relationship between drug and receptor is based on work done by which of the following?
   a   Paul Ehrlich
   b   John Langley
   c   William Withering
   d   Paracelsus
   e   Emil Fischer.

3 Which of the following bond types can be broken by energy levels normally present in biological tissues?
   a   van der Waals
   b   ionic (electrostatic)
   c   hydrogen
   d   covalent
   e   a, b, and c.

4 Which is/are true regarding receptors?
   a   can be located in the nucleus
   b   can be located in the mitochondrion
   c   can be located in the cell membrane
   d   can be located in the cell cytosol
   e   all of the above.

5 Which of the following is/are classified as ligand-gated ion channel ligands?
   a   cyclic-AMP
   b   inositol triphosphate
   c   acetylcholine
   d   GABA
   e   c and d above.

6 Which of the following is/are second messengers that transduce G protein membrane receptors?
   a   cyclic-AMP
   b   1,2-diacylglycerol
   c   inositol triphosphate
   d   all of the above
   e   guanosine triphosphate.

7 Successful generation of second messengers results in which of the following?
   a   phosphorylation of certain enzymes
   b   an amplification cascade
   c   activation of protein kinases
   d   all of the above
   e   a and c only.

8 Rapid desensitization of β receptors is believed to involve which of the following?
   a   functional uncoupling of the receptor from its G protein
   b   no change in receptor number
   c   increased degradation of receptor
   d   increase in receptor number
   e   a and b above.

9 Sensitization of β receptors can involve which of the following?
   a   development of myasthenia gravis
   b   chronic exposure to thyroid hormone (e.g., thyroxin)
   c   reduction of receptor number
   d   increased sequestration into endosomes
   e   none of the above.

10 Which of the following endogenous peptides play an important role in analgesia by interacting with opioid receptors?
   a   enkephalins
   b   β-endorphin
   c   dynorphin
   d   all of the above
   e   none of the above.

Chapter 6

Dose–response relationship

BACKGROUND

As mentioned in the previous chapter, the concept of biological receptors mediating the effect of drugs provided a useful conceptual framework to understand the action of most drugs. In fact, the foundation of receptor pharmacology is the dose–response curve, a graphical representation of the observed effect of a drug as a function of its concentration at the receptor site.

As drug development became of greater importance during the first half of the twentieth century, a more quantitative and analytical foundation was needed to assess drug potency per se as well as comparative drug potency. The standardization and quantification of technique and experimental design, and the rigorous application of statistical analysis, have provided pharmacodynamics with a necessary solid base.

The individual most associated with the development of early quantitative expressions of drug–receptor interactions is Alfred Joseph Clark. Clark published most of his proposals between the world wars based on his studies of atropine and the cholinergic system. Clark proposed that drugs combined with receptors in proportion to their concentration and then dissociated from the receptors in proportion to the concentration of the drug–receptor complexes. In essence, Clark envisioned that the interaction between drug and receptor was analogous to the reversible adsorption of a gas to a metal surface and, therefore, follows the law of mass action. This relationship can be illustrated in a hyperbolic curve, referred to as a Langmuir adsorption isotherm, when depicted using arithmetic scales on both coordinates (Figure 6.1).

Mathematically, the interaction between drug and receptor can be represented by the following basic relationship:

$$[X] + [R] \leftrightarrow [XR] \rightarrow E$$

where [X] is the concentration of drug at the receptor, [R] is the concentration of free receptors, and [XR] is the concentration of the drug–receptor complex. Because the law of mass action states that the velocity of a chemical reaction is proportional to the concentration of the reacting substances, the dissociation constant, K_d, of a drug–receptor complex is expressed by the following relationship:

$$K_d = [X][R]/[XR]$$

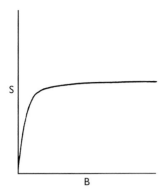

Figure 6.1 Typical Langmuir isotherm: S, concentration of substance adsorbed; B, total concentration of substance.

Source: A. Albert (1979), *Selective Toxicity: The Physico-Chemical Basis of Therapy*, 6th ed. London: Chapman & Hall. Reprinted with permission.

The above two equations indicate, therefore, that the fraction of all receptors that is combined with a drug is a function of both drug concentration and the dissociation constant of the [XR] complex. K_d is, therefore, basically an indication of strength of binding and can be determined by many methods but these are beyond the scope of this book.

From the basic drug–receptor relationship just described it may be apparent that there are several implicit assumptions: (1) that the magnitude of the pharmacological effect (E) is directly proportional to [XR]; and (2) that the maximal effect (E_m) occurs when the drug (X) occupies 100 percent of the receptors. These assumptions embody the classical receptor theory developed by Clark. Although the validity of these assumptions has been justifiably questioned from time to time (e.g., some experimental data indicate that maximal effect can be achieved with less than 100 percent occupancy, leaving "spare receptors"), the Clark "occupancy" model has, nevertheless, found wide validation and provided the framework for subsequent development of concepts such as agonism, antagonism, affinity, and efficacy.

MEASUREMENT

Experimentation on isolated organs offers several advantages in quantifying drug effects including:

(1) the drug concentration in the tissue is usually known;
(2) there is reduced complexity and ease of relating dose and effect;
(3) it is possible to circumvent compensatory physiological responses that may partially cancel the primary effect in the intact organism (e.g., the heart rate increasing action of norepinephrine cannot easily be demonstrated in the intact animal because a simultaneous compensatory response occurs that slows heart rate); and
(4) the drug effect may be examined over its full range of intensities.

Disadvantages include:

(1) unavoidable tissue injury during dissection;
(2) loss of physiological regulation of function in the isolated tissue; and
(3) the artificial milieu imposed on the tissue.

Obviously, some drug effects that are being studied require use of the whole animal (e.g., sedation).

Characterization of ligand interaction with tissue receptors can also be carried out by studying concentration–binding relationships. The analysis of drug binding to receptors aims to determine the affinity of ligands, the kinetics of interaction, and the characteristics of the binding site itself. In studying the affinity and number of such binding sites, use is made of membrane suspensions of different tissues. This approach is based on the expectation that binding sites will retain their characteristic properties during cell homogenization.

In the case of binding studies, the drug under study is radiolabeled (enabling low concentrations to be measured quantitatively), added to the membrane suspension, and allowed to bind to receptors. Membrane fragments and medium are then separated by filtration over filter discs and the amount of drug bound is determined by measuring the radioactivity remaining on the dried filter disc. Binding of the ligand increases in proportion to concentration as long as a significant number of free binding sites remain. However, as binding sites approach saturation, the number of free sites decreases and the increment in binding is no longer proportional (i.e., linear) to the increase in concentration and a hyperbolic relationship develops.

The law of mass action describes the hyperbolic relationship between binding and concentration. The relationship is characterized by the drug's affinity and maximum binding. Affinity is expressed as the equilibrium dissociation constant and corresponds to that ligand concentration at which 50 percent of the binding sites are occupied (K_d). Maximum binding (B_{max}) is the total number of binding sites per unit weight of membrane homogenate (e.g., mg protein) represented by the upper limit of the curve.

The differing affinity of various ligands for a binding site can be demonstrated quite elegantly by binding assays. Although simple to perform, these binding assays pose the difficulty of correlating binding site data with pharmacological effect; this is particularly difficult when more than one population of binding site is present (a not unusual situation). In addition, receptor binding must not be implied unless it can be demonstrated that (1) binding is saturable (*saturability*); (2) the only substances bound are those possessing the same pharmacological mechanism of action (*specificity*); and (3) binding affinity of various ligands correlates with their pharmacological potency (see later discussion). Although binding assays provide information about the affinity of ligands, they do not provide evidence as to whether a ligand is an agonist or an antagonist (discussed later).

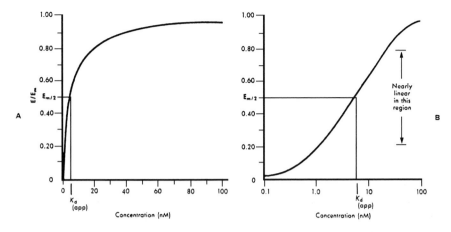

Figure 6.2 Concentration–response curve for graded response: (A) arithmetic scale; (B) log concentration scale. K_d(app) is arbitrarily taken to be 4.5 nM.

Source: T. M. Brody, J. Larner, K. P. Minneman and H. C. Neu (eds) (1994), *Human Pharmacology: Molecular to Clinical*, 2nd ed. St Louis, MO: Mosby. Reprinted with permission.

GRAPHICAL REPRESENTATION

Graded response

In pharmacology, it is conventional to plot the dependent variable, response or effect, against the independent variable, dose (total amount) or dosage (e.g., mg/kg body weight). This can be done by expressing dose on either an arithmetic or a logarithmic scale (Figure 6.2).

However, there are practical difficulties associated with fitting pharmacological data with appreciable scatter to a curved arithmetic line (Figure 6.2A). For example, a plot of arithmetic dose reaches a maximal asymptote value when the drug occupies all of the receptor sites. In addition, the range of concentrations needed to fully depict the dose–response relationship is usually too wide to be useful in the format shown.

Most dose–response data are routinely transformed, therefore, to a nearly straight line by plotting dose on the x-axis on a logarithmic scale (Figure 6.2B). The result is essentially a linear relationship between approximately 20 and 80 percent of the maximum response. Depicting the data in this manner allows a more accurate determination of a drug's ED_{50} (i.e., the concentration of a drug required to produce 50 percent of the maximal response possible and conventionally used as a criterion for drug comparison).

A binding constant for ligand attaching to receptor or inhibitor constant for an enzyme reaction may also be determined. These quantities are usually expressed in terms of the dissociation constant of the ligand–receptor complex (K_d) or enzyme-inhibitor complex (K_i). For the ligand–receptor interaction this constant is equal to the ligand concentration at which 50 percent of the receptors are occupied by the ligand and it is assumed, although this is not always correct, that the measured response has fallen to half its maximum value. For typical drug–receptor interactions,

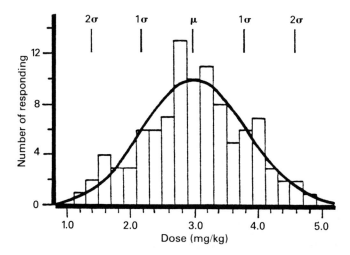

Figure 6.3 Quantal effects. Typical set of data after administration of increasing doses of drug to a group of subjects and observation of minimum dose at which each subject responds. Data shown are for 100 subjects: dose increased in 0.2 mg/kg of body weight increments. Mean (μ) (and median) dose is 3.0 mg/kg; standard deviation ($\bar{v}$) is 0.8 mg/kg. Results plotted as histogram (bar graph) showing number responding at each dose; smooth curve is normal distribution function calculated for μ of 3.0 and $\bar{v}$ of 0.8.

Source: T. M. Brody, J. Larner, K. P. Minneman and H. C. Neu (eds) (1994), *Human Pharmacology: Molecular to Clinical*, 2nd ed. St Louis, MO: Mosby. Reprinted with permission.

the dissociation constants are generally on the order of 10^{-7} to 10^{-10} M (i.e., generally in the nanomolar range).

The measurement of the reversible binding of a radioactive ligand to a receptor preparation (radioligand binding) has greatly increased our understanding of receptors, and, provided it is understood that the binding occasionally may have to be discounted because it is an artifact of the preparation, the knowledge gained has been of great value in identifying, quantifying, and in some cases isolating a receptor. Two of the greatest challenges in pharmacology are (1) to link binding data with pharmacological effect and (2) to understand in molecular terms how the signal is transduced in a given cell to produce a given response.

Quantal response

The data plotted in Figure 6.2 represent a graded response. That is, the response occurs in gradations in proportion to the number of receptors occupied. However, drug responses can also be classified as quantal. That is, the observable response is described on an all-or-none basis. Figure 6.3 depicts a quantal drug response in which the number of individuals responding becomes the dependent variable in response to the minimum dose required. Because the shape of the histogram (i.e., the bell curve), in this example, is in reasonably good agreement with that of a normal or gaussian distribution, statistical parameters for normal distribution can be used to predict variability of drug response in the general population.

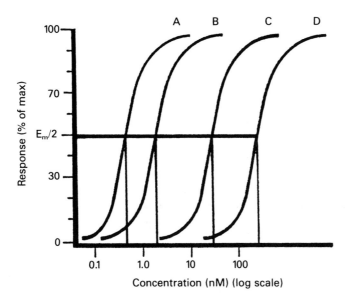

Figure 6.4 Schema of log concentration–response curves for a series of agonists (A, B, C, and D). Note that all the drugs are shown having the same maximum response. The most potent drug produces $E_m/2$ at the lowest concentration; thus drug A is the most potent. Concentration of each drug needed to produce 50 percent of maximum response (ED_{50}) also shown. Concentration values are arbitrary.

Source: T. M. Brody, J. Larner, K. P. Minneman and H. C. Neu (eds) (1994), *Human Pharmacology: Molecular to Clinical*, 2nd ed. St Louis, MO: Mosby. Reprinted with permission.

AGONISTS

The term agonist (derived from the Greek word meaning "to contend" or "to act") was introduced by J. Reuse in 1948 and refers to compounds that activate receptor-based processes via reversible interactions based upon the laws of mass action described earlier. An example of typical log concentration–response curves for a series of agonist drugs that bind to the same receptor type is shown in Figure 6.4. In this schema, the *x*-axis reflects the relative affinity of four agonists for the receptor type in question. Affinity is a chemical property, mandated by chemical forces (see Chapter 5) that cause the drug to associate with the receptor. It should be obvious from the relationship of the four agonists that agonist A has greater affinity for the receptor than the other agonists. In other words, it takes less of agonist A to produce a given effect than agonists B, C, or D. In fact, we can quantify this difference by determining the respective ED_{50} values (in this case agonist A is approximately 20–30 times more potent than D). Potency is, therefore, a comparative term and is most appropriately used when comparing agonists that interact with the same receptor type.

As mentioned earlier, there are several assumptions made in the classic Clark occupancy model. While these assumptions may be true in some cases, there are many exceptions. One of the main problems is that sometimes there is a nonlinear relationship between occupancy and response. In order to explain this seemingly anomalous situation Ariens (1954) and Stephenson (1956) introduced the terms "intrinsic activity" and "efficacy," respectively. These terms refer to inherent qualities of the drug, independent of concentration, that modulate the effect. Today, the terms are commonly used interchangeably and are operationally synonymous (some authors have, in fact, combined the terms into a new hybrid, namely, "intrinsic efficacy"). These terms have been treated functionally as a proportionality constant that quantifies the extent of change imparted to a receptor upon binding an agonist. Thus, the amplitude of the signal for each receptor type is a product of the efficacy of the agonist and its concentration at the receptor site.

While the x-axis reflects an agonist's affinity for the receptor type, the y-axis provides us with information regarding the efficacy of the agonist. That is, how high will its maximal effect go? In essence, does the drug do anything? For drug development companies this is an important question since the 1962 Kefauver–Harris amendments to the Federal Food, Drug, and Cosmetics Act require proof of efficacy before a new drug can be marketed. Affinity and efficacy characterize an agonist.

In Figure 6.4 all four agonists produce the same level of maximal response. Therefore, although the agonists differ in their affinity for the receptor, they can be equally efficacious if given in adequate amounts. In summary, agonist D can produce the same effect as agonist A but its lesser affinity for the receptor must be compensated for by increasing its concentration in the vicinity of the receptor; in essence, increasing its probability of a "hit."

There are situations in which agonists can have a relationship the reverse of that described above. Figure 6.5 depicts three agonists that have the same affinity for the

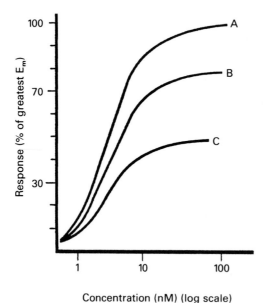

Figure 6.5 Series of agonists that vary in efficacy (E_m) at essentially constant potency. Drug A is the most efficacious and drug C the least. Concentrations are arbitrary but in therapeutic plasma concentration range for many drugs.

Source: T. M. Brody, J. Larner, K. P. Minneman and H. C. Neu (eds) (1994), *Human Pharmacology: Molecular to Clinical*, 2nd ed. St Louis, MO: Mosby. Reprinted with permission.

receptor type (i.e., the same ED_{50}) but not the same efficacy. In this schema agonist A is approximately 2.5 times more efficacious than agonist C. Therefore, agonist C may be thought of as a partial agonist. Partial agonists, in fact, have a dual effect since they can also have antagonistic properties. That is, in the presence of agonists with greater efficacy they can reduce their effectiveness (i.e., they have mixed agonist–antagonist properties depending on the situation). Interestingly, because all three agonists have the same ED_{50} they are equally potent, by definition. It should be obvious, therefore, that simply knowing a drug's potency is not the whole story.

ANTAGONISTS

Antagonists are compounds that can (partially) diminish or prevent (totally) agonistic effects and are usually classified as competitive, noncompetitive, or allosteric. Competitive antagonists have the capacity to bind to the same set of receptors as an agonist (i.e., also have affinity) but do not possess efficacy. Because agonist and antagonist compete for the same receptor binding site, it is possible for an agonist to reassert its efficacy if its concentration is sufficiently increased to compensate for the antagonist present.

An example of such competitive displacement is illustrated in Figure 6.6. This figure illustrates a typical parallel shift to the right of the original agonist curve in the presence of a competitive antagonist. The magnitude of the shift to the right on the x-axis is an index of the relative affinity of the antagonist with no change in maximal

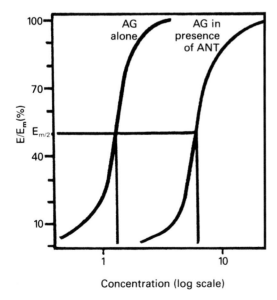

Figure 6.6 Competitive antagonism, where both the agonist (AG) and the antagonist (ANT) compete to bind reversibly to the same subtype of receptor sites.

Source: T. M. Brody, J. Larner, K. P. Minneman and H. C. Neu (eds) (1994), *Human Pharmacology: Molecular to Clinical*, 2nd ed. St Louis, MO: Mosby. Reprinted with permission.

response. Competitive antagonists with high affinity for the receptor will produce a greater shift to the right than weaker compounds since higher concentration of the agonist is required to successfully compete. Note that the ultimate potential efficacy of the agonist is not diminished in the presence of a competitive inhibitor. Such is not the case when noncompetitive or allosteric inhibition occurs.

NONCOMPETITIVE AND ALLOSTERIC INHIBITORS

Noncompetitive antagonism can occur if the antagonist binds to the same site as the agonist but does so irreversibly or pseudo irreversibly (i.e., very slow dissociation but no covalent binding). It also causes a shift in the dose–response curve to the right but does cause depression of the maximal response (not shown).

Some noncompetitive antagonists do not interact with the agonist receptor binding site but, rather, interact with a different site on the receptor molecule such that the receptor is altered. This is sometimes referred to as allosteric inhibition. The impact of allosteric inhibition on agonist action is shown in Figure 6.7. In this case, the response to the agonist is plotted in the absence or presence of increasing concentrations of the allosteric noncompetitive antagonist. The result is a decrease in both the slope of the agonist dose–response curve and the maximum effect produced by the agonist. If high enough concentrations of the noncompetitive antagonist are used, the agonist effect can be abolished even though it may be occupying the receptor. Therefore, in contrast to competitive antagonism, the effect of an allosteric noncompetitive antagonist cannot be reversed by simply increasing agonist concentration since the law of mass action does not apply.

It may be useful at this point to acknowledge the fact that there are other types of antagonisms involving drug effects. Physiological antagonism involves those compensatory biological mechanisms that exist to maintain our homeostasis. For example,

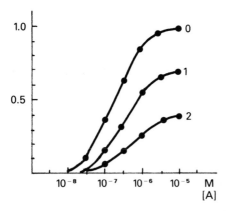

Figure 6.7 Concentration–effect curves of: (0) A in the absence of B; (1) A in the presence of B; and (2) A in the presence of three times the amount of B used for curve 1.

Source: E. Mutschler and H. Derendorf (eds) (1995), *Drug Actions: Basic Principles and Therapeutic Aspects.* Boca Raton, FL: CRC Press. Reprinted with permission.

if we inject a sufficient amount of norepinephrine to increase blood pressure, baroreceptors located in the carotid arteries will be activated and heart rate slowed via cardiovascular centers in the brain. Chemical antagonism occurs when a substance reduces the concentration of an agonist by forming a chemical complex (see Chapter 8). Pharmacokinetic antagonism is present when one drug accelerates the metabolism or elimination of another (e.g., enzyme induction by phenobarbital as described in Chapter 3).

SELECTED BIBLIOGRAPHY

Albert, A. (1979) *Selective Toxicity, The Physico-Chemical Basis of Therapy,* 6th ed. London: Chapman & Hall.

Brody, T. M., Larner, J., Minneman, K. P. and Neu, H. C. (eds) (1994) *Human Pharmacology: Molecular to Clinical,* 2nd ed. St Louis, MO: Mosby.

Clapham, D. E. (1993) Mutations in G protein-linked receptors: novel insights on disease. *Cell* 75: 1237–1239.

Mutschler, E. and Derendorf, H. (eds) (1995) *Drug Actions: Basic Principles and Therapeutic Aspects.* Boca Raton, FL: CRC Press.

Pratt, W. B. and Taylor, P. (1990) *Principles of Drug Action. The Basis of Pharmacology,* 3rd ed. New York: Churchill Livingstone.

Smith, C. M. and Reynard, A. M. (eds) (1995) *Essentials of Pharmacology.* Philadelphia: W. B. Saunders.

Stephenson, R. P. (1956) Modification of receptor theory. *Br. J. Pharmacol.* 11: 379–393.

QUESTIONS

1 The individual most associated with the early *quantitative* expressions of drug receptor interactions is which of the following?
   a A. J. Foyt
   b A. J. Clark
   c Paul Ehrlich
   d Claude Bernard
   e William Withering.

2 The "occupancy" model of drug–receptor interaction is based upon which of the following?
   a Fick's law
   b Le Chatelier's principle
   c the law of mass action
   d the law of diminished returns
   e none of the above.

3 Most pharmacological dose–response curves are plotted on which of the following?
   a arithmetic scale
   b linear scale
   c logarithmic scale
   d nonlinear scale
   e Gaussian curve.

4 Quantal drug responses refer to which of the following?
 a percent maximal response
 b log of percent maximal response
 c number of individuals responding
 d number of receptors occupied
 e a and c above.

5 When a series of agonist dose–response curves are plotted on a log scale the x-axis reflects which of the following?
 a intrinsic activity (efficacy)
 b lipophilicity
 c potency
 d the number of receptors occupied
 e affinity.

6 Which of the following is/are true regarding competitive inhibitors?
 a cause a shift to the right of the agonist dose–response curve
 b cause a shift to the left of the agonist dose–response curve
 c bind to the same receptors as the agonist
 d bind to allosteric receptor sites
 e a and c above.

7 Which of the following is/are true regarding allosteric inhibitors?
 a bind to the same sites as agonists
 b can be displaced by increasing concentration of agonist
 c have significant intrinsic activity
 d probably produce conformational change in the agonist receptor
 e a and d above.

8 A graded dose–response curve for a series of agonists can provide which of the following data?
 a ED_{50}
 b potency
 c affinity
 d intrinsic activity
 e all of the above.

9 Which of the following factors contribute to a β-agonist's response?
 a concentration at the receptor site
 b K_d
 c intrinsic activity
 d signal transduction
 e all of the above.

10 Activation of baroreceptors (blood pressure) is an example of which of the following?
 a pharmacokinetic antagonism
 b allosteric antagonism
 c physiological antagonism
 d chemical antagonism
 e none of the above.

Chapter 7

Drug toxicity

BACKGROUND

Toxicology is the field of science that focuses on the deleterious effects of chemicals (i.e., xenobiotics) on biological systems. Pharmacology has a rather positive image, being concerned with the treatment of disease by natural products, structural modifications of natural products, and the production of synthetic drugs designed for the treatment of a particular disease. In contrast, toxicology is sometimes regarded in a negative way. Toxicology and pharmacology are, however, complementary and the thought processes involved in each are often similar (i.e., toxicokinetics, toxicodynamics, receptors, and dose–response).

Among the tens of thousands of chemicals produced each year are those developed for medicinal purposes. Although the actual percentage that drugs represent is quite small, the medical armamentarium that has evolved over the years also numbers in the thousands. Therefore, the possibility of drugs producing toxic effects is a constant concern and represents the other side of the therapeutic coin. It is estimated that each year approximately 2 million hospitalized patients have serious adverse drug reactions, and about a hundred thousand have fatal adverse drug reactions. If this estimate is correct, then more people die annually from medication errors than from highway accidents, breast cancer, or AIDS.

Every year, 17 million prescription errors occur, such as the wrong drug or the wrong dose. One recent survey of pharmacists found that approximately 16 percent of physician's prescriptions were illegible. Medical abbreviations can also be a problem. For example, the physician may mean to write "QD" (once-a-day) and accidentally write "QID" (four times daily). Similarly, since some drugs such as insulin are prescribed in units (U), if written hastily the U can be misinterpreted as a zero (0). A prescription for 100 U could, therefore, result in 1000 units being delivered. Drug errors can also happen when a doctor prescribes a medication with a name similar to another drug. The potential for medication mix-ups has increased dramatically over the past two decades as more and more drugs—each with one or more generic and brand names—have flooded the market. There are more than 15,000 drug names in general use in the United States. With only 26 letters in the alphabet, some of these names will inevitably sound alike.

For example, soon after the new arthritis drug Celebrex entered the market, the FDA received 53 reports of dispensing errors that occurred when it was mistaken for the antiseizure drug Cerebyx or the antidepressant drug Celexa. Other commonly confused drugs include Flomax (used to treat an enlarged prostate) and Fosamax (osteoporosis), Adderall (attention deficit disorder) and Inderal (hypertension or other heart problems), Lamisil (fungal infections) and Lamictal (epilepsy), Prilosec (acid reflux) and Prozac (depression). The problem of drug misidentification due to name similarity has become such a problem that a nonprofit organization has been founded to address the issue. The Institute for Safe Medication Practices independently reviews errors reported through the U.S. Pharmacopoeia's Medication Errors Reporting System and publicizes the findings in the media.

Fingl and Woodbury in 1966 cogently summarized the significance of drug side effects: "Drug toxicity is as old as drug therapy and clinicians have long warned of drug-induced diseases. However with the introduction into therapeutic practice of drugs of greater and broader efficacy, the problem of drug toxicity has increased, and it is now considered the most critical aspect of modern therapeutics. Not only is a greater variety of drug toxicity being uncovered, but the average incidence of adverse effects of medication is increasing, and unexpected toxic effects occur relatively frequently."

The incidence of drug toxicity in the general population is unknown. However, there have been reports that 5–10 percent of hospitalized patients report some drug side effects. Fortunately, life-threatening toxicity from drugs is relatively rare. On the other hand, drug toxicity may manifest itself via seemingly innocent forms. For example, in 1996 the FDA warned that dietary supplements such as Herbal Ecstasy also pose "significant health risks." Many of the labels on these products do not list ingredients, such as the cardiovascular stimulant ephedrine (as mentioned previously).

Most cases of human lethality from drugs are due to either accidental or intentional overdose. An example of the former occurred in 1994 in one of the nation's most prestigious cancer institutes. In that case, a dosage error in an experimental chemotherapy regimen resulted in the death of one patient and the crippling of another. The error revolved around ambiguous dosage guidelines of whether 4000 mg of the anticancer drug (times the patient's body surface in square meters) was intended as the daily dosage or as the cumulative, 4-day dose. Unfortunately, it was the latter.

Accidental poisoning sometimes has assumed the character of a genuine disaster. An example is poisoning by the fungus *Claviceps purpurea*. This fungus grows as a parasite in grain, particularly rye, and causes the malady known as ergotism. The fungus produces the highly toxic alkaloid known as ergot (from which LSD is derived). In the past, this type of epidemic has killed thousands of people who ingested the fungus with their bread. There are detailed accounts of such calamities. For example, in the year 992 an estimated 40,000 people died of ergotism in France and Spain. As recently as the 1950s similar outbreaks were still occurring.

One of the most significant historic figures in the development of the science of toxicology was the Swiss physician Paracelsus (1493–1541), mentioned in Chapter 1, who recognized the requirement for appropriate experimentation and gave the discipline a scientific foundation. One of the important distinctions that Paracelsus made was between the therapeutic and toxic properties of chemicals, and he appreciated the fact that these characteristics are generally manifested by dose. Today, his views remain an integral part of the structure of pharmacology and toxicology.

Paracelsus promoted a focus on the "toxicon," the primary toxic agent, as a chemical entity, as opposed to the Grecian concept of the mixture or blend. This concept initiated by Paracelsus became a lasting contribution embodied in a series of corollaries: (1) experimentation is essential in the examination of responses to chemicals; (2) one should make a distinction between the therapeutic and toxic properties of chemicals; (3) the properties are sometimes but not always indistinguishable except by dose; and (4) one can ascertain a degree of specificity of chemicals and therapeutic or toxic effects.

These principles led Paracelsus to introduce mercury as the drug of choice for the treatment of syphilis, a very prevalent malady of the day, but led to his famous trial. Nevertheless, the practice of using mercury for syphilis survived for 300 years. The use of a heavy metal as a therapeutic agent presages the "magic bullet" (arsphenamine) of Paul Ehrlich and the introduction of the therapeutic index. In addition, in a very real sense, this was the first sound articulation of the dose–response relationship, a bulwark of pharmacology and toxicology.

Another important contributor to the development of toxicology was the Spanish physician Orfila (1787–1853). He was one of the first scientists to make systematic use of test animals and autopsy material. Orfila was the first to treat toxicology as a separate scientific subject and was also responsible for the development of numerous chemical assays for detecting the presence of poisons, thus providing an early foundation for forensic toxicology. In 1815 Orfila published the first major work dealing with the toxicity of natural agents.

As mentioned earlier, Paracelsus recognized the correlation of dose with toxicity. In fact, his statement that "all substances are poisons; there is none which is not a poison. The right dose differentiates a poison and remedy" is the most frequently quoted declaration in the field of toxicology. However, as we shall see there are a number of other factors that can influence the toxic manifestations(s) of a drug. The major factors include dose, the underlying genetic makeup of an individual (both within a given gender and between), the age of the individual, the presence of underlying pathology, and the status of one's immune system.

DOSE

In view of the fact that most, but not all, toxic reactions to drugs are related to dose, this subject is the most logical to begin with. Fortunately, many of the principles that we have discussed previously can be applied to questions dealing with the dose (dosage)–response relationship. Although there are numerous potential parameters that can be used to measure drug toxicity, a traditional standard in industry deals with lethality. In experimental animals it is obviously all-or-none and is easily quantifiable. While there are serious reservations about this approach, and attempts are under way to limit its application (see Chapter 15), it is, nevertheless, still utilized to a certain extent. The basic relationship between pharmacology and toxicology on the basis of dose–response is shown in Figure 7.1.

In Chapter 6 the concept of a dose–response relationship was introduced (equivalent to the concentration–response curves seen in Figure 6.2). In that context we were concerned with drug effectiveness (i.e., efficacy) as the response. In the present context we are concerned with drug toxicity. When comparing Figure 7.2 in this chapter with Figure 6.2B we can see that the same type of typical sigmoidal curve is produced when plotting drug dosage versus percent mortality.

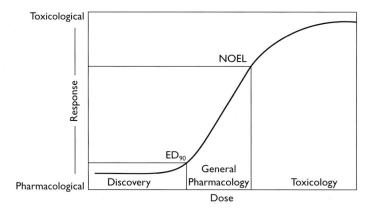

Figure 7.1 Representation of departmental responsibility in the evaluation of a drug dose–response curve. ED_{90}, efficacious dose that produces 90 percent of the intended effect; NOEL, no toxicological effect level.

Figure 7.2 A typical dose–responsive curve where the percentage response or mortality is plotted against the log of the dosage.

Source: J. A. Timbrell (1991), *Principles of Biochemical Toxicology*, 2nd ed. London: Taylor & Francis.

Once a drug's dose–response relationship for lethality has been established there are several ways in which this information can be utilized. For example, from the data in Figure 7.2 we can obtain a numerical index of toxicity analogous to the way we obtained a numerical index of effectiveness in Chapter 6. If you remember, we chose to select the ED_{50} as a standard index of effectiveness. In the present example, if we apply the same method our drug can be seen to have an LD_{50} of 100 mg/kg.

The LD_{50} is a routinely utilized index (although not the only one) defined as the dosage of a substance that kills 50 percent of the animals over a set period of time following an acute exposure. During drug development, multiple routes of administration are usually examined that generally, but not always, yield different LD_{50} values. For example, the LD_{50} of procaine when administered orally is approximately 10-fold higher than when given intravenously. On the other hand, the LD_{50} of isoniazid is almost identical when given by five different routes.

The examples that have been utilized for determining both ED_{50} (in Chapter 6) and LD_{50} values in this chapter have been based upon visual inspection of graphical data. In actuality, in the pharmaceutical industry acute LD_{50} as well as ED_{50} values are obtained by employing one or more of several statistical formulas/methods (e.g., Litchfield and Wilcoxon). These analyses provide a more accurate determination of the value in question.

Standing alone, the LD_{50} provides us with insufficient information to evaluate a drug's potential usefulness. However, if we compare its LD_{50} to its ED_{50} we can obtain some measure of the margin of safety that exists for the drug. By convention, calculation of the LD_{50}/ED_{50} ratio yields what is referred to as the therapeutic index (TI) of the drug. Obviously, the higher a drug's TI, the greater the margin of safety.

If a drug's TI is 2.0 or less, however, the compound will probably be difficult to use clinically in patients without encountering significant toxicity. An example of a drug with a TI close to 2.0 is the cardiac drug digoxin (an early toxic effect is vomiting). Other drugs with a relatively low TI are anticancer drugs and the antiasthma drug theophylline. The use of drugs with relatively low TIs can be justified on the basis of risk vs. benefit. It should be pointed out that since no drug has a single toxic effect and many drugs have more than one therapeutic effect, the possibility exists for a given drug to have numerous therapeutic indices or toxic effects (i.e., spectra) other than lethality.

Sometimes, in addition to lethality, some other aspect of drug toxicity can be measured. In this situation one could then determine a TD_{50} (toxic dose producing the effect in 50 percent of the population) as well as an ED_{50} and an LD_{50}. In this situation the data are often plotted in a comparative fashion using probit analysis. It is not necessary that you understand the underlying mathematical transformation of biological data to a probit analysis. Suffice it to say that it is merely a tool to enable the data to be plotted as a straight line. By definition, the 50 percent value is probit 5.

When expressing efficacy and toxicity data using probit analysis, comparison of the data is facilitated. This is illustrated in Figure 7.3. In this case we can see that the TI for the drug in question is approximately 18, while the ratio of toxicity for a nonlethal toxic effect (e.g., gastric irritation) to efficacy is approximately 2.4. By obtaining those types of data we can now express toxicity in a quantitative manner. It should also be emphasized that there is a continuum of side effects that could conceivably be plotted between lines A and C.

However, one caveat should be mentioned at this point. If you examine Figure 7.3 closely, you will observe that the lines for lethality and efficacy do not exactly follow the same slope. In cases where the mortality/toxicity dose–response curves follow a shallower slope, the TI will necessarily be lower in the lower dosage range. This is

Figure 7.3 Comparison of dose–response curves for efficacy (A), toxicity (B), and lethality (C). The effective, toxic, or lethal dosage for 50 percent of the animals in the group can be estimated as shown. This graph shows the relationship between these parameters. The proximity of the ED_{50} and TD_{50} indicates the margin of safety of the compound. (Probits are units of standard deviation, where the median is probit 5.)

Source: J. A. Timbrell (1991), *Principles of Biochemical Toxicology*, 2nd ed. London: Taylor & Francis.

particularly significant in hyperresponsive individuals who respond to lower dosage (see later). Therefore, in cases where efficacy and toxicity lines do not parallel each other, a more conservative index of safety can be ascertained by determining the LD_1/ED_{99} ratio, which is sometimes referred to as the margin of safety or the certain safety factor.

In addition to providing information relative to a drug's TI, an LD_{50} value can also have utility when comparing the toxicity between drugs. Table 7.1 illustrates this point. In comparing the LD_{50} values of a number of drugs we can see that they can vary by several orders of magnitude. But what do these data mean? Perhaps one way to put the data in perspective is to apply a classification system based upon acute lethality.

Table 7.1 Approximate oral LD_{50} values for a variety of drugs in the rat

Compound	LD_{50} (mg/kg)
Ethanol	13,600
Acetaldehyde	1900
Amitriptyline	530
Digitoxin	24
Protoveratrine	5

Source: M. A. Hollinger (1995), *CRC Handbook of Toxicology*, Chapter 22. Boca Raton, FL: CRC Press.

Table 7.2 Toxicity classification system

Toxicity rating	Commonly used term	LD_{50} single oral dosage in rat
1	Extremely toxic	< 1 mg/kg
2	Highly toxic	1–50 mg/kg
3	Moderately toxic	50–500 mg/kg
4	Slightly toxic	0.5–5 g/kg
5	Practically nontoxic	5–15 g/kg
6	Relatively harmless	> 15 g/kg

Table 7.2 presents a toxicity classification system based upon an LD_{50} single oral dose in rats. In applying this system to the drugs listed in Table 7.1 we can see that these drugs would be classified from almost nontoxic to highly toxic. However, it must be emphasized that caution should be exercised when using such classification systems to communicate risk information.

Classification based solely upon lethality can communicate a false sense of security because other determinants of toxicity are not addressed in such a classification system. For example, a teratogenic substance such as thalidomide could be classified as "slightly toxic" based upon its LD_{50} but "highly toxic" on the basis of producing fetal malformations. Therefore, classification schemes must always be assessed with their inherent limitations in mind.

It should also be borne in mind that it is difficult to extrapolate the LD_{50} of a drug for a particular population of an animal species to other populations of that species, under slightly different conditions. Obviously then, extrapolation to a different species, for example man, gives extremely uncertain results in predicting teratogenic effects. Furthermore, comparison of LD_{50} values determined in various laboratories often shows significant variability. For example, in an interesting study, when the LD_{50} of a test drug was determined in rats by 65 laboratories worldwide, the variation in reported LD_{50} was more than 10-fold.

Toxicologists and pharmacologists routinely divide the exposure of experimental animals to drugs into four categories: acute, subacute, subchronic, and chronic. Acute exposure is defined as exposure to a drug for less than 24 hours, and examples of typical exposure routes are intraperitoneal, intravenous, and subcutaneous injection, oral intubation, and dermal application. While acute exposure usually refers to a single administration, repeated exposures may be given within a 24-hour period for some slightly toxic or practically nontoxic drugs. Acute exposure by inhalation refers to continuous exposure for less than 24 hours, most frequently for 4 hours. Repeated exposure is divided into three categories: subacute, subchronic, and chronic. Subacute exposure refers to repeated exposure to a drug for 1 month or less, subchronic for 1 to 3 months, and chronic for more than 3 months.

In some cases, drug exposure may be followed for the lifetime of the animal. In these situations clinical chemistry measurements can be made as well as pathological examination of post-mortem samples. Chronic studies can be carried out in animals at the same time that clinical trials are undertaken (see Chapter 14).

The importance of chronic testing can be illustrated by an experience that occurred with an antiviral drug (a nucleoside analog) being developed for the treatment of hepatitis. In this particular case, a delayed toxic liver reaction occurred months after treatment was begun and, in fact, continued to manifest itself even after administration of the drug was discontinued. Initial short-term clinical tests had missed the toxicity. Development of the antihepatitis drug was halted when five of 15 patients being tested died suddenly from liver failure.

In certain cases, drug toxicity has manifested itself under circumstances that are even more bizarre and could not have been reasonably anticipated. For example, daughters of mothers who took diethylstilbestrol (DES) during pregnancy have a greatly increased risk of developing vaginal cancer in young adulthood, some 20–30 years after their in utero exposure to DES.

For all of the four types of duration-based toxicity testing just described, the selection of dosages, species, strain of animal, route of exposure, parameters measured, and numerous other factors are extremely important. Although the types of data generated by acute, subacute, subchronic, and chronic toxicity tests can be useful, there are other types of tests that address more specific toxicity questions. For example, reproductive studies determine the effect of a drug on the reproductive process; mutagenicity tests determine whether a drug has the potential to cause genetic damage; carcinogenicity tests may reveal the appearance of neoplastic changes; and skin sensitization can be useful in determining a drug's irritancy.

A pharmaceutical company developing a drug or a contract research company that specializes in such testing typically carries out toxicity tests. In either case, the conduct of toxicity studies must adhere to strict guidelines codified in national regulatory requirements. Of particular importance is the necessity to carry out the studies in compliance with a system known as Good Laboratory Practice (GLP). Violation of these guidelines can jeopardize the successful approval of the drug.

GENETICS

Other than dose, perhaps the most important determinant in influencing our response to drugs (both toxic and therapeutic) is our underlying genetic makeup. This area of pharmacology has been traditionally referred to as pharmacogenetics and has helped to explain drug responses previously referred to as *idiosyncratic* (i.e., occurring for no known reason). The genetic component is pervasive in influencing drug toxicity because it affects almost every phase of pharmacodynamics and pharmacokinetics. From the membranes in our small intestine to the detoxifying enzymes in the liver and systems beyond, there is a succession of genetically regulated factors. You can probably think of many yourself.

The influence of genetic factors is readily apparent when comparing "normal" differences in drug toxicity within a species, between genders of the same species, as well as strain differences within the same species. In addition, there are also examples of drug toxicity related to "abnormal" genetic expression. We will consider significant aspects of both situations in this section.

With regard to species, there are numerous examples of the widely disparate response of different species to a drug. For example, the LD_{50} of ipomeanol ranges from 12 mg/kg in the rat to 140 mg/kg in the hamster. This variability in species response can have significant ramifications when drugs undergo preclinical trials. For example, rats are relatively insensitive to the teratogenic effect of thalidomide, while New Zealand White rabbits more closely reflect the human condition. Unfortunately, this fact was not known at the time of the thalidomide disaster when early teratogenic testing in the rat proved negative.

While differences in drug toxicity between species may not be surprising, the more subtle expression of strain differences within a given species can also be significant. For example, the duration of hexobarbital sleeping time to a given dose in mice of the A/NL strain is approximately 48 minutes while in the SWR/HeN strain it is approximately 18 minutes. Therefore, strain selection by a pharmacologist/toxicologist can also be a significant factor in preclinical evaluation of a drug's action.

Perhaps the best place to begin analyzing the influence of genetic expression on a population's comparative response to a drug is to apply some basic statistical principles. To begin with, we need to appreciate the concept of frequency distribution as it applies to natural phenomena. For example, assume for the moment that we could obtain 100 genetically "normal" college students of a given gender. We could then administer a fixed dose of drug X and measure some response, such as sedation. If we plotted the frequency of individuals responding against the intensity of sedation (i.e., light drowsiness, heavy drowsiness, and sleep) we would, theoretically, obtain a frequency distribution curve similar to that shown in Figure 7.4.

In analyzing Figure 7.4 we can see that it can be arbitrarily divided into three sections. The ascending limb of the curve represents those individuals who are hyporeactive (i.e., light drowsiness). The crown of the bell represents the most frequent

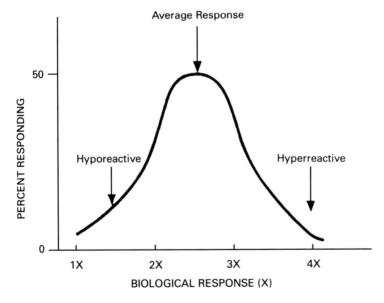

Figure 7.4 Typical frequency distribution of a population response to an equivalent dose of a biologically active agent. This type of response represents the variability that occurs within biological systems and is the basis for the concept of dose response in pharmacology and toxicology. This figure demonstrates that within any population, both hyporeactive and hyperreactive individuals can be expected to exist and must be addressed in a risk assessment.

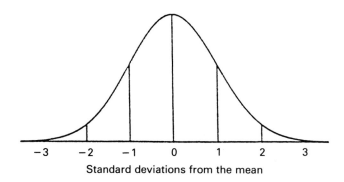

Figure 7.5 Typical frequency distribution with the demarcations of standard deviations from the mean.

number of responders who comprise the average (i.e., heavy drowsiness). The descending limb of the curve reflects those individuals manifesting greater responsiveness (i.e., sleep). Assuming no other significant variable (e.g., nutritional status, etc.) the most likely explanation for the variability in response is the collective effect of the genetic factors already mentioned.

However, we can take our analysis of the student's response to the drug one step further and attempt to quantify where individuals are within the group's distribution. The statistical expression standard deviation is a measure of how wide the frequency distribution is for a given group. For example, if someone says, "My cat is a lot bigger than average," what does this mean? The standard deviation is a way of saying precisely what "a lot" means.

Without going into the mathematics of computing a standard deviation, one can conveniently think of it as the average difference from the mean. This can be graphically depicted as shown in Figure 7.5. In any true normal distribution, 68.27 percent of all the responders fall in the interval between 1 standard deviation above the mean and 1 standard deviation below it. Applied to Figure 7.4 this would correspond to approximately those individuals showing a biological response between 2X and 3X. In addition, the range within ±3 standard deviations encompasses 99.7 percent of a normally distributed population. Obviously, the standard deviation within a population can be narrow or wide, depending upon whether the corresponding frequency distribution is narrow or wide.

In some cases the variability in response to a drug within the normal population can be quite significant and present a therapeutic challenge. For example, the anticoagulant drug warfarin (also known as coumadin) shows a 20-fold range in the dose required to achieve controlled anticoagulant therapy in humans. Obviously, care must be exercised in administering this drug since a number of people can be predicted to experience excessive bleeding episodes while others will be refractory to a given dose. The relative sensitivity or resistance to the anticoagulant action of warfarin is due to altered expression of vitamin K epoxide reductase. This enzyme is the site of drug action (inhibition) and is critically involved in the regeneration of reduced vitamin K used in the synthesis of important coagulation proteins.

As mentioned earlier, in addition to the variability imposed by genetic factors within the "normal" population there are also examples of genetically mediated drug

Number of
individuals

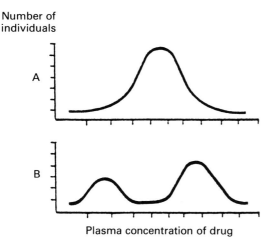

Plasma concentration of drug

Figure 7.6 Frequency distribution curves showing (A) the normal variability in plasma concentration when a fixed dose of drug X is administered to a large population of patients; and (B) a bimodal distribution typical of a pharmacogenetic alteration when drug Y is administered under the same conditions.

toxicity outside this constraint. In these situations the population distribution curve becomes bimodal (or sometimes multimodal), indicating statistically separate populations that can be more or less sensitive for a given parameter and have their own frequency distribution. An example of a bimodal distribution in drug metabolism is shown in Figure 7.6B. In this situation the left- and right-hand curves represent fast and slow metabolizers, respectively, of a hypothetical drug.

Genetic modification of enzyme activity associated with the detoxification of certain drugs is a significant factor in pharmacogenetics. A classical example is *N*-acetylation polymorphism (i.e., variation in a particular type of conjugation reaction), originally discovered in tuberculosis patients treated with isoniazid. Because of patient variability in response to isoniazid, plasma concentrations were determined at a specific time following a fixed dose of the drug. It was found that patients could be separated into two distinct populations based upon remaining isoniazid plasma levels. These two groups are referred to as "slow" and "rapid" acetylators and correspond to the frequency distribution curves shown in Figure 7.6B.

Since the discovery of this phenomenon with isoniazid over 40 years ago, nearly a dozen related drugs and chemicals have been found to be similarly influenced by genetic variation in this acetylase enzyme. Therefore, the likelihood of a "slow" acetylator encountering such a chemical/drug has increased. DNA amplification assay techniques of samples obtained from leukocytes, single hair roots, buccal epithelia, or other tissue have been developed that can be used to predict the acetylation phenotype of an individual. The availability of such information could, theoretically, be used to assess workers at high risk for toxicity (e.g., chemical workers exposed to arylamines normally inactivated by acetylation).

N-Acetylation polymorphism varies considerably depending upon racial genetic predisposition; 45 percent of the United States population (Caucasian and African-American) are slow acetylators and 55 percent are rapid, whereas 90 percent of

Orientals are fast acetylators. Separation of individuals into either "rapid" or "slow" acetylators is determined by variation at a single autosomal locus and constitutes one of the first discovered genetic polymorphisms of drug metabolism. In general, Eskimos are fast acetylators, while Jews and white North Africans are slow. The half-life of the acetylation reaction for isoniazid in fast acetylators is approximately 70 minutes, whereas in the slow acetylators this value is in excess of 3 hours.

Another example of a genetically predisposed toxic reaction to drugs is a condition known as primaquine sensitivity (primaquine is an antimalarial drug). This is a genetic alteration of the X chromosome that affects approximately 10 percent of African-American males as well as darker-hued Caucasian ethnic groups including Sardinians, Sephardic Jews, Greeks, and Iranians. Manifestation of the disorder is excessive hemolytic anemia in the presence of oxidizing drugs such as primaquine or some 50 other known drugs. The hemolytic anemia occurs at approximately one-third the normal dose.

The mechanism of hemolysis relates to the paucity of glucose-6-phosphate dehydrogenase (G6PDH) in their erythrocytes. Under normal circumstances this deficiency may not express itself. However, in the presence of oxidative stress within the erythrocytes, their capacity to generate the antioxidant-reduced glutathione (GSH) is compromised due to inadequate G6PDH (see the following simplified reaction sequence). The result is oxidative damage to the red blood cells (membranes, hemoglobin, etc.) culminating in death due to failure to replenish NADPH and, hence, GSH.

$$G6P + G6PDH \rightarrow \text{6-phosphogluconolactone} + NADPH$$

$$2NADPH + GSSG \rightarrow 2GSH + 2NADP$$

If one were to plot the frequency distribution for erythrocyte G6PDH in the general population a trimodal distribution would be revealed. This would reflect: (1) males and females not carrying the affected gene; (2) males carrying the affected gene; and (3) heterozygous females. Hemolysis is often of intermediate severity in the latter group since they have two populations of red blood cells, one normal and the other deficient in G6PDH. Approximately 400 million people carry the trait for G6PDH deficiency, and approximately 300 enzymic variants are known.

Another important example of "abnormal" gene expression occurs in the syndrome known as succinylcholine apnea. This malady expresses itself with a frequency of approximately 1 in 6000 and involves serum cholinesterase variants called "atypical cholinesterase." Plasma cholinesterase is capable of hydrolyzing a number of drugs including cocaine and heroin, but its most important clinical importance is inactivating the muscle relaxant succinylcholine. Normally, this drug is given to reduce skeletal muscle rigidity and facilitate operative procedures and its duration of action is a matter of minutes. However, in the presence of an atypical enzyme the action of an ordinary dose of succinylcholine can last for approximately an hour.

Expression of the atypical enzyme can be monitored in humans by exposing their serum samples to a substrate (benzoylcholine) and a competitive inhibitor (dibucaine) and measuring the percent inhibition of benzoylcholine hydrolysis. In the presence of the atypical enzyme, dibucaine produces less inhibition of substrate hydrolysis due to lower affinity of the atypical serum cholinesterase for benzoylcholine. The result is a trimodal distribution reflecting 20, 60, and 80 percent inhibition (i.e., the so-called dibucaine number).

The most obvious manifestation of genetic expression is gender identity. In addition to the obvious differences between males and females there are also differences in genetic expression that affect drug toxicity. We have mentioned previously that after consuming comparable amounts of ethyl alcohol, women have higher blood ethanol concentrations than men, even after correcting for body weight and body water content. Much of the first-pass metabolism of ethanol occurs in gastric tissue even before it reaches the liver. The first-pass metabolism of ethanol in women in this organ is approximately 50 percent less than in men because of the presence of lower alcohol dehydrogenase activity in the female gastric mucosa. This largely explains the increased hyperresponsiveness of women to the acute effects of alcohol.

In addition to differences in metabolic transformation between genders, there are also examples of gender differences in routes of excretion that can influence xenobiotic toxicity. For example, 2,6-dinitrotoluene-induced hepatic tumors occur with a greater frequency in males of some rodent species. This is because the biliary excretion of the glucuronide conjugate of the carcinogen is favored in males, where it is hydrolyzed by intestinal microflora, reabsorbed, transported to the liver, forms a reactive metabolite (see later discussion), binds to DNA, and causes a mutation. In females, urinary excretion predominates and results in greater clearance. Male mice are also more susceptible to chloroform-induced kidney damage. Endocrine status obviously plays an important role since castration diminishes the effect while androgens restore it. Testosterone may be mediating this effect by enhancing the formation of a toxic metabolite.

AGE

Pharmacokinetic as well as pharmacodynamic differences can exist between infant, adult, and geriatric populations. This is because of the many physiological changes that take place during one's life span. The changes that principally affect drug toxicity include (1) liver metabolic function, (2) renal elimination, and (3) body composition. Although we know that differences can exist in drug effects due to age, drug screening is still generally not carried out in neonates, infants, or extremely old animals.

Liver metabolism of drugs is typically reduced at the extremes of age. Hepatic drug-metabolizing and glucuronidation conjugation enzymes are generally present in significantly decreased amounts in the newborn infant due to incomplete genetic expression. In fact, the unique physiology of the newborn, particularly premature infants, can lead to clinical disorders such as gray baby syndrome. This pediatric entity is due to inadequate glucuronidation of excessive doses of the antimicrobial agent chloramphenicol. The syndrome usually begins 2 to 9 days after treatment is started. It is characterized by cyanosis producing an ashen-gray color.

At times of physiological change, corresponding alterations can occur in pharmacokinetics. This can be reflected in variability in response and the need for dosage adjustment. Unusual, paradoxical pharmacodynamic differences can occur in children, for example. While antihistamines and barbiturates generally sedate adults, these drugs may cause some children to develop hyperexcitable behavior. Conversely, the use of stimulants such as methylphenidate in adolescents may stabilize attention deficit disorder in some children. These unusual responses may be due to differences between receptors and transduction pathways in the two age groups and may reflect the imbalance toward excitation in the young brain.

As noted earlier, variation in kidney function can affect drug toxicity. Regardless of whether renal function is normalized to body weight or body surface area, it is lower in the neonate compared to the adult. As the infant matures, renal blood flow increases as a consequence of increased percent of the cardiac output going to the kidneys as well as decreased peripheral vascular resistance. Renal plasma flow increases approximately eight-fold within 1–2 years of birth.

In addition to renal blood flow, development of the glomerulus results in an increase in glomerular filtration rate (GFR). Adult values for GFR are generally reached within 2.5–5 months of age. For drugs eliminated almost entirely by glomerular filtration, such as the antibiotic gentamicin, significant reductions in half-life occur within the first several weeks of life. In summary, developmental changes affecting presentation of the drug via renal blood flow as well as processing by glomerular filtration contribute to relatively rapid changes in the elimination kinetics of drugs cleared by the kidneys.

Decline in physiological function as part of the normal aging process can also lead to altered drug disposition and pharmacokinetics as well as altered pharmacodynamic response to drugs. This field of study is often referred to as geriatric pharmacology. It should be appreciated in discussing this area, however, that physiological changes in the elderly are highly individualized.

Among the factors that can influence pharmacokinetic changes in older people are decreased percentage of total body water, increased percentage of body fat, decreased liver mass and blood flow, decreased cardiac output, and reduced renal function. For example, total body water decreases by 10–15 percent between 20 and 80 years of age. Coincidentally, the fat portion of body weight increases from midlife averages of approximately 18 percent for men and 33 percent for women to 36 and 48 percent respectively for individuals aged 65 and over. As a result, the volume of distribution for water-soluble drugs decreases with age, whereas that for fat-soluble drugs increases.

After 40 years of age, liver mass decreases at a rate of approximately 1 percent per year, in addition to a reduction in blood flow (40–50 percent), resulting in a diminished ability to metabolize drugs. However, since hepatic drug metabolism varies widely among individuals, there are no absolute age-related alterations in this regard. Cardiac output also decreases by approximately 1 percent per year beginning at 30 years of age and contributes to the decrease in hepatic blood flow. Glomerular filtration rate, renal plasma flow, and tubular secretory capacity also become reduced.

Reduced total body water in conjunction with elevated body fat in the geriatric population can lead to alterations in drug distribution and, hence, pharmacokinetic and possible toxic effects. As mentioned earlier, lipid-soluble drugs such as the tranquilizer valium will have a potentially larger volume of distribution in a typical elderly person, while water-soluble drugs such as acetaminophen, alcohol, and digoxin (a drug used to treat congestive heart failure) will have a smaller volume of distribution. Therefore, the geriatric population will generally be more sensitive to the effects of alcohol consumption because a given dose will be concentrated in a smaller compartment. Similarly, the dose of digoxin will probably have to be monitored particularly carefully in order to avoid toxicity since it has a relatively low TI.

In view of the fact that several aspects of kidney function decline with age (e.g., 35 percent reduction in GFR by the seventh to eighth decade), it should not be surprising that the rate of elimination of those drugs primarily dependent upon the kidney is reduced. Unlike hepatic clearance, the GFR reduction leads to predictable, directly proportional decreases in the clearance of drugs dependent on the kidney for excretion. In order to minimize toxicity for drugs frequently prescribed in the geriatric population, such as lithium carbonate (used in manic depression), chlorpropamide (used in maturity-onset diabetes), and digoxin, it may be necessary to assess renal drug clearance including GFR (i.e., creatinine clearance; see Chapter 3). Determinations are usually achieved using either normograms or mathematical equations adjusting for age, body weight, and gender.

Changes in pharmacodynamic responses in the elderly have been less well studied than pharmacokinetic changes. However, drug responses can be altered due to factors such as age-related changes in receptors and transduction pathways. For example, reduced sensitivity of β-receptors to β-agonists in the hearts of the elderly may be the result of reduced formation of the second-messenger cyclic adenosine monophosphate. The fact that the elderly are more prone to experience depression after taking valium, despite a larger volume of distribution for this drug, also suggests that altered tissue sensitivity at the receptor/transduction level may play a role.

ALLERGY

Drugs play an important role in allergic reactions because some are used to treat allergic responses while others can actually cause them. Drug-induced allergic reactions are responsible for approximately 6 to 10 percent of all adverse drug reactions. Although an estimated 5 percent of the population are allergic to one or more medications, approximately 15 percent of the population believe themselves to have medication allergies or have been incorrectly described as having a medication allergy.

It might be appropriate, at this time, to expand upon a caveat alluded to previously in this chapter. In the section dealing with dose, it was indicated that most toxic reactions to drugs generally follow a conventional dose–response relationship (the Paracelsus dictum). The word *most* was used intentionally because allergic reactions to drugs do not really follow a clear-cut dose–response relationship. This is basically because many allergic reactions can involve the explosive release of mediators in response to minute levels of the drug, bee venom, or environmental toxin—akin to an all-or-nothing effect. The classic example of a drug that can cause a whole-body allergic response is penicillin (see later discussion). The same principle holds true for environmental toxins. An example in humans is chronic beryllium disease (CBD). CBD is an allergic lung disorder caused by exposure to beryllium, primarily in mining, that has been demonstrated to be not strictly dependent on beryllium concentration. It should be pointed out, however, that putative exceptions such as these to the dose–response rule are not universally accepted. A further list of distinguishing characteristics between various types of drug side effects is shown in Table 7.3.

Table 7.3 Distinguishing characteristics of toxic, idiosyncratic, and allergic responses to drugs

	Toxic response	Idiosyncratic response	Allergic response
Occurrence			
Incidence in population	In all subjects, if dose high enough	Only in genetically abnormal subjects	Varies widely
Incidence among drugs	All drugs	Few drugs	Many drugs
Circumstance	Prior exposure unnecessary	Prior exposure unnecessary	Prior exposure essential
Dose–response relationship	Dose related	Dose related	Independent of dose; erratic relationship
Mechanism	Drug–receptor interaction	Drug–receptor interaction	Through antigen–antibody reaction; specific antibody formed in response to first dose of antigen
Effect produced	Determined by drug–receptor interaction; depends on eliciting drug	Determined by drug–receptor interaction; depends on eliciting drug	Independent of eliciting drug; determined by mediators released by antigen–antibody complex
Effect antagonized	By specific antagonists	By specific antagonists	By antihistamines, epinephrine, or anti-inflammatory steroids, such as cortisone

As mentioned earlier, the reason for the lack of clear correlation between dose and response in allergic reactions has to do with the underlying mechanism(s). This will be described in more detail later. Suffice it to say at this point that allergic responses can involve explosive mediator release in response to minute quantities of drug, in much the same way that one well-placed canon shot at the mountain can start an avalanche of snow.

Normally, we consider the immune system as playing a vitally important role in protecting us against the invasion of pathogenic organisms. This protective function is accomplished via the formation of antibodies in response to antigenic determinants residing on the bacteria or viruses. Similarly, antibody formation is also the underlying factor in immune disorders such as "hay-fever," which serves no apparent useful function. In both cases, the immune system is responding to relatively large molecules of many thousands, if not millions, of daltons. How, then, do drugs whose molecular weight usually ranges between 250 and 500 daltons achieve antigenicity?

We now know, based upon the pioneering work of Landsteiner, that certain drugs or metabolites can bind to endogenous proteins (carriers). In this context the binding ligand is referred to as a hapten. The resulting hapten–protein complex can be sufficiently different in nature that it is perceived by the body to be foreign and becomes an antigenic determinant, or epitope.

A classic example of a drug that forms haptenic derivatives is penicillin. Penicillin and its structural analogs are widely used antibiotics that are, unfortunately, responsible for more allergic reactions than any other class of drug (1–10 percent of the population). Although all four types (see later discussion) of allergic reactions have been observed with penicillin, type I anaphylactic reactions, which can occur with a frequency of 1/15,000 patients, may be life-threatening.

Among the metabolites that can be formed during penicillin metabolism are those containing penicilloyl groups. These particular metabolites have been shown to bind to endogenous protein. Studies in humans have shown that the antibodies most often associated with sensitivity in penicillin-treated patients are specific for the penicilloyl groups.

Like most immune responses, a characteristic feature of drug allergy is that a response occurs only after a sufficient interval follows initial exposure. This period of sensitization is normally on the order of 7–10 days and represents the requisite time for antibody synthesis. The manifestations of drug allergy are numerous. They may involve various organ systems and range in severity from minor skin irritation to death. The pattern of allergic response differs in various species. In humans, involvement of the skin (e.g., dermatitis, urticaria, and itching) and the eyes (e.g., conjunctivitis) is most common, whereas in guinea pigs, bronchoconstriction leading to asphyxia is most common. It may be useful, at this time, to consider the various types of allergic responses that have been ascribed to drugs. They are summarized in Figure 7.7.

Type I, or immediate immune, response involves the body's production of immunoglobulin E (IgE) antibodies in lymphatic tissue that bind to the surface of mast cells and basophils and prime them for action. The antibodies are produced in B lymphocytes during the period of sensitization. Sensitization occurs as the result of exposure to appropriate antigens through the respiratory tract, dermally, or by exposure via the gastrointestinal tract. Subsequent cross-linking of the antibodies

Figure 7.7 Mechanisms of stimulation of immune responses.

Source: J. A. Timbrell (1989), *Introduction to Toxicology*. London: Taylor & Francis. Adapted from W. C. Bowman and M. J. Rand (1980), *Textbook of Pharmacology*, 2nd ed. Oxford: Blackwell Scientific.

with the hapten–protein complex results in the release of preformed, granule-stored mediators (e.g., histamine, heparin, and tryptase) as well as newly generated mediators (e.g., leukotrienes, prostaglandins, and cytokines).

These mediators can produce a number of effects including bronchiolar constriction, capillary dilatation, or urticaria (i.e., hives). In severe episodes of type I reactions a life-threatening anaphylaxis can develop in humans due to extreme bronchoconstriction and precipitate hypotension. Epinephrine is the principal drug used in the acute management of these critical effects since it achieves (1) an elevated blood pressure via activation of alpha receptors in peripheral resistance blood vessels and (2) relaxation of bronchiolar smooth muscle via activation of β_2 receptors in the lung. Relief from the dermatological problem (i.e., hives) is also achieved via vasoconstriction of capillaries in the skin that reduce permeability, and, hence, fluid accumulation. Penicillin is a classic example of a drug that can cause a type I reaction.

Type II, or cytotoxic immune, responses can be complement-independent or complement-dependent in nature. In the former case, IgG antibodies bind to antigens attached to the surface of normal cells (e.g., erythrocytes, platelets, etc.). Cytotoxic cells (macrophages, neutrophils, and eosinophils) then attach to the crystallizable fragment (Fc) portion of the antigen, release cytotoxic granules, and lyse the cell.

The complement system is a series of approximately 30 serum proteins that promote the inflammatory response. In complement-dependent responses, after IgG antibodies bind to the cell-surface antigens, complement fixes to complement receptors on the target cell membrane, inducing lysis. Drugs such as methyldopa and quinidine may cause hemolytic anemia and thrombocytopenia, respectively, via type II responses.

Type III hypersensitivity reactions also involve immunoglobin G. The distinguishing feature of type III reactions is that, unlike type II reactions, in which immunoglobin production is against specific tissue-associated antigen, immunoglobin production is against soluble antigen in the serum. Hence the term serum sickness is often used. The formation of circulating immune complexes composed of a lattice of antigen and immunoglobin may result in widely distributed tissue damage in areas where immune complexes are deposited. The most common location is the vascular endothelium in the lung, joints, and kidneys. The skin and circulatory system may also be involved. Pathology occurs from the inflammatory response initiated by the activation of complement. Macrophages, neutrophils, and platelets attracted to the deposition site contribute to the tissue damage. Examples of drugs that can cause serum sickness include sulfonamides, penicillins, and certain anticonvulsants.

Type IV, or cell-mediated, response involves a delayed reaction to the antigenic material. Contact dermatitis is an example of a type IV response. Sensitization occurs when the antigen penetrates the epidermis and forms a complex with a protein carrier that subsequently migrates to local lymph nodes where activated, memory T lymphocytes are expressed. No serum antibodies are formed. When these activated T lymphocytes subsequently encounter the original antigenic material, they release lymphokines which then activate inflammatory cells such as macrophages and neutrophils, resulting in erythema and the formation of papules and vesicles. The infiltration of these cells into an internal organ can produce an analogous response. An example is believed to be halothane-induced hepatitis, the mechanism of which will be described in more detail in a subsequent section on covalent binding.

ANTIHISTAMINES

As mentioned earlier, one of the principal mediators involved in certain allergic reactions (e.g., type I anaphylactic) is histamine. Histamine is an endogenous substance that is synthesized, stored, and released primarily from tissue mast cells and circulating basophils. The actions of histamine are mediated by at least three distinct receptor subgroups: H_1, H_2, and H_3. Of these, H_1 receptors mediate the major actions in humans related to allergic responses. A list of some of the principal actions of histamine in humans is shown in Table 7.4.

Histamine is formed in vivo via the decarboxylation of the amino acid L-histadine. As indicated previously, it is stored in an inert, ionically bound complex with

Table 7.4 Principal effects of histamine related to allergic reactions in humans

Organ/tissue	Effects	Receptor subtype
Cardiovascular	Decreased peripheral resistance	H_1, H_2
	Increased permeability of postcapillary venules	H_1
Respiratory	Increased contraction of bronchiolar smooth muscle	H_1
Skin	Increased pain and itching	H_1

Figure 7.8 Comparison of "old" and "new" antihistamine structures with histamine.

proteoglycans, such as heparin and chondroitin sulfate, within granules at its site of synthesis. Histamine is distributed throughout the body. However, the greatest concentrations in humans occur in the skin, lungs, and gastrointestinal mucosa. It is the latter site that is the locus of action of H_2 blockers, such as cimetidine (introduced during the 1970s), to inhibit gastric acid secretion in cases of acid indigestion or ulcers. The H_1 and H_2 receptors have been cloned and shown to belong to the superfamily of G-protein-coupled receptors. H_3 receptors are believed to play a role in histaminergic neurons in vivo. To date, no H_3 agonist or antagonist has found clinical use.

Agents generally referred to as antihistamines are those that antagonize the action of histamine at H_1 receptors. They act in a competitive manner and are primarily used in situations such as urticaria, hay fever, and insect bites. They are available for both local and oral administration. At the time of the development of the first antihistamines in the 1940s, they were hailed as the cure for the common cold.

The original antihistamines bore a relatively close structural similarity to histamine (Figure 7.8). One of the most significant structure–activity relationships is the ethylamine side chain present as a substituted derivative in chlorpheniramine, a common component in over-the-counter (OTC) preparations. Newer, second-generation antihistamines such as terfenadine (subsequently withdrawn from the market for drug interaction problems), loratadine (Claritin), and fexofenadine (Allegra) show more significant structural divergence.

Antihistamines differ primarily in terms of their potency, selectivity of action, and side effects. The newer second-generation H_1 blockers, loratadine and fexofenadine, for example, are more specific for H_1 receptor antagonism than the older generation, which can also block cholinergic and muscarinic receptors. In addition, the second-generation drugs do not cross the blood–brain barrier as readily and are, therefore, generally devoid of sedative properties (hence the term nonsedating antihistamines).

Several of the older generation antihistamines are used exclusively for situations that do not involve an allergic reaction. For example, some demonstrate significant antiemetic, antimotion sickness, antiparkinsonian, antitussive, and local anesthetic actions (some H_1 antagonists are more potent than procaine). They can be found in many OTC products, particularly for the relief of symptoms from the common cold and allergies, as well as by prescription. The effectiveness of the agents in the treatment of motion sickness and Parkinson's disease may be attributed to their anticholinergic actions.

One of the interesting aspects of the marketing of first-generation antihistamines has to do with their propensity to induce sedation. The ethanolamines (e.g., diphenhydramine) are particularly prone to cause sedation. While this is generally an undesirable side effect that has been basically eliminated in newer generation drugs, this property does have commercial value. For example, most OTC sleeping aides contain older generation antihistamines that are quite useful because of their tendency to produce sedation.

IMMUNE-RELATED DRUG EFFECTS

The past decade has seen an increasing number of indications that human exposure to substances suppressing the immune system results in an increased incidence of infections and neoplastic disorders. In this regard, the most provocative theory regarding the etiology of AIDS relates to a proposed immunotoxicity of drugs of abuse rather than the human immunodeficiency virus (i.e., the so-called Duesenberg hypothesis). While this is a "radical" theory and not generally accepted, we do know of studies of transplant patients who have received long-term treatment with immuno-suppressants, such as glucocorticoids or azathioprine (to prevent organ rejection), showing a marked increase in the incidence of tumors.

Apart from the process of haptenization discussed earlier, certain drugs are also capable of modifying the antigenic potential of endogenous molecules, without binding. In unknown ways the tissue becomes modified and is recognized as foreign and induces an autoimmune disorder. Table 7.5 lists drugs that can give rise to a syndrome known as systemic lupus erythematosus (SLE). SLE is characterized by skin eruptions, arthralgia, leukopenia, and fever.

A particularly good example of a drug inducing SLE is the vasodilator hydralazine, sometimes used for the treatment of hypertension. The drug-induced lupus syndrome

Table 7.5 Drugs known to produce systemic lupus erythematosus

Practolol	(β-adrenergic receptor blocker)
Chlorpromazine	(antipsychotic)
Hydralazine	(antihypertensive)
Isoniazide	(antibacterial agent)
Diphenylhydantoin	(anticonvulsant)
Ethosuximide	(anticonvulsant)

usually occurs after at least 6 months of continuous treatment and its incidence is related to dose, gender, and race. In one study, after 3 years of treatment with hydralazine, drug-induced lupus occurred in 10.4 percent of patients who received 200 mg daily, 5.4 percent who received 100 mg daily, and none who received 50 mg daily. The incidence is approximately four times higher in women then in men, and the syndrome is seen more commonly in Caucasians than in African-Americans.

PRIMARY MECHANISMS OF DIRECT DRUG-INDUCED CELL INJURY

Advances in techniques used in the biological sciences (e.g., histopathology, electron microscopy, subcellular fractionation, and analytical methods) have provided the framework for identifying mechanisms of toxicity at the cellular level. One of the underlying principles driving this type of inquiry is the concept of a "biochemical lesion," first proposed by Rudolf Peters in 1931. In essence, the term biochemical lesion refers to the initial metabolic alteration produced by a xenobiotic that is ultimately expressed in morphological change.

While antihistamine-induced sedation may be a side effect that can have a commercial "spin" put on it, there are several more fundamental toxic effects at the cellular level that can jeopardize cellular function as well as produce cell death. Although any organ or tissue may be a target for a toxic drug effect as a result of differences in anatomical structure (e.g., blood–brain barrier), blood flow (e.g., liver and kidney), oxygen tension (e.g., lung), and highly specialized binding affinity (e.g., adriamycin in the heart), there are several primary mechanisms that can produce cellular damage.

The principal mechanisms underlying the primary events of drug toxicity include (1) covalent binding, (2) lipid peroxidation, and (3) oxidative stress. The dividing line between these types of mechanisms is not always clear. For example, a reactive intermediate may cause death via covalent binding while the necrotic cells may release toxic oxidative products. The reverse scenario is also conceivable.

Covalent binding

In Chapter 5 the four major types of chemical bonds involved in drug–receptor interaction were described. One of these is the covalent bond. Being practically irreversible, covalent binding is of great toxicological significance because it results in the permanent alteration of endogenous molecules. In Chapter 3 it was indicated that certain drugs could undergo bioactivation (often catalyzed by the P450 system), yielding metabolites with the capacity to form covalent bonds with endogenous macromolecules. Covalent adduct formation is common with electrophilic metabolites (molecules containing an electron-deficient atom) interacting with endogenous electron-rich atoms (nucleophiles). Nucleophilic atoms are abundant in biological macromolecules such as proteins and nucleic acids.

Protein function is impaired when conformation or structure is altered by interaction with such toxic metabolites. Many proteins contain critical moieties, particularly thiol (SH) groups, that are essential for catalytic activity or assembly of macromolecular

Figure 7.9 The metabolism of halothane and its proposed involvement in liver toxicity. Pathway 1 (oxidative) and pathway 2 (reductive) are both catalyzed by cytochrome P450.

Source: J. A. Timbrell (1991), *Principles of Biochemical Toxicology*, 2nd ed. London: Taylor & Francis.

complexes. These proteins are sensitive to covalent modification of their thiol groups, enzymes involved in metabolism, Ca^{2+} pumps, and transcription factors.

The covalent binding of highly active drug metabolites to DNA could conceivably cause nucleotide mispairing during replication. For example, covalent binding to the reactive N at the 7 position of guanine could result in pairing of the adduct-bearing guanine with adenine rather than cytosine, leading to the formation of an incorrect codon and the insertion of an incorrect amino acid into protein. Such a sequence of events is known to occur with aflatoxin 8,9-oxide in the liver.

An example of a drug that can undergo metabolic activation with subsequent tissue injury is the widely used anesthetic agent halothane. There are believed to be two types of hepatic damage that halothane can produce, depending upon whether an oxidation or a reduction pathway is involved. Oxidative dehalogenation is the primary mechanism in humans, while reductive dehalogenation predominates in the rat, but covalent binding is a common feature. Halothane hepatitis in humans is a rare (1 in 20,000) but severe form of liver necrosis associated with repeated exposure to this volatile anesthetic.

Halothane, as the name implies, contains halogen atoms within its molecular structure (e.g., three F, one Br, and one Cl). Within the human liver, halothane undergoes a dechlorination reaction that leads to the production of an unstable free radical intermediate (Figure 7.9). A free radical is a molecule or molecular fragment that contains one or more unpaired electrons in its outer orbital shell and is highly electrophilic. Most of the free radical formed in the human liver is trifluoroacetylchloride.

Some of this free radical covalently binds to specific liver protein and elicits an immune response. This scenario is supported by data obtained in human subjects. Serum samples from patients suffering from halothane hepatitis contain antibodies directed against neoantigens formed by the trifluroacetylation of liver proteins. In addition, the administration of radiolabeled halothane to a patient undergoing a transplant operation resulted in the detection of covalent binding in liver protein.

The principal antigenic proteins seem to be associated with the smooth endoplasmic reticulum. This is not particularly surprising since it is the probable site of metabolite formation via P450. Trifluoroacyl adducts have also been detected on the outer surface of hepatocytes, although it is not clear how they arrive there. In halothane-induced hepatitis the number of exposures does seem to be important, with about four being optimum.

Perhaps the best-studied example of drug toxicity resulting from covalent binding involves the widely used analgesic drug acetaminophen. Under normal circumstances the drug poses little risk. However, if extremely large amounts are taken, the liver's capacity to detoxify it via sulfation and glucuronidation is exceeded, while, coincidentally, there is increased formation of a toxic metabolite. The result is necrosis of liver and kidney cells, and death.

The mechanism of acetaminophen toxicity has been studied extensively in experimental animals. Oxidation of acetaminophen in the liver via cytochrome P450 results in the formation of a cytotoxic electrophile, N-acetyl-p-benzoquinoneimine (NAPQI), that binds to hepatic protein. In the kidney, the formation of a one-electron oxidation product, namely N-acetyl-benzosemiquinoneimine radical, occurs via prostaglandin H synthase. This free radical binds to renal proteins and damages the renal medulla.

Evidence from rodent studies indicates that NAPQI binds covalently with cysteinyl sulfhydryl groups yielding 3-(cystein-S-yl) acetaminophen protein adducts (3-Cys-A) on more than 15 proteins. Studies in humans indicate a similar pathogenesis. The primary target for NAPQI covalent binding appears to be a 58-kDa binding protein. This protein may function as an electrophile sensor that signals the nucleus that an electrophile is present and that alterations in cellular homeostasis are necessary. The NAPQI adduct may also function as a hapten and elicit an immunological response.

The final example of covalent binding does not really involve a drug but, rather, chemical warfare agents known as organophosphates. Diflurophosphate (DFP) is probably the most extensively studied compound of this class. DFP functions by irreversibly inhibiting esterases such as acetylcholinesterase via alkylphosphorylation to become covalently bound. The result is an accumulation of acetylcholine at cholinergic synapses, both in the periphery and in the CNS, with the attendant exaggeration of cholinergic effects (see Chapter 11).

Lipid peroxidation

As indicated earlier, some drugs are bioactivated to reactive intermediates that interact with cellular constituents. One specific type of reactive substance mentioned previously is the free radical. Free radicals are highly reactive chemical species containing, in the outermost or bonding orbital, a single unpaired electron. As a result, this is an extremely reactive electrophilic species with a very short half-life. Free radicals seek other electrons to make a new pair. A free radical may collide with another free radical to create a stable electron pair (a process termed annihilation) or it may obtain the transfer of another electron from a compound more susceptible to electronic donation, thus eliminating the original free radical but replacing it with another (perpetuation). Free radicals cause cellular damage when they pull electrons from components of normal cells of the body.

An example of free radical formation is molecular oxygen, which can accept electrons from a variety of sources to produce reactive oxygen species (ROS) such as the superoxide radical, the hydroxyl radical, and the nitric oxide radical. The superoxide anion radical is formed when one electron is taken up by one of the 2p orbitals of molecular oxygen. Certain drugs and other xenobiotics have the capacity to undergo so-called redox cycles, whereby they provide electrons to molecular oxygen and form superoxide.

The generation of free radicals in mammalian cells is continuous and occurs as a result of both normal and abnormal cellular activity and also environmental perturbations. It has been estimated that every single one of our body's cells suffers approximately 10,000 free radical "hits" per day. Over a typical 70-year life span, the body generates an estimated 17 tons of free radicals. DNA is a probable target, which may partially explain the higher frequency of mutations in the elderly. In addition to DNA, cell membranes, proteins, and fats are also being targeted by free radicals.

Polyunsaturated fatty acids such as those present in lipid biomembranes are particularly susceptible to free radical action because of their state of unsaturation. When exposed to superoxide or other reactive radicals such as trichloromethylperoxy or hydroxyl, for example, a chain reaction known as lipid peroxidation occurs, resulting in a breakdown in membrane structure and function. After the breakdown has been initiated by the free radical attack, lipid fragmentation is self-propagating due to the successive formation of a series of highly reactive lipid breakdown products. Therefore, lipid peroxidation not only destroys lipids in cellular membranes but also generates endogenous free radicals and electrophiles. These substances can readily react with neighboring molecules, such as membrane proteins, or diffuse to more distant molecules such as DNA. Although lipid peroxidation may be a critical mechanism for the cellular injury induced by some drugs, it is not a comprehensive mechanism underlying all toxic drug effects.

Oxidative stress

Since mitochondria are the site of high oxidative metabolism, they are under continual oxidative stress. In fact, it has been estimated that approximately 2 percent of mitochondrial O_2 consumption generates ROS. The mitochondrial electron transfer chain is one of the main sources of ROS in aerobic cells, due to electron leakage from energy-transducing sequences leading to the formation of superoxide radicals.

The generation of the superoxide anion radical is but the first of four steps in the complete reduction of oxygen to water. Successive steps include the sequential generation of hydrogen peroxide, formed through the dismutation of superoxide via superoxide dismutase (SOD), and the hydroxyl radical. The hydroxyl radical is one of the most powerful and most reactive oxidants that exist. It reacts immediately with any available biological substance. For example, it is believed to play a role in the toxicopathology produced by the anticancer drugs bleomycin (lung) and doxorubicin (heart) as well as the antibiotic nitrofurantoin.

As mentioned previously (Chapter 3) reduced glutathione (GSH) plays an important role as an antioxidant. Oxidative stress is believed to play a key role in a number of neurological disorders, including neuronal degeneration. As discussed in Chapter 11, the central nervous system possesses a very high rate of aerobic metabolism and thus would be expected to generate considerable ROS. Recent research suggests that GSH plays a vital role in protecting the CNS by functioning as a free-radical scavenger. Figure 7.10 shows possible roles for GSH in neurological disease. However, it

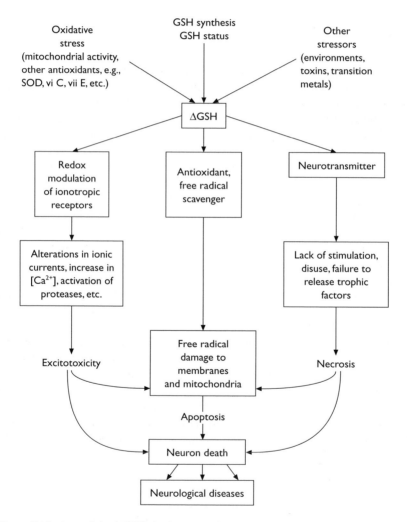

Figure 7.10 A model of GSH depletion and neurological disease. GSH is known to play an analogous role in other tissues.

Source: C. A. Shaw (ed.) (1998), *Glutathione in the Nervous System*. Washington, DC: Taylor & Francis. Reprinted with permission.

should be kept in mind that a similar role for GSH as a free-radical scavenger in other tissues is well documented.

There are three classes of enzymes known to provide protection against reactive oxygen species: the catalases and peroxides, which react specifically with hydrogen peroxide, and the superoxide dismutases (a family of enzymes). If the protective capacity of superoxide and catalase is inadequate, then superoxide anions and hydrogen peroxide can react to form hydroxyl radicals. Oxidant stress, followed by depletion of cellular reducing agents (e.g., thiols, pyridine nucleotides—NADP and NADPH) as well as ATP depletion and elevated intracellular Ca^{2+}, can lead to cell necrosis. Cells can sometimes avoid this disordered decay by activating a controlled catabolic process that brings about an ordered disassembly and removal of the cell, called apoptosis.

APOPTOSIS

Drugs such as alkylating agents and doxorubicin can produce DNA damage. DNA damage is potentially mutagenic and carcinogenic; therefore, apoptosis (otherwise called programmed cell death) of cells with damaged DNA is an important self-defense of the body against drug-induced oncogenesis. In addition, catecholamines such as epinephrine and norepinephrine, as well as cocaine, are also believed to induce cardiomyopathy, at least partially, via apoptosis. A lack of apoptotic cell death is associated with cancer, while its inappropriate occurrence is associated with pathologies such as autoimmune and neurodegenerative diseases.

The apoptotic process is mediated by the caspase family of cysteine protease. Caspases are implicated both in the induction and execution of the death sentence. Apoptosis can be induced by (1) activation of "death" receptors, such as Fas, which recruits procaspase 8 via adaptor proteins and promotes its autocatalytic activation, and (2) the release of cytochrome C from mitochondria by DNA damaging drugs and other chemotherapeutic agents (Figure 7.11).

In summary, damage to the mitochondria causes release of the protein Apaf–1 from their membrane as well as leakage of cytochrome C from the organelle. The released cytochrome C and Apaf–1 bind to molecules of caspase 9. The resulting complex of cytochrome C, Apaf–1, caspase 9, and ATP is called the apoptosome. Caspase is one of a family of over a dozen caspases. They are all proteases and they get their name because they cleave proteins, mostly each other, at aspartic acid (Asp) residues. Caspase 9 cleaves and, in so doing, activates other caspases. The sequential activation of one caspase by another creates an expanding cascade of proteolytic activity (similar to blood clotting), which leads to digestion of structural proteins in the cytoplasm, degradation of chromosomal DNA, and phagocytosis of the cell.

TERATOGENESIS

From the time that humanity has been capable of leaving records, "monsters" resulting from biological malformations appear to have been of considerable interest. In early cave paintings, for example, monsters are portrayed frequently. Recent painters have also utilized this theme by using congenitally malformed models in their work

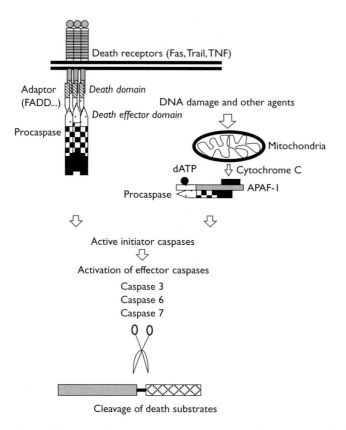

Figure 7.11 Activation of the caspase proteases during apoptosis. Caspases are implicated in both the induction and execution of the apoptotic process. Following the apoptotic stimuli, initiator caspases (caspase 8 or 9) are activated by autocatalysis. The initiator caspases then activate the effector caspases (caspase 3, 6, and 7), which are responsible for most of the protein cleavage during apoptosis.

Source: C. Szabo (ed.) (2000), *Cell Death: The Role of PARP*. Boca Raton, FL: CRC Press. Reprinted with permission.

(e.g., the painting of a phocomelic infant by the nineteenth-century Spanish painter Francisco de Goya in the Louvre).

The condition of phocomelia was so rare prior to 1961 that no photographs were available and Goya's painting was used in medical texts for illustration. The term phocomelia is derived from the Greek words for "seal" and "limb." It is characterized by the hands or feet growing directly from the main joint, like the flippers of a seal.

Early attempts to explain congenital malformations followed two basic premises. Either they were of prophetic significance (a belief held by the Babylonians) or they were manifestations of the "wrath of God." A "modern" twist on this kind of thinking occurred in Iraq in 1965. In this situation, a mother and newborn child were put to death following a family "trial" since the infant was born with a well-developed "tail." The assertion was that the mother must have indulged in obscene sexual practices with a monkey.

In mammals, the first report of induction of congenital malformations attributed to extrinsic factors is a single observation in 1921. This report linked a dietary deficiency of a "fat soluble factor" with rudimentary limb development in pigs, subsequently determined to be vitamin A. It was not until 1929 that X-rays were shown to affect embryonic development.

Chemically related teratogenesis was not finally accepted until 1935 when anophthalmia (failure in eye development) was reported in piglets born to sows fed a vitamin A-deficient diet throughout pregnancy. Further studies of teratogenesis followed in the 1940s, but it was not until 1948 that nitrogen mustard and trypan blue were implicated as positive chemical teratogens. Rubella had been identified as a teratogen in 1941.

In Chapter 2 the significance of the placental transfer of drugs from the maternal circulation into the fetus was discussed. At that time, the prototypic teratogen thalidomide was discussed along with several contemporary drugs such as alcohol and cocaine. By the time that thalidomide was finally removed from the market and the medicine cabinets, it had caused severe deformities in approximately 10,000 children in 46 countries.

Interestingly, almost 40 years after its removal from the market, thalidomide is experiencing a renewed interest in its clinical utility. Based upon observations made in 1964 by an Israeli physician treating a leprosy patient with a painful condition known as erythema nodosum leprosum (ENL), thalidomide is being used as a sedative; the drug is alleviating the pain symptoms of this painful condition. Thalidomide has become the drug of choice for the treatment of ENL according to the World Health Organization. Celgene, the company that holds the rights to thalidomide, received approval to market the drug in 1998.

Thalidomide has also been reported to display efficacy in the treatment of advanced cases of multiple myeloma, which are notorious for being resistant to chemotherapy. The prevailing hypothesis is that thalidomide possesses an antiangiogenesis capacity that can starve rapidly dividing cells from developing the additional blood supply that is necessary for their growth. Celgene has also provided the drug, under FDA approval, to treat more than 70 forms of cancer and various skin, digestive, and immunological disorders. Thalidomide may also be useful in treating AIDS-associated cachexia (wasting).

In this section we consider some of the underlying principles related to embryotoxicity. A teratogen is an agent that induces structural malformations, metabolic or physiological dysfunction, psychological or behavioral alterations, or deficits in the offspring, either at birth or manifested during the postnatal period. While it is known that approximately 25 percent of malformations are due to genetic transmission and chromosomal aberrations, the incidence of drug-induced teratogenic effects is not known with precision and estimates vary widely. However, because this toxic potentiality exists, teratogenic assessment of new drugs is required by all regulatory agencies around the world.

In order for a teratogen to express its toxicity it must be administered at a sufficient dose to a genetically susceptible animal when the embryo is in a susceptible stage of development. Based upon material presented in this chapter, the reader should already recognize the obvious implications of (1) the dose–response relationship as well as (2) the influence of an organism's genotype on drug toxicity. With regard to the latter,

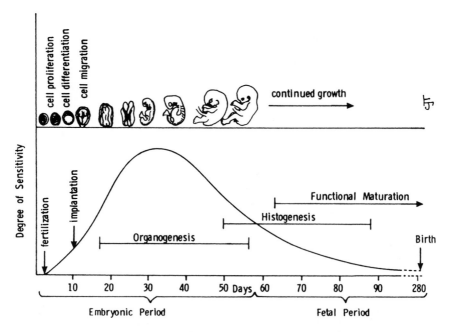

Figure 7.12 The stages of mammalian embryogenesis indicating the periods of greatest susceptibility to teratogens.

Source: J. A. Timbrell (1991), *Principles of Biochemical Toxicology*, 2nd ed. London: Taylor & Francis.

Table 7.6 Comparison of maximum periods of teratogenic sensitivity for various organs/systems in humans

Organ/system	Days following fertilization
Brain	15–60
Eye	15–40
Genitalia	35–60
Heart	15–40
Limbs	25–35

Note
The period of susceptibility in humans occurs primarily in the first 60 days of pregnancy, at a time when a woman might not be aware of her pregnancy.

humans, monkeys, and rabbits appear to produce a toxic metabolite from thalidomide while other species, such as rats and mice, do not. This explains why screening for teratogenicity in the rat proved negative for thalidomide.

In humans, the period during which drugs can affect the morphological development of embryonic organs is relatively short. It is largely completed by the end of organogenesis (approximately 56 days following fertilization; Figure 7.12). The sequence of embryonic events during the period of organogenesis is such that each organ/system undergoes a critical state of differentiation during which it is sensitive to chemical toxicity (Table 7.6; Figure 7.13).

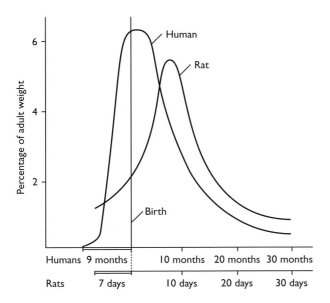

Figure 7.13 The brain growth spurt expressed as first-order velocity curves during development in humans and rats. Growth is measured as the percentage of adult weight.
In humans, the brain growth spurt commences during early gestation, peaks around
birth, and continues in early postnatal life. In rats, the growth curve ascends
gradually during the latter part of gestation and peaks around the middle of the
postweaning period. Unit scale: months in humans and days in rats.

Source: E. L. Abel (ed.) (1996), *Fetal Alcohol Syndrome: From Mechanism to Prevention*. Boca Raton, FL: CRC
Press. Reprinted with permission.

These periods of sensitivity are referred to as "toxic" or "target" windows. For
example, the window for thalidomide in the human is as little as one dose between
the 20th and 35th day of gestation. If a drug produces a toxic effect in the fertilized
egg prior to differentiation beginning, the effect is usually all-or-none and the embryo
fails to reach the differentiation stages.

Although new drugs are screened for teratogenicity, usually in two species, animal
experiments give only an approximation of possible effects in the human. One of the
reasons for this is that the period of gestation is contracted (e.g., 21 days in rat and
mouse and 32 days in rabbit). Therefore, the "target windows" for some organ
systems in some species are sometimes no longer than a 24-hour period.

The number of drugs reported to be teratogenic in laboratory animals approximates
1000. Therefore, a working hypothesis within the field is that all chemicals are capable of providing some embryotoxic effect under the appropriate conditions of dose,
developmental stage, and species selection. The number of drugs generally considered
to have teratogenic potential in humans is on the order of several dozen.

The teratogenic effects reported cover a wide spectrum including bleeding problems, deafness, discoloration of teeth, masculinization of female offspring, and cleft
palate. The major classes of drugs implicated include hormones (e.g., glucocorticoids
and progestins with androgenic activity), folic acid antagonists, oral anticoagulants,
antibiotics, alkylating anticancer agents, and anesthetic gases. Unfortunately, there

are undoubtedly other more subtle toxic effects upon brain development affecting intelligence, motor skills, and behavior that are more difficult to ascertain. However, recent data relating to subtle changes in intelligent quotients (IQs) in children exposed to cocaine in utero are alarming.

Using a meta-analysis, a statistical procedure in which effects from differing studies are pooled to provide a better estimate of the effect, a study of the effect of prenatal cocaine exposure on IQ was carried out. The investigators reported a decrease of 3.26 IQ points in the cocaine-exposed group. (For more details of the study design consult Lester *et al.* in the Bibliography at the end of this chapter.) The societal cost of such children is difficult to assess since estimates of the number of cocaine-exposed children ranges from 45,000 to more than 375,000 per year in the United States. These figures predict that the number of children affected by this 3.26-point deficit in IQ is estimated to be between 1688 and 14,062. The added costs of the special educational services required of this population has been estimated to be between $4 million and $35 million per year or more.

In response to concerns about the adverse effects of alcohol, the Congress of the United States passed the Federal Beverage Labeling Act of 1988. The law requires that all containers of alcoholic beverages display the following warning. **Government Warning**: (1) According to the Surgeon General, women should not drink alcoholic beverages during pregnancy because of the risk of birth defects; and (2) Consumption of alcoholic beverages impairs your ability to drive a car or operate machinery and may cause health problems. This legislation was in response to several reports during the 1970s that described a syndrome suitably titled as fetal alcohol syndrome (FAS).

FAS is characterized by a triad of features: (1) pre and/or postnatal growth deficiency; (2) specific pattern of craniofacial malformations; and (3) evidence of central nervous system dysfunction. Reports of at least two dozen autopsies have appeared in the literature and cover a wide range of neuropathology. The CNS deficits of FAS appear to be long-lasting, since recent studies have shown that they persist in young adults born with FAS, even if other symptoms such as growth retardation and facial characteristics have become diminished. Studies carried out during the 1990s indicate that implementation of the beverage warning label achieves only a modest reduction for underage drinkers (pregnant women under the age of 21). Older pregnant women were even less aware of the label and gave it less heed.

FAS is now considered to be a leading cause of mental retardation in the general population. Figure 7.13 shows the comparison between brain growth spurt in humans and rats. It should be noted that brain development characterized by accelerated synaptogenesis, neuronal proliferation, and myelination commences prenatally during the third trimester in humans and continues into early postnatal life.

It appears likely that the distinctive FAS facial dysmorphology is related to first-trimester alcohol exposure. The clinical data are derived from cases of FAS in populations of women reporting heavy alcohol consumption during this period. This is alarming since a majority of women who abuse alcohol may not know they are pregnant for the first 4 to 6 weeks of gestation.

One of the particularly perplexing aspects of drug-induced teratogenesis is that it may not express itself for considerable time. Concern over subtle effects on brain development was indicated earlier; decrements in cognitive development can be difficult to discern and may not manifest themselves for decades. Other drug-induced

Table 7.7 CNS depressants associated with neonatal withdrawal syndrome

Opiates/narcotics
  Methadone
  Heroin
  Codeine
  Pentazocine (Talwin)
  Propoxyphene (Darvon)
  Other narcotics

Other drugs
  Alcohol
  Barbiturates
  Bromine
  Chlordiazepine (Librium)
  Diazepam (Valium)
  Diphenhydramine (Benadryl)
  Ethchlorvynol (Placidyl)

Source: E. L. Abel (ed.) (1996) *Fetal Alcohol Syndrome: From Mechanism to Prevention.* Boca Raton, FL: CRC Press. Reprinted with permission.

teratogenic effects can also have a substantial latent period. During the 1950s, hormones were often given to pregnant women in an attempt to prevent premature labor. As mentioned previously, one of the agents used in this regard was the synthetic estrogenic compound diethylstilbestrol (DES). Following its use during this period, some daughters of treated mothers developed an increased incidence of cervical and vaginal carcinomas approximately 20 years later. An unfortunate aspect of the DES tragedy is that the drug did not prove efficacious in preventing miscarriages.

Conversely, drugs can express nonteratogenic effects upon delivery. This is particularly true if the mother has been exposed to CNS depressants of licit or illicit drugs. These types of drugs are particularly prone to produce withdrawal symptoms (Table 7.7).

Recent teratogens

During the 1980s, two drugs used to treat different types of skin diseases were found to be teratogenic. The drugs, generic names are isotretoin and etretinate, respectively, and they are synthetic retinoids (i.e., derivatives of vitamin A). Isotretoin (Accutane) was prescribed for the treatment of acne while etretinate was prescribed for psoriasis.

Isotretoin was recognized as an animal teratogen before it was first marketed in September 1982. It was therefore classified as Category X, contraindicated for use during pregnancy. A statement to that effect was included in the package insert. All physicians did not heed this warning, and 9 months later human teratogenicity was reported to the FDA in June 1983. By the late 1980s approximately 78 babies were reported with birth defects.

Exposure to isotretoin during the first few weeks of exposure results in a characteristic group of birth defects. These include facial abnormalities such as missing ears or ears developing below the chin as well as cardiac and brain malformations. A prospective follow-up study revealed a relative risk of 25.6 percent for the defects associated with isotretoin embryopathy.

Human birth defects have also been observed after prenatal exposure to etretinate. Of particular significance in the case of this drug is that measurable serum concentrations have been documented more than 2 years after cessation of therapy, suggesting a remarkable example of tissue sequestration. Therefore, the risk of teratogenicity may exist for an extended period of time.

The Bendectin story

Although numerous drugs have been shown to have the capacity to induce teratogenic toxicity, there is an example of a drug falsely accused. In 1979, a report appeared in the literature estimating an 80 percent increase in the prevalence of congenital heart disease among children of women who recalled use in early pregnancy of Bendectin, an antinausea medication. Prior to this date, 10–25 percent of pregnant women were exposed to Bendectin and over the years the drug was used in as many as 33 million pregnancies. The scientific evidence available pointed to the safety of Bendectin (the relative risk was calculated as being 0.89 with 95 percent confidence limits of 0.7 and 1.04).

In 1983, Merrell Dow Pharmaceuticals, Inc. voluntarily removed Bendectin from the market because of the many product liability suits pending. However, subsequent in-depth analysis of epidemiological and scientific data indicated that the therapeutic use of Bendectin had no measurable teratogenic effects. Nevertheless, despite the overwhelming scientific evidence, a number of jury decisions were rendered against the company (providing an argument for tort reform).

A generation of pregnant women has been without access to this highly effective drug. As a result, hospital admissions for excessive vomiting in pregnancy per thousand live births rose by 50 percent in 1984. An estimate of excess hospital costs attendant to these admissions over the years 1983–1987 in the United States was $73 million.

SELECTED BIBLIOGRAPHY

Abel, E. L. (ed.) (1996) *Fetal Alcohol Syndrome: From Mechanism to Prevention*. Boca Raton, FL: CRC Press.

Aldridge, W. N. (1996) *Mechanisms and Concepts in Toxicology*. London: Taylor & Francis.

Brody, T. M., Larner, J., Minneman, K. P. and Neu, H. C. (eds) (1994) *Human Pharmacology: Molecular to Clinical*, 2nd ed. St. Louis, MO: Mosby.

Ecobichon, D. J. (1997) *The Basis of Toxicity Testing*, 2nd ed. Boca Raton, FL: CRC Press.

Hardman, J. G., Limbird, L. L. and Gilman, A. G. (eds) (2001) *Goodman and Gilman's The Pharmacological Basis of Therapeutics*, 10th ed. New York: McGraw-Hill.

Klassen, C. D. (ed.) (2001) *Casarett and Doull's Toxicology: The Basic Science of Poisons*, 6th ed. New York: McGraw-Hill.

Lester, B. M., LaGasse, L. L. and Seifer, R. (1998) Cocaine exposure and children: the meaning of subtle effects. *Science* 282: 633–634.

Niesink, R. J. M., De Vries, J. and Hollinger, M. A. (eds) (1996) *Toxicology: Principles and Applications*. Boca Raton, FL: CRC Press.

Raje, N. and Anderson, K. (1999) Thalidomide—a revival story. *New Engl. J. Med.* 341: 1606–1609.

Rama Sastry, B. V. (ed.) (1995) *Placental Toxicology*. Boca Raton, FL: CRC Press.

Rama Sastry, B. V. (ed.) (1996) *Placental Pharmacology*. Boca Raton, FL: CRC Press.

Szabo, C. (ed.) (2000) *Cell Death: The Role of PARP*. Boca Raton, FL: CRC Press.

Timbrell, J. A. (1991) *Principles of Biochemical Toxicology*, 2nd ed. London: Taylor & Francis.

QUESTIONS

1   Which of the following is generally credited with developing the early concept of the dose–response relationship?
   a   August Busch
   b   Paul Ehrlich
   c   Orafilla
   d   Paracelsus
   e   Oneacelsus.

2   The type of allergic reaction most likely to cause death in humans is which of the following?
   a   type I
   b   type II
   c   type III
   d   type IV
   e   type A.

3   A chemical feature common to first-generation antihistamine drugs is which of the following?
   a   three benzene rings
   b   halogenation
   c   ethylamine side chain
   d   sulfuration
   e   a and c.

4   A "hapten" is which of the following?
   a   a serum protein that binds to a drug
   b   a plasma protein that binds to a drug
   c   a drug–lipid complex
   d   twice a "hapfive"
   e   a drug or metabolite that binds to endogenous protein.

5   Antihistamine drugs that block H_2 receptors are most effective against which of the following?
   a   combining of antigen with antibody
   b   reducing acid indigestion
   c   blocking release of leukotrienes from mast cells
   d   relieving bronchiolar smooth muscle contraction
   e   blocking release of histamine from mast cells.

6 The type of antibodies (immunoglobulins) principally involved in type I drug-induced allergy is which of the following?
   a   IgA
   b   IgI
   c   IgG
   d   IgE
   e   IgK.

7 Which of the following produces the most prompt alleviation of bronchoconstriction in the airway and hypotension that occurs in anaphylaxis?
   a H_1 blockers
   b H_2 blockers
   c   epinephrine
   d   leukotrienes
   e   histamine.

8 In the human, which of the following is the period of gestation when a fetus is most susceptible to a teratogenic effect?
   a   first trimester
   b   second trimester
   c   third trimester
   d   at implantation
   e   there is equal sensitivity throughout gestation.

9 Subchronic administration of a test drug to animals generally involves which of the following?
   a   repeated daily injections for less than a month
   b   repeated daily injections for more than 3 months
   c   repeated daily injections for 1–3 months
   d   weekly injections for less than 3 months
   e   weekly injections for 1–3 months.

10 Drug X has an ED_{50} of 10 mg/kg and an LD_{50} of 10 g/kg. Which of the following is its TI (therapeutic index)?
   a   0.1
   b   1.0
   c   10.0
   d   100.0
   e   1000.0.

Chapter 8

Treating drug overdose

BACKGROUND

As indicated in the preceding chapter, the exact incidence of drug side effects is not known with certainty. However, we do know that among the millions of cases of human poisonings, pharmaceuticals are most frequently involved in fatalities. According to the 1998 Annual Report of the American Association of Poison Control Centers Toxic Exposure Surveillance System, analgesics, antidepressants, stimulants and street drugs, cardiovascular drugs, and sedative/hypnotics/antipsychotics were responsible for 264, 152, 118, 118, and 89 deaths, respectively. Most of the people who die are adults, and the deaths often result from intentional rather than accidental exposure.

Ingestion is the most likely route of exposure for human poisoning, occurring in 75 percent of the cases. Accidental ingestion is most likely in children under the age of 5 (60 percent) while intentional ingestion is most likely between 18 and 64 years (6.2 percent) and between 13 and 17 years (2.2 percent). Fifty to 60 percent of intentional poisonings in adults are poly-drug exposures.

ASPIRIN

The pattern of drug ingestion hazards parallels the substances required to have child-resistant closures by the Poison Prevention Packaging Act (PPPA) of 1970. Before 1972 aspirin was the drug most frequently associated with childhood poisoning, a fact that contributed to the passage of the PPPA. Under the provisions of the act, regulations were issued that require special child-resistant packaging for any aspirin-containing preparations for human use in a dosage intended for oral administration. The regulation also covered liquid preparations containing more than 5 percent by weight of methyl salicylate, other than those packaged in pressurized spray containers.

The special packaging regulations were devised to protect children less than 5 years of age from serious personal injury or illness resulting from handling, using, or ingesting dangerous drugs. The law required vendors to follow a specific protocol to test the special packaging for its effectiveness with children as well as adults. The child-resistant effectiveness is required to be not less than 85 percent without a demonstration and not less than 80 percent after a demonstration of the proper means of opening the package. Adult-use effectiveness was also required, being not less than 90 percent.

Analyzing the number of aspirin-associated deaths after implementation of the program can assess the effectiveness of the program. Between 1972 and 1989 the total number of deaths in the children under 5 years of age category, as a result of aspirin intoxication, decreased from 46 to 2. It has been estimated that a total of 500 to 620 child deaths have been saved since the PPPA went into effect, from the early 1970s through to 1989. Remarkably, there were no reported childhood deaths due to aspirin in 1998.

IRON SUPPLEMENTS

The most likely cause of unintentional pediatric fatalities reported between 1983 and 1990 was iron supplements, representing approximately 30 percent of all deaths (16 of 53). From 1986 to 1995, over 110,000 such pediatric incidents were reported, including 33 deaths. The children who died had swallowed possibly as few as five to as many as 98 tablets. Antidepressants represented an additional 18.9 percent (10 of 53) of fatalities in the pediatric population between 1983 and 1990.

Iron is an essential nutrient that is sometimes lacking in people's diets. For that reason, physicians often recommend iron for people with certain health conditions, such as iron-deficiency anemia. Some iron products are available without a prescription, either as single-ingredient iron pills or in combination with vitamins or other minerals, including pediatric vitamins with iron. Drugs that contain iron and folic acid are available by prescription and are principally used by women during pregnancy.

Two-year-olds account for the majority (53.7 percent) of ingestions of prescription drugs. Once again, the most frequently ingested is ferrous sulfate. In more than 75 percent of cases surveyed, non-child-resistant packages or no containers at all were involved in the ingestion. Although parent's prescriptions account for approximately 54 percent of the ingestions, nearly 30 percent involve grandparent's medications. Factors responsible for the ineffectiveness of child-resistant closures include consumer noncompliance and violations of the PPPA by the dispensing pharmacist.

The FDA has proposed that manufacturers be required to wrap high-potency iron tablets and capsules individually, such as in blister packaging—the type that makes it necessary to punch out each tablet or dosage unit. The FDA believes that the time and dexterity needed to remove tablets from unit-dose packaging would discourage a youngster, or at least limit the number of tablets a child would swallow. The unit-dose packaging requirement would apply to products that contain 30 mg or more iron per dosage unit.

AGE-RELATED DRUG POISONING

Intentional poisoning in adolescents (11–17 years of age) is one of the 10 leading causes of death and loss of productive years of life in the United States. Alcohol use and abuse obviously play a large role in fatal injuries in this age group. However, drug-related fatalities following the use of antidepressants represented nearly one-half of those reported between 1989 and 1991.

It has been estimated that adult aspirin poisonings are approximately 10 percent accidental, about 10 percent planned suicides, and approximately 80 percent impulsive suicidal gestures. The fatal toxic dose is generally in the range of 20–30 g (60–90 adult tablets) in reported cases. Much larger amounts have been ingested without fatality, however, and the potency varies with the specific preparation. The pharmacodynamics also change somewhat with the use of enteric-coated tablets, which delay absorption. The degree of intoxication varies with the serum salicylate level. The lethal blood concentration of salicylate is approximately 500 mg/kg per 24 hours for 2 or more days.

Poisoning in the geriatric population is an ongoing public health concern. In the majority of patients older than 64 years of age, accidental poisoning due to dementia and confusion, improper use or storage of a product, and therapeutic errors is the rule. However, approximately one in 10 is intentional with suicidal intent. Interestingly, elderly females are approximately three times more likely to commit suicide with drugs than males (who prefer carbon monoxide).

As mentioned previously, there are a number of theoretical changes that can occur in the elderly that influence a drug's pharmacokinetics. For aspirin, the two most important alterations in pharmacokinetics that accompany aging are decreases in serum albumin and a decreased glomerular filtration rate. Following absorption, aspirin rapidly deacetylates to salicylate, its circulating form, and is predominantly (80–90 percent) bound to albumin. Circulating albumin concentrations decrease approximately 10 percent with age. Therefore, in the presence of other drugs that can displace salicylate or a high initial dose, the binding capacity of albumin can be exceeded, thus contributing to elevated free blood levels. Probably of more significance is the association of decreased creatinine clearance with aging. On the average, the elimination time of salicylate in healthy elderly people, mean age 77 years, is 1.5 times the rate of younger people with a mean age of 21 years.

MANAGEMENT TRENDS

The principal therapies employed for the treatment of drug overdose are shown in Table 8.1. They can be divided into three major categories: (1) initial decontamination; (2) measures to enhance elimination; and (3) specific antidotes. During the past several years there has been a change in emphasis within some of these categories. In any event, they are all used within the broader context of appropriate supportive care.

INITIAL DECONTAMINATION

During the period from 1983 to 1991 there has been a continual decline in the use of syrup of ipecac to induce emesis. Ipecac contains a number of plant alkaloids including emetine. It induces emesis through stimulation of the chemoreceptor trigger zone in the brain and local irritation of the gastrointestinal tract. The latency period for

Table 8.1 Various therapies provided in human drug exposure cases

Initial decontamination	Specific antidote administration
Dilution	Naloxone
Irrigation/washing	N-Acetylcysteine (oral)
Activated charcoal	Atropine
Cathartic	Deferoxamine
Ipecac syrup	Ethanol
Gastric lavage	Hydroxycobalamin
Other emetic	N-Acetylcysteine (IV)
Measures to enhance elimination	Pralidoxime (2-PAM)
Alkalinization (with or without diuresis)	Fab fragments
Hemodialysis	Pyridoxine
Forced diuresis	Dimercaprol (BAL)
Hemoperfusion (charcoal)	Methylene blue
Exchange transfusion	Cyanide antidote kit
Acidification (with or without diuresis)	EDTA
Hemoperfusion (resin)	Penicillamine
Peritoneal dialysis	

Note
Each category in decreasing frequency of use.

the induction of emesis by ipecac ranges from approximately 5 to 20 minutes, with a single dose successfully inducing vomiting in approximately 85 percent of patients. Contraindications for the use of ipecac include the presence of coma or convulsions, the ingestion of corrosive substances, and an impaired gag reflex.

While ipecac has been decreasing in popularity in emergency rooms, there has been a corresponding increase in the use of activated charcoal (AC) to adsorb the drug. AC is an inert, nonabsorbable, odorless, tasteless, fine black powder that has a high adsorptive capacity. When AC is administered after emesis or lavage, it binds residual drug within the lumen of the gastrointestinal tract and reduces its absorption. A cathartic can be coadministered with AC to prevent constipation.

Normally, AC is mixed with water and administered orally or by nasogastric tube. For optimal binding, a charcoal to drug ratio of 10:1 is recommended. The success with which AC prevents absorption depends upon the nature of the drug as well as the time between ingestion and administration of AC. With regard to the latter factor, simultaneous administration of AC with aspirin results in nearly 60 percent being adsorbed while a 3-hour delay achieves only 9 percent of the drug being adsorbed.

ENHANCED ELIMINATION

Most techniques used for enhancing the elimination of drugs from the body utilize facilitated renal excretion or extracorporeal (outside of the body) techniques. Attempts to increase renal excretion of a drug will be successful only if that drug is substantially excreted via the kidneys to a significant extent. Unfortunately, there are relatively few drugs that have significant renal excretion following an acute overdose.

Table 8.2 Hemodialysis (HD) and hemoperfusion (HP) in drug overdose

Carbamazepine	HP preferred
Ethylene glycol, methanol	HD preferred
Lithium	HP not effective
Theophylline	Both HP and HD effective
Salicylates	HD indicated for acute overdose
Valproic acid	HD preferred

Source: K. R. Olson and B. Roth (1997), *Update on Management of Patient With Poisoning or Drug Overdose*, Northbrook, IL: American College of Chest Physicians. Reprinted with permission.

Among the drugs that can be managed in this way are the weak acids phenobarbital and acetylsalicylic acid, the weak bases phencyclidine and amphetamine, and the ion lithium.

Enhanced renal excretion is usually achieved by fluid diuresis, in which excess fluid is administered to increase urine flow. Forced diuresis is generally reserved for cases of mild to moderate severity. In some cases, fluid diuresis is supplemented by ionized diuresis (discussed previously in Chapter 3). By the appropriate raising or lowering of urine pH, the degree of ionization of acidic and basic drugs, respectively, is increased and they can be "trapped" in the urine.

Extracorporeal strategies for treating drug overdose include dialysis and hemoperfusion. Dialysis is usually carried out on blood (hemodialysis) while peritoneal dialysis is used infrequently. For hemodialysis to be effective, the dialyzing membrane must be permeable to the drug and the drug should equilibrate rapidly between the circulating plasma and the dialysis fluid. Hemodialysis and hemoperfusion are usually reserved for cases of severe drug intoxication (e.g., deep and prolonged coma), ingestion of known lethal doses, or the presence of lethal blood concentrations of the drug. Table 8.2 lists some of the drugs that have been treated with hemodialysis and hemoperfusion in drug overdose.

It should be kept in mind that these procedures are invasive, requiring cannulation of a large vessel (usually the femoral vein), systemic anticoagulation, and pumping the blood through the dialysis machine. Complications can include laceration of the cannulated vessel, air embolism, hypovolemia, and thrombocytopenia (depletion of platelets). It should also be pointed out that neither of these procedures is effective for drugs with a high degree of tissue binding (i.e., a large volume of distribution).

Generally, hemodialysis is easier to perform and is associated with fewer complications. It is ideal for low-molecular-weight, polar, water-soluble molecules such as alcohol, salicylate, or lithium. Hemoperfusion is used for drugs that are poorly soluble in water or relatively higher in protein binding.

Hemoperfusion differs from hemodialysis in that the blood is passed over a resin or charcoal column. The drug becomes bound to the column and the "clean" blood returned to the body. Hemoperfusion units have adsorptive surface areas of several thousand square meters while hemodialysis devices have an effective dialysis surface limited to several square meters. Obviously, relatively sophisticated technology is required for these procedures and there is the need to prevent clotting in the circuit, which can produce complications.

ANTIDOTAL THERAPY

Naloxone is a drug structurally related to the opioid class of analgesics such as morphine. Naloxone has virtually no intrinsic activity but can compete for opioid receptors. By reversibly competing for the μ and κ opioid receptors in the brain and spinal cord, it can reverse the sedation and respiratory depression associated with an overdose of morphine-like drugs.

One of the most important developments in the field of antidotes has been the utilization of N-acetylcysteine. This sulfhydryl-containing compound is specifically used in drug toxicity cases (e.g., acetaminophen) in which an electrophilic drug metabolite binds to critical cellular macromolecules after saturating intracellular GSH pools (discussed in Chapter 7). By providing exogenous SH groups for electrophilic attack, endogenous sites are protected.

In adults, hepatotoxicity may occur after ingestion of a single dose of acetaminophen (10–15 g); doses of 20–25 g or more are potentially fatal. Severe liver damage occurs in 90 percent of patients with plasma concentrations of acetaminophen in excess of 300 μg/ml at 4 hours or 45 μg/ml at 15 hours after ingestion of the drug. Administration of N-acetylcysteine is recommended if less than 36 hours has elapsed since ingestion of acetaminophen, although the antidote is most effective if administered within 10 hours.

As mentioned previously, one of the major sources of pediatric drug poisoning relates to the ingestion of maternal iron preparations taken for the treatment of iron-deficiency anemias. An agent useful in the treatment of iron poisoning is the drug deferoxamine. This particular drug is a member of an antidotal class of drugs known as chelating agents (from the Greek *chele*, meaning crab's claw).

Chelating agents act by forming stable complexes with inorganic ions. There are naturally occurring chelators in the body such as hemoglobin, which complexes with iron. The therapeutic use of exogenous chelating agents is based upon their differential tendency to form various chelate complexes. In essence, each chelating compound has a stability constant for each inorganic ion. Fortunately, the chelating constant of hemoglobin for iron, for example, is greater than that of deferoxamine. Therefore, when deferoxamine is used clinically, it preferentially removes excess iron without disrupting biologically indispensable iron complexes.

Another novel antidotal strategy is the development of antibody fragments to certain drugs. For example, treatment of life-threatening digoxin intoxication with digoxin-specific Fab antibody fragments has been found to be useful. Patients with life-threatening digoxin poisoning who receive intravenous digoxin antibody fragments demonstrate an immediate decrease in free digoxin serum concentrations due to binding to the antibody fragment, and favorable changes in cardiac arrhythmias within 30 minutes of administration. This area of research could prove fruitful for the future development of similar strategies for other drugs.

In 1995, scientists at Scripps Research Institute reported the development of a "vaccine" that elicits antibodies to cocaine. The nature of the antigen is a cocaine analog bound covalently to a protein with a Monty Python-like name, keyhole limpet hemocyanin. Administration of the complex resulted in a reduction of the psychoactive response to subsequently administered cocaine. In experiments in rats, the antibodies bound cocaine in the bloodstream and prevented the drug from crossing the blood–brain barrier. A potential clinical application would be to immunize cocaine abusers

Table 8.3 Comparative serum concentrations (mg/ml) of drugs at therapeutic and toxic levels

Drug	Therapeutic	Toxic
Digoxin	0.0010–0.0022	>0.0025
Diphenylhydantoin	10–20	>25
Phenobarbital	15–30	>40
Procainamide	4–8	>10
Theophylline	10–20	>20

Source: T. M. Brody (1994), Issues in therapeutics. In *Human Pharmacology: Molecular to Clinical* (eds) T. M. Brody, J. Larner, K. P. Minneman and H. C. Neu, Chapter 7. St Louis, MO: Mosby.

trying to abstain from the drug. However, because of the short duration of these foreign antibodies in the body, and the fundamental behavioral pathology of drug addiction, immunization may have greater benefit in treating cocaine overdose rather than treating drug addiction itself.

TOXICOLOGICAL TESTING

Toxicological testing of blood, urine, and gastric contents is frequently ordered for patients with suspected drug overdoses. In view of the fact that 10–15 drugs account for more than 90 percent of all drug overdoses, most laboratories limit the number of drugs tested to the common drugs of abuse and therapeutic agents. These include alcohols, barbiturates/sedatives, antiepileptics, benzodiazepines, antihistamines, antidepressants, antipsychotics, stimulants, narcotics, cardiovascular drugs, and OTC analgesics. A comparison of therapeutic and toxic serum levels of selected drugs is shown in Table 8.3. As can be seen, in certain cases the differences can be relatively small.

A toxicology screen utilizes various methodologies to identify and quantify the drugs most frequently used or abused by the poisoned patient. Drug quantitation in serum is used to monitor the course of the patient, to diagnose whether toxicity is occurring but not yet clinically apparent, to establish a prognosis, and to determine whether extreme methods of drug elimination will be necessary.

ROLE OF THE POISON CONTROL CENTER

There are over 100 regional poison centers in the United States that are members of, or are certified by, the American Association of Poison Control Centers. Poison control centers serve several functions including: (1) providing expert information and consultation to the public and health professionals; (2) providing public education programs; (3) providing regional professional education programs; (4) interacting with care providers and analytical toxicology laboratories to improve the management of the poisoned patient; and (5) collecting data on poisonings.

Most of the calls received by poison control centers are managed by poison information specialists who are registered nurses, pharmacists, or other health-related professionals. In general, when a poison control center is called regarding drug ingestion it will want to know the following: (1) the type of ingested drug; (2) the age of the victim; (3) the estimated dose and time taken; and (4) the victim's condition.

SELECTED BIBLIOGRAPHY

Dolgin, J. G. (2001) Human clinical toxicology. In CRC *Handbook of Toxicology*, 2nd ed. (eds) M. Derelanko and M. A. Hollinger, pp. 957–999. Boca Raton, FL: CRC Press.

Kalant, H. and Roschlau, W. H. E. (eds) (1989) *Principles of Medical Pharmacology*, 5th ed. Toronto: B. C. Decker.

Litovitz, T. L., Klein-Schwartz, W., Caravatti, E. M., Youniss, J., Crouch, B. and Lee, S. (1999) 1998 Annual Report of the American Association of Poison Control Centers Toxic Exposure Surveillance System. *Am. J. Emerg. Med*. 17: 435–487.

Melmon, K. L., Morrelli, H. F., Hoffman, B. B. and Nierenberg, D. W. (eds) (1992) *Clinical Pharmacology Basic Principles in Therapeutics*, 3rd ed. New York: McGraw-Hill.

QUESTIONS

1 Which of the following is/are most frequently associated with pediatric drug poisoning?
   a   iron supplements
   b   birth control pills
   c   vitamin C
   d   a and b above
   e   all of the above.

2 With regard to deaths from aspirin poisoning which of the following is/are true?
   a   some are accidental
   b   some are planned suicides
   c   some are impulsive suicide gestures
   d   the fatal dose is in the range of 2–3 grams
   e   a, b, and c above.

3 Which of the following is/are employed for the treatment of drug overdose?
   a   specific antidotes
   b   measures to enhance elimination
   c   measures to enhance metabolism
   d   a and b above
   e   all of the above.

4 Which of the following is/are true regarding initial decontamination treatment in drug poisoning over the past 10–15 years?
   a   there has been an increase in the use of ipecac
   b   there has been a decrease in the use of ipecac
   c   there has been an increase in the use of activated charcoal
   d   there has been a decrease in the use of activated charcoal
   e   b and c above.

5 Which of the following is/are extracorporeal treatments for drug overdose?
   a   ionized diuresis
   b   hemodialysis
   c   retrograde iontophoresis
   d   hemoperfusion
   e   b and d above.

6 Which of the following is/are considered antidotal treatments?
   a   deferoxamine
   b   naloxone
   c   N-acetylcysteine
   d   antibody fragments
   e   all of the above.

7 Chelating agents act by which of the following antidotal mechanisms?
   a   enhancing glomerular filtration rate
   b   providing increased levels of SH groups
   c   decreasing renal reabsorption
   d   increasing hepatic P450
   e   forming stable complexes with inorganic ions.

8 Which of the following is/are true with regard to most laboratory testing for drugs?
   a   they are required to test for at least 100
   b   they are required to test for at least 200
   c   they usually test for about 10–15
   d   they usually test for about 3
   e   none of the above.

9 N-Acetylcysteine is useful in which of the following drug overdoses?
   a   aspirin
   b   deferoxamine
   c   acetaminophen
   d   digoxin
   e   a and c above.

10 Antibody fragments provide a provocative relatively new method to deal with poisoning by which of the following drugs?
   a   acetaminophen
   b   morphine
   c   aspirin
   d   antidepressants
   e   digoxin.

Part 3

Drugs that replace, cure, or treat symptoms

Chapter 9

Hormones

BACKGROUND

Regulation of the body's homeostasis is partially under the control of the endocrine system. This is a system whereby specialized tissues or glands elaborate hormones (from the Greek "to urge on") into the bloodstream for distribution within the body, where they regulate organ and cellular function in a "feedback" relationship. Without this constant feedback, the human body would be a disorganized mob of 50 trillion cells. Endocrine transmission is relatively slow and diffuse. In comparison, neuronal transmission is rapid and discrete, sometimes delivering a specific signal to an individual cell.

The modern history of endocrine research can be traced back to Claude Bernard's introduction of the term "milieu interieur." A notable advance in endocrine research was initiated by the invention of radioimmunoassay by Berson and Yalow in 1967. However, to understand how low concentrations of circulating hormones affect the function of their target cells, the equally important concept of cell surface receptors was introduced, together with the idea of signal transducers that transmit the information from the receptors to the cell interior. Much of our current understanding of cellular biochemistry and cell physiology results from the significant expansion of research stemming from these early endocrine and metabolic studies.

Hormones are exceptionally potent chemicals that operate at concentrations so low that they can be measured only by the most sensitive analytical methods. Their concentrations are typically expressed as parts per trillion, one thousand times lower than parts per billion. This magnitude of dilution can be dramatized by thinking of a drop of gin dissolved in a train of tank cars containing tonic. It has been calculated that one drop in 660 tank cars would approximate one part in a trillion; such a train would be 6 miles long.

The hypothalamus-pituitary, thyroid, parathyroid, pancreas, adrenals, ovary, and testes are considered to be the principal endocrine glands producing hormones. A more complete list of the major endocrine hormones and their primary gland of origin is shown in Table 9.1.

As indicated in Table 9.1, the endocrine hormones can be divided into two major chemical classes: (1) the peptides and amino acid derivatives; and (2) the cholesterol-based steroid compounds. In general, the former are believed to interact primarily with membrane-associated receptors, while the latter are more lipophilic and are able to gain entrance into target cells. In any event, overactive or underactive endocrine

Table 9.1 Principal endocrine hormones

Hormone	Secreted by
Peptide or amino acid derivative	
Insulin	Pancreas
Glucagon	Pancreas
Somatostatin	Pancreas
Thyroid hormones (T_3 and T_4)	Thyroid
Antidiuretic hormone (ADH)	Pituitary
Oxytocin	Pituitary
Adrenocorticotropic hormone (ACTH)	Pituitary
Thyroid-stimulating hormone (TSH)	Pituitary
Luteinizing hormone (LH)	Pituitary
Follicle-stimulating hormone (FSH)	Pituitary
Growth hormone (GH)	Pituitary
Prolactin	Pituitary
Gonadotropin-releasing hormone (GnRH)	Pituitary
Luteinizing-hormone releasing hormone (LHRH)	Pituitary
Thyrotropin-releasing hormone (TRH)	Pituitary
Parathyroid hormone	Parathyroid
Melatonin	Pineal
Calcitonin	Thyroid
Catecholamines	Adrenals
Steroid	
Estrogens	Ovary, adrenals
Progesterone	Ovary, testes, adrenals
Testosterone	Testes, ovary, adrenals
Cortisol	Adrenals
Corticosterone	Adrenals
Aldosterone	Adrenals

glands may produce syndromes that require treatment with drugs and/or surgery or hormone replacement, respectively.

Hormones can be exploited for a variety of therapeutic and diagnostic purposes. However, when considering the clinical applications of hormones, one usually thinks first of their use in replacement therapy. It is the latter aspect of endocrine pharmacology that this chapter is primarily concerned with. However, when significant pharmacological aspects of glandular products exist over and above replacement roles they will be presented. In a number of instances, the development of synthetic hormone analogs has achieved significant improvements over natural hormones in terms of potency, selectivity, and usefulness.

As mentioned in Chapter 1, perhaps the purest form of drug therapy is the replacement of inadequate amounts of an endogenous substance such as a hormone. Any gland that normally secretes a hormone is a potential target for hypofunctioning. Classical examples include Addison's disease (adrenal cortex), dwarfism (anterior pituitary), juvenile-onset insulin-dependent diabetes (pancreas), and hypothyroidism (thyroid).

When the appropriate hormone is given to replace a physiological inadequacy it is given as a pharmaceutical preparation at a "physiological" dose. If the appropriate dose is given, no undesired side effects should be expected. However, when hormones are given at supraphysiological levels, referred to as "pharmacological" doses, side effects are relatively common and are usually extensions of their physiological properties. This is a particular concern with adrenal glucocorticoids, which are often used in high doses to suppress serious cases of chronic inflammation or the rejection of transplanted organs.

As mentioned earlier, there are a number of physiological disorders related to glandular hypofunction that require pharmacological intervention. However, the underlying principles of therapeutics are essentially the same. That is, determine the correct replacement dose and deliver the hormone in a manner that most accurately reproduces its normal physiological pattern of release. Among the endocrine replacement disorders, the most prevalent in the world is diabetes mellitus, which serves as our prototype.

DIABETES MELLITUS

The word diabetes is derived from the Greek word of the same spelling, which signifies the copious urine production associated with the affliction (i.e., a siphoning). However, diabetes mellitus should be distinguished from diabetes insipidus, which also produces excess urine production because of a deficiency of antidiuretic hormone (vasopressin). Mellitus is the latinized Greek word for "honeyed" and reflects the increased concentration of glucose in the urine. Although diabetes has a name that suggests both its symptoms and its nature, physicians were nonetheless unable to stem its debilitating effects until the twentieth century.

Diabetes mellitus has been diagnosed in approximately 14 million people in the United States. Of these, 10–20 percent are classified as having insulin-dependent, juvenile-onset (type 1) while the remainder have non-insulin-dependent, maturity-onset (type 2). However, the situation can be somewhat more complex than these straightforward definitions in that type 1 can occur at any age and type 2 can require the use of insulin. At the present time, there is a serious increase in type 2 diabetics, particularly among the young.

Generally, in the case of type 1, there is inadequate production of insulin, which eventually becomes absolute. It is an autoimmune disease that kills pancreatic beta cells. If left untreated, the body will starve because glucose cannot gain access into key body organs. Type 1 diabetics are typically underweight. Death will occur from ketoacidosis due to the unregulated production of acidic lipid breakdown products. In the case of type 2 diabetes, there is often a "relative" lack of adequate insulin production since these individuals are characterized by target-cell "resistance" to the hormone. In fact, their circulating insulin levels may be normal or even elevated. Type 2 has a genetic component. Both types of diabetes mellitus are managed by diet and exercise, to achieve caloric control, as well as exogenous insulin. Oral hypoglycemic drugs that either increase release of endogenous insulin or increase sensitivity at peripheral receptors may also be used to treat type 2 patients.

HISTORY OF INSULIN

Of all the hormones, perhaps insulin possesses the most interesting history in endocrine pharmacology. Diabetes mellitus itself has been recognized as a clinical entity for at least 2000 years. However, the discovery of insulin, and its utilization in treating diabetes mellitus, required a combination of circumstances that illustrate the scientific method. For example, the symptoms of the disorder had to be recognized, a hypothesis based upon relevant physiological knowledge had to be constructed, appropriate experiments needed to be carried out dealing with both glandular extirpation and extract replacement, and the application of these observations to the human clinical condition had to be assessed. Finally, the utilization of modern genetic engineering has resulted in the synthetic production of the hormone for treatment, thus rendering patients less susceptible to shortages of animal preparations.

In 1889, Austrian scientists Joseph von Mering and Oskar Minkowski observed that if experimental animals were pancreatectomized they developed symptoms identical to diabetes mellitus (e.g., loss of weight, and copious urine production containing glucose) and speculated that an unknown substance in the pancreas could be the missing factor. Support for this hypothesis was based upon the general concept of the physiological function of endocrine secretions as well as the specific observation of a correlation between pancreatic β-cell damage and diabetes symptoms. Therefore, by the beginning of the twentieth century it was widely believed that some type of "internal secretion" of the pancreas played a significant role in the control of carbohydrate metabolism. In 1909, the German scientist Georg Zuelzer developed the first pancreatic extract in an attempt to treat diabetes, but the side effects were too severe to allow further studies.

Despite the widely held belief of pancreatic secretion, early attempts to prove the existence of the missing factor were widely disparate and inconclusive. For example, the early administration of pancreatic extracts to human diabetics would sometimes reduce glycosuria, while in other cases the results would be life-threatening. The latter was probably the result of the presence of toxic contaminants and subsequent immunological responses to them. However, by 1919 a somewhat more regular hypoglycemic effect was achieved in experimental animals by the intravenous injections of aqueous solutions of ground fresh pancreas. It only remained for Frederick Grant Banting to appear on the scene and complete the discovery process.

In 1920, the 22-year-old Banting accepted a demonstratorship in surgery and anatomy at Western University in London, Ontario. One of Banting's responsibilities involved lecturing on carbohydrate metabolism to medical students. It was in the process of preparing for these presentations that his curiosity was stimulated regarding the relationship of pancreatic islets of Langerhans cells to diabetes.

Upon returning to his alma mater (University of Toronto) the following year, Banting enlisted the support of J. J. R. Macleod, a professor of physiology, to carry out research on his theories relating to the functional relationship between the pancreas and diabetes. It was Banting's hypothesis that previous attempts to use pancreatic extracts were doomed to failure, or achieved mediocre success at best, because they were heterogeneous in nature. That is, they contained material from both acinar cells (e.g., digestive enzymes) and β-cells (presumably containing insulin). In order to circumvent this problem, Banting's strategy was to ligate the pancreatic duct in dogs, keep them alive while their acinar cells degenerated, and then remove the remaining pancreatic tissue for the preparation of an extract. Banting began his work, assisted by Charles Best, in May 1921.

Within 2 months, Banting and Best had succeeded in preparing saline extracts of atrophied pancreas that they administered by intravenous injection to depancreatectomized dogs. Over the course of the next 6 months Banting and Best accumulated data substantiating that their extract could reduce hyperglycemia in diabetic dogs, most notably with a dog named "Marjorie." Although their saline extracts continued to produce side effects, it was decided that a clinical test in humans was merited.

On January 11, 1922, a 14-year-old severely diabetic boy named Leonard Thompson received a 15-ml saline extract at the Toronto General Hospital. He appeared at the hospital with a blood glucose of 550 percent (normal being approximately 90 percent) and he was excreting 3–5 liters of urine per day. After initial failures during the first week and a half, a series of injections begun on January 23 produced immediate results including significantly decreased glycosuria and ketoacidosis, as well as a general feeling of improvement on the part of the patient. The research team initially feared that some unknown factor may have caused the youngster's amazing recovery, so they withheld insulin for 10 days to determine whether this was indeed so. Once off the insulin, Thompson's condition deteriorated and he displayed all of the classic symptoms of diabetes. Insulin injections were resumed and the boy's health improved.

For the first time in history there was clear, unambiguous clinical evidence, in humans, that symptoms of diabetes mellitus could be controlled with the exogenous administration of the active factor of the pancreas—insulin. Thus, replacement therapy with the newly discovered hormone, insulin, had arrested what was clearly an otherwise fatal metabolic disorder. From that point forward, diabetes mellitus (type 1) became a manageable disease by pharmacological intervention.

Following the treatment of Leonard Thompson, events proceeded rapidly toward the commercial production of insulin. A formal agreement was signed with Eli Lilly and Company on May 29, 1922, for the isolation and processing of insulin from animal sources (pigs and cows). By the end of June, Lilly was producing potent batches of pig insulin that were sent to Toronto for testing, and by the autumn an improved method for producing large quantities of even purer insulin was developed. By the end of 1923 insulin was being widely used clinically and Banting and Macleod's work was rewarded with a Nobel prize in physiology and medicine.

On the human side, Banting was outraged that the Nobel Committee decided to split the award with Macleod, whom he had grown to dislike, and had slighted Charles Best, who had assisted Banting throughout the entire research process. In an honorable display, Banting gave half of his $40,000 share of the award to Best (compare to $950,000 awarded for the equivalent prize in 2001). Not to be outdone, Macleod gave half of his award to James Collip, a biochemist who had also worked closely on the project.

The first commercial insulins, obtained from animals such as cows and pigs, were very impure acidic solutions. The pancreases were collected after slaughter and cooled to −20°C. The frozen glands were chopped up and the insulin extracted with acidified ethanol and water. Then came purification by salting-out, pH adjustment, and crystallization. Later, insulins were further purified using ion-exchange chromatography.

By this means, contaminants were reduced by as much as 20 percent to less than 1 ppm, and concentration was increased from 1 to 100 units per ml.

Animal insulins are still available, but the trend is clearly toward the use of human insulins (produced semisynthetically from porcine insulin or via recombinant technology in *Escherichia coli*), which were introduced in the early 1980s. Animal insulins, although they work in humans, are not structurally identical to human insulin. Porcine insulin differs in one amino acid while bovine insulin differs in three amino acids. While these differences may be small, they may nevertheless be sufficient to induce antibody formation and subsequent allergic reactions. Human insulins are structurally identical to endogenous insulin and are basically devoid of antigenicity. Today, several types of insulin preparations are available, differing primarily in their onset and duration of action. Since diabetics differ in their "brittleness," i.e., difficulty in maintaining appropriate glycemic control, some products may not be appropriate for all patients all the time.

For almost a decade there was a continuing dispute over the exact nature of insulin's chemical composition until it was finally accepted that the hormone was in fact a protein. Sanger established the amino acid sequence of insulin in 1960, and this led to the complete synthesis of the protein in 1963, and to the elucidation of its three-dimensional structure in 1972. Insulin was the first hormone for which a radioimmunoassay was developed (1978) and the first to be produced by genetic engineering (given to human volunteers in the summer of 1980).

THE THYROID GLAND

Hypothyroidism

The thyroid gland, which is anatomically located in the neck, is an organ that sequesters iodine (obtained from the diet) from the bloodstream. Uptake, organification, and release of thyroid hormones are largely regulated by thyroid-stimulating hormone (TSH) released from the anterior pituitary. Within the thyroid follicular cells there occurs a sequence of events that results in the formation of iodinated tyrosine that couples to form the principal hormones of the thyroid gland, namely triiodothyronine (T3) and thyroxine (T4). T4 is converted into T3 in the body. The former is the magical hormone responsible for the metamorphosis of the tadpole into a mature frog. T3 and T4 act to regulate TSH release by feedback inhibition. These hormones play decisive roles in regulating cellular metabolism throughout the body.

Hypothyroidism, known as myxedema in adults, when severe, is the most common disorder of the thyroid gland. Worldwide, hypothyroidism is most often the result of endemic iodine deficiency. In nonendemic areas, where iodine is sufficient in the diet, chronic autoimmune thyroiditis (Hashimoto's thyroiditis) accounts for the majority of cases. This disorder is primarily characterized by high levels of circulating antibodies against a key enzyme (thyroid peroxidase) in the processing of iodine in the thyroid gland. Blocking antibodies directed at the TSH receptor may also be present. Thyroid destruction may also occur via apoptotic cell death.

Hypothyroidism at birth is known as cretinism and is the most common preventable cause of mental retardation in the world. The incidence of cretinism is approximately

Table 9.2 Principal symptoms of hypothyroidism

Fatigue
Cold intolerance, cold skin
Constipation
Bradycardia, excessive menstrual bleeding
Impaired growth of skeletal tissues
Impaired growth, development, and function of the CNS
Impaired synthesis of protein
Impaired absorption of carbohydrates and amino acids
Impaired lipid metabolism (hypercholesteremia)
Impaired gonadal function
Impaired cardio renal function (diminished peripheral resistance and glomerular filtration rate)
Impaired overall tissue metabolism (basal metabolic rate)

1 per 4000 births. Diagnosis and early intervention with thyroid hormone replacement prevents the development of cretinism. Failure to achieve timely intervention results in irreversible damage to the developing central nervous system as well as other changes. The child is dwarfed, with short extremities, inactive, uncomplaining, and listless. The face is puffy and expressionless, and the enlarged tongue may protrude through the thickened lips of the half-opened mouth. Screening of newborn infants for deficient function of the thyroid is carried out in most industrialized nations. The principal symptoms of hypothyroidism are shown in Table 9.2.

Failure of the thyroid to produce sufficient thyroid hormone is the most common cause of hypothyroidism and is known as primary hypothyroidism. Secondary hypothyroidism occurs much less often and results from diminished release of TSH from the pituitary. Treatment of hypothyroidism is achieved by the replacement of thyroid hormone, primarily T4. A synthetic preparation of T4 is available, levothyroxine (Synthroid®), which has been a popular choice for hypothyroidism because of its consistent potency and prolonged duration of action. No toxicity occurs when given in physiological replacement doses. Desiccated animal thyroid is also available at a lesser cost. Overdoses cause symptoms of hyperthyroidism and can be used as a guide in clinical management. Hypothyroidism is not cured by the daily intake of thyroid hormone; it is a life-long regimen.

Hyperthyroidism

While hypofunction of the thyroid gland is relatively common, hyperfunction is an uncommon illness affecting less than 0.25 percent of the population. It is more prevalent among females than males (8:1) and usually occurs in middle age; it rarely occurs in children or adolescents. Hyperfunction of the thyroid gland is known as Graves' disease, after the Irish physician who was one of the first to fully describe the syndrome.

The leading cause of Graves' disease occurs when there is a defect in the immune system that causes the production of autoantibodies to TSH receptors located on the surface of thyroid cells. These antibodies act as agonists to stimulate the thyroid, causing it to enlarge (goiter formation), with the overproduction of thyroid hormones

Table 9.3 Symptoms of Graves' disease

Protruding eyes	Fatigue	Changes in sex drive
Weight loss	Muscle cramps	Heart palpitations
Increased appetite	Tremors	Blurred or double vision
Nervousness	Frequent bowel movements	
Restlessness	Menstrual irregularities	
Heat intolerance	Goiter	
Sweating	Rapid heart rate	

(T3 and T4). The underlying etiology is unknown but may have a genetic or immune basis. Typical symptoms of Graves' disease are shown in Table 9.3.

The primary treatment for Graves' disease is to control the overactive thyroid gland. There are three standard regimens for treating Graves' disease but the choice of treatment varies from country to country and from physician to physician. The selection of which treatment to use is predicated on factors such as age, degree of illness, and patient preference. The treatment of choice among endocrinologists is radioactive iodine (I^{131}, a beta emitter). Because the thyroid gland concentrates iodine, this nuclide is taken up and irradiates the thyroid tissue that produces T3 and T4. Its advantages include ease of administration, effectiveness, and economics. Disadvantages include delayed effect, overdose, and it cannot be used in pregnant women. Young patients with relatively small glands and mild disease can sometimes be treated with drugs.

Antithyroid drugs such as propylthiouracil (PTU) and methimazole inhibit the iodination of tyrosyl residues as well as the coupling of monoiodotyrosine and diiodotyrosine into T3 and T4. In addition, PTU inhibits the peripheral conversion of T4 to T3. Unfortunately, there is a very high relapse rate with these drugs and a cure is very infrequent, if at all. The final alternative is thyroidectomy. In this case it is very difficult to determine exactly how much is to be excised. Not surprisingly, a consequence of surgery is the production of a hypothyroid individual who will require daily levothyroxine for the remainder of their life.

THE ADRENAL CORTEX

The adrenal glands are located anatomically above the kidneys. They comprise a three-layer cortex and a medulla. The medulla is the source of catecholamines such as epinephrine, the "fight-or-flight" hormone. The cortex is the source of aldosterone, the primary mineralocorticoid that is involved in the regulation of sodium reabsorption in the kidneys. In addition, the cortex is also the source of steroids known as glucocorticoids, of which cortisol is the principal endogenous representative. Synthesis and release of cortisol is under the control of adrenocorticotropic hormone (ACTH).

Cortisol helps to maintain homeostasis by regulating numerous enzymes throughout the body by affecting gene expression subsequent to binding to a cytosolic receptor and transport to the nucleus. During periods of stress, cortisol plays an important role in increasing blood glucose levels and elevating blood pressure. Clinically, cortisol

Table 9.4 Comparison of pharmacologic properties of glucocorticoids

Compound	Anti-inflammatory potency	Na$^+$-retaining potency	Duration of action
Cortisol	1	1	Short
Cortisone	0.8	0.8	Short
Prednisone	4	0.8	Intermediate
Prednisolone	4	0.8	Intermediate
Betamethasone	25	0	Long
Dexamethasone	25	0	Long

and its derivatives are used for replacement theory in the management of Addison's disease (hypofunctioning of the adrenal cortex) as well as for their anti-inflammatory and immunosuppressant properties.

The anti-inflammatory property of cortisol and its derivatives is probably the main pharmacological effect of this group of drugs used in therapy, since inflammation is a common denominator in tissue injury regardless of etiology. Once the anti-inflammatory property of cortisol was discovered during the 1940s, great effort was expended in separating the anti-inflammatory potency of cortisol (the desired effect) from its inherent mineralocorticoid potency (the undesirable effect). A comparison of the endogenous glucocorticoids (cortisol and cortisone) and several contemporary derivatives is shown in Table 9.4.

As can be seen, chemists have successfully achieved, over the succeeding decades, an excellent separation of the anti-inflammatory effect from the salt-retaining effect. In addition, compounds have also been developed that possess a prolonged duration of action (short; 8–12-hour biological half-life vs. long; 36–72-hour biological half-life). The increase in anti-inflammatory potency and the extended duration of action are primarily the result of (1) decreased binding to plasma globulin (30 percent vs. 5 percent free) and (2) decreased metabolism, respectively.

The main clinical uses of glucocorticoids are for physiological replacement therapy in adrenal insufficiency (where approximately 10–20 mg of cortisol equivalent/day is administered) as well as a wide range of nonendocrine, inflammatory disorders, and immunosuppression (e.g., organ transplants). In the latter cases, pharmacological doses (exceeding approximately 10–20 mg of cortisol equivalent/day) may be needed for prolonged periods of time. In these situations, toxicity may manifest itself in the affected patients. Side effects are basically an extension of the normal physiological effects of the glucocorticoids on the body (primarily involving carbohydrate, protein, and fat metabolism).

As mentioned earlier, endogenous glucocorticoids are stress hormones. Their task is to provide glucose from the liver, and replenish this substrate via catabolic effects on skeletal muscle and adipose tissue. The increased breakdown of skeletal muscle protein provides amino acids for gluconeogenesis in the liver. Blood glucose becomes elevated, a condition that can exacerbate glycemic control in diabetics. The breakdown of adipose tissue can sometimes cause a redistribution of fat to certain areas of the body such as the upper middle back producing a "buffalo hump." Chronic administration of glucocorticoids can also produce a potentially life-threatening condition resulting from adrenal insufficiency. Pharmacologic doses will cause the hypothalamus, and hence the anterior pituitary, to cease production of ACTH via feedback inhibition.

Chronic suppression of the pituitary–adrenal axis presents a condition that must be managed properly upon withdrawal of therapy in order to avoid acute adrenal insufficiency. There have been several strategies developed to meet this scenario including (1) the use of glucocorticoids with less than a long duration of action (to allow the pituitary to periodically "escape") and (2) gradually tapering off of the glucocorticoids to allow the pituitary–adrenal axis to recover its normal production of cortisol.

While work was being carried out in France during the 1970s on discovering glucocorticoid antagonists, a compound was discovered that proved to be a very potent antagonist to progesterone. It was given the developmental code identification of RU-486. The potential application of a potent progesterone antagonist was readily apparent. Progesterone is necessary for the maintenance of the decidualized endometrium (i.e., keeping the implanted fertilized egg alive). The subsequent administration of RU-486 to women in their first trimester of pregnancy proved it to be a powerful abortifacent. When used in conjunction with a prostaglandin (PGF$_2$alpha), expulsion of the developing fetus generally occurs within 4 hours in 95 percent of cases. Obviously, this type of drug is surrounded by considerable controversy. Acceptance as an abortifacent in Europe still exceeds that in the United States.

Cushing's disease

Cushing's syndrome is a hormonal disorder caused by prolonged exposure of the body's tissues to high levels of the adrenal hormone cortisol. Dr Henry Cushing first described a woman with signs and symptoms of this disease in 1912. In 1932 he was able to link the adrenal overproduction of cortisol to an abnormality in the pituitary. It is a relatively rare disorder with a frequency estimated at 1–5/100,000 people per year primarily in the age range 20 to 50 years. It is caused primarily by pituitary adenomas that secrete increased amounts of ACTH. ACTH can also be produced outside the pituitary. This is called ectopic ACTH production. In addition, noncancerous tumors of the adrenal glands, called adrenal adenomas, can release excess cortisol into the blood. When the source of excess cortisol production is a tumor of the adrenal gland itself, then it is not dependent on ACTH.

Symptoms vary, but they are usually the same as glucocorticoid overdose (described previously). Most people have upper body obesity, rounded face, increased fat around the neck, and thinning arms and legs. Children tend to be obese with slowed growth rates. Other characteristic symptoms include severe fatigue, weak muscles, high blood pressure, and high blood sugar (exacerbating diabetes). Irritability, anxiety, and depression are common.

Treatment of Cushing's disease depends upon its etiology and can include surgery, radiation therapy, or drugs. Drugs such as mitotane (*o,p'*-DDD) are used to treat adrenal carcinoma when surgery is not possible. It causes adrenal inhibition by an unknown mechanism. Mitotane was discovered when it was observed that the *o,p'* isomer of the insecticide DDD caused severe damage to the adrenal cortex in dogs.

BIRTH CONTROL HORMONES

Probably the most widely used hormone preparations in the world are those used in healthy women who are not suffering from a disease. These are, of course, birth control pills, which usually contain derivatives of estrogen and progesterone. While they can be used in certain gynecologic disorders with efficacy, the vast majority of prescriptions are written to prevent pregnancy. Their development introduced a new era in society; a virtually 100 percent effectiveness, replacing IUDs (intrauterine devices), condoms, creams, jellies, and diaphragms.

It had been known for a long time that alteration of the normal endocrine status in female experimental animals could disrupt their ability to become pregnant. During the normal monthly reproductive cycle there is a sequential elaboration of estrogen and progesterone by the ovaries. This prepares the endometrial lining of the uterus for implantation of a fertilized egg and nourishment of it. Successful implantation and continuation of pregnancy therefore depends not only on the presence of appropriate hormones but also on exquisite timing between preparation of the endometrium and arrival of the egg. Alteration of the hormonal milieu out of the norm can result in failed pregnancy.

As mentioned earlier, physiologists had noted that altering either estrogen or progesterone levels in experimental animals could impact on pregnancy. However, this was little more than a laboratory curiosity since there was no practical way to take advantage of the situation—pure estrogen and progesterone were of limited supply, extremely expensive, and had ultrashort half-lives (> 90 percent first-pass metabolism). What was needed was some type of breakthrough in the extremely difficult synthetic processes for the formation of these steroids.

The breakthrough occurred when a species of Mexican yam was discovered that normally produced a compound that could be used as a precursor in steroid synthesis. Many laborious steps were thereby circumvented, allowing the synthesis of relatively large amounts of estrogen and progesterone at significantly reduced cost. The availability of the final product also allowed chemists to study structure–activity relationships aimed at developing new derivatives. One of these was a progesterone derivative called norethynodrel.

Norethynodrel was first used in clinical studies to treat female infertility. Ironically, initial studies demonstrated that, in fact, fertility was decreased by virtue of blocked ovulation. Analysis of the early batches of norethynodrel revealed the presence of a contaminant with estrogenic potency, namely mestranol. When mestranol was removed in subsequent batches, treatment with pure norethynodrel led to more breakthrough bleeding and less consistent inhibition of ovulation. Mestranol was thus reincorporated into the preparation, and this combination was employed in the first large-scale clinical trial of combination oral contraceptives. In late 1959, Enovid® (norethynodrel and mestranol) was the first "pill" approved by the FDA for use as a contraceptive agent in the United States. Today's combination preparations have an effectiveness of approximately 99.9 percent with "perfect use," and can contain various progestins other than norethynodrel, as well as the estrogen ethinyl estradiol, which has largely replaced mestranol. Ethinyl estradiol differs from endogenous estrogen only in the presence of an ethinyl group on carbon 17 of the steroid nucleus. Table 9.5 shows a comparison of the relative effectiveness of various contraceptive methods when used typically.

Table 9.5 Percent of accidental pregnancies in first year of typical use

Progesterone implants	0.09
Vasectomy	0.15
Depo-Provera	0.30
Tubal sterilization	0.40
Copper IUD	0.80
The Pill	2.00
Mini-Pill	3.00
Condoms	12.00
Diaphragm and spermicidal	18.00
Spermacide alone	21.00
Withdrawal	21.00

Early combination preparations contained relatively high doses of the progestin and estrogenic components. Untoward effects of early hormonal contraceptives fell into several major categories: adverse cardiovascular effects, including hypertension, myocardial infarction, hemorrhagic or ischemic stroke, and venous thrombosis and embolism; breast, hepatocellular, and cervical cancers; and a number of endocrine and metabolic effects. Once a dose relationship was realized (particularly with the estrogenic component) with the side effects, doses were decreased. Today's preparations contain approximately 90 percent less of the progestin and 80 percent less of the estrogen than the original preparations, while still maintaining effectiveness. They are available in a variety of fixed-dose, biphasic, and triphasic combinations that vary in their estrogen and progestin content throughout the cycle, the goal being to use the smallest total hormone content possible that is still effective.

The current consensus is that the contemporary low-dose preparations pose minimal risks in women who have no predisposing risk factors and, in fact, may provide certain beneficial health effects (e.g., protection against endometrial and ovarian cancer). Oral contraceptive pills have been associated with increased risk for myocardial infarction, stroke, and venous thromboembolism. However, studies have been published that suggest that these risks are minimal in appropriately chosen low-risk women.

Stroke is a very uncommon event in childbearing women, occurring in approximately 11 per 100,000 women over a 1-year period of time. Therefore, even a doubling of this risk with oral contraceptive pills would have minimal effect on attributable risk. The estimated risk of myocardial infarction associated with oral contraceptive pill use in nonsmokers is 3 per million women over 1 year. The estimated risk of venous thromboembolism attributable to oral contraceptive pills is less than 3 per 10,000 women per year. However, the risk may be increased in women who smoke or have other predisposing factors to thrombosis or thromboembolism. In fact, it should be emphasized that the risk of serious cardiovascular side effects is particularly marked in women over 35 years of age who are heavy smokers (e.g., more than 15 cigarettes per day). Additionally, the literature suggests that there may be an increased risk of breast cancer associated with long-term oral contraceptive pill use in women under the age of 35. However, because the incidence of breast cancer is so relatively low in this population, the attributable risk of breast cancer from birth control pill use is small.

Following the recognition that combination birth control pills were associated with adverse thrombolic events, alternatives to combination contraceptives were developed to avoid or minimize side effects. For example, the "Mini" pill was developed in the 1970s. This product is a progestin-only product taken daily. Its contraceptive effectiveness is approximately 97 percent. Its mechanism of action is apparently due to changing the motility of the oviduct, putting the endometrium out of phase, and increasing the thickness of vaginal mucus (the vast majority of women continue to ovulate which differentiates them from users of combination pills where ovulation is blocked). Variations on progestin-only preparations include silastic implants (effective up to 5 years), depo-deposition intramuscularly (effective 2–3 months), and a progestin-containing IUD.

PARKINSON'S DISEASE

Although replacement therapy is classically exemplified by the treatment of hypofunctioning endocrine glands, there is an important neurological disorder that can be successfully treated with a replacement strategy. Parkinson's disease is a clinical syndrome characterized by slowness of movement, muscular rigidity, resting tremor, and an impairment of postural balance. In the absence of therapy, death frequently results from complications of immobility.

The syndrome is the result of an 80–90 percent loss of dopaminergic neurons, and the attendant neurotransmitter (dopamine), in the substantia nigra region of the brain. These neurons normally project into a region of the basal ganglia where they inhibit firing of cholinergic neurons. These cholinergic neurons, in turn, form excitatory synapses onto other neurons that project out of the basal ganglia. The net result is that the cholinergic neurons are without their normal inhibition. The loss of dopaminergic neurons and their dopamine suggested to researchers that replacement of the neurotransmitter could restore function. However, dopamine is highly polar and does not cross the blood–brain barrier. So a different strategy had to be devised.

Dopamine is synthesized in the terminals of dopaminergic fibers originating with the amino acid tyrosine and, subsequently, L-dihydroxyphenylalanine (L-dopa or levodopa), the rate-limiting metabolic precursor of dopamine. Fortunately, L-dopa is significantly less polar than dopamine and can gain entry into the brain via an active process mediated by a carrier of aromatic amino acids. Although L-dopa is itself basically pharmacologically inert, therapeutic effects can be produced by its decarboxylation to dopamine within the CNS.

In clinical practice, L-dopa is conventionally administered in combination with a peripherally acting *inhibitor* of aromatic L-amino acid decarboxylase (e.g., carbidopa). If L-dopa is administered alone, the drug is largely decarboxylated by enzymes in the intestinal mucosa and other peripheral sites. Inhibition of peripheral decarboxylase by carbidopa markedly increases the fraction of orally administered L-dopa that remains unmetabolized and available to enter the brain (i.e., its bioavailability).

Dopamine receptor agonists are also available for therapy in Parkinson's disease. The strategy of using dopamine agonists early as monotherapy or in combination with levodopa to delay long-term levodopa complications is gaining wider acceptance.

However, levodopa combined with carbidopa remains the most effective symptomatic treatment for Parkinson's disease.

Although replacement therapy is basically limited to endocrine disorders, it still plays an important therapeutic role in clinical pharmacology. The number of people requiring replacement therapy for diabetes and hypothyroidism alone makes insulin and thyroid hormone among the most commonly prescribed drugs in the United States. For example, the drug Synthroid® is taken daily by 8 million people to correct hypothyroidism, and its share of the market is worth $600 million per year. As more information is discovered about the role of other endogenous substances in the body, new examples of replacement therapy will occur.

QUESTIONS

1 Which of the following is/are true regarding the endocrine system?
   a   composed of specialized tissues or glands
   b   hormones are released into the bloodstream
   c   transmission is rapid throughout the body
   d   all of the above
   e   a and b.

2 In normal replacement therapy of a hypofunctioning gland, which of the following will apply?
   a   a pharmacological dose is most advantageous
   b   a physiological dose will not be sufficient to compensate
   c   a pharmacological dose is the only way to cure the disease
   d   a physiological dose is generally most appropriate
   e   a physiological dose is the only way to cure a disease.

3 Which of the following occurs with insulin-dependent, juvenile-onset, type 1 diabetes?
   a   overactivity of the beta cells of the pancreas
   b   elevated blood insulin levels
   c   increase in body weight
   d   reduced blood glucose levels
   e   decrease in body weight.

4 Which of the following is/are the cause of death in untreated insulin-dependent, juvenile-onset, type 1 diabetes?
   a   excess blood glucose
   b   excess urine formation
   c   kidney failure
   d   ketoacidosis
   e   none of the above.

5 Which of the following is/are true regarding insulin?
   a   it is a low-molecular-weight steroid
   b   it is produced in the alpha cells of the pancreas

    c   it is used in type 1 diabetes
    d   it is always used in type 2 diabetes
    e   a and c.

6 The first commercial insulin preparations were obtained from which of the following?
    a   slaughtered pigs
    b   human cadavers
    c   slaughtered cows
    d   slaughtered sheep
    e   a and c.

7 Which of the following is/are true of today's insulin preparations?
    a   differ in onset and duration of action
    b   are primarily produced by recombinant technology
    c   are less antigenic since they are based upon human insulin
    d   offer no advantage over bovine or porcine insulin
    e   a, b, and c above.

8 Hypofunctioning of which gland is particularly significant in neonates?
    a   adrenal
    b   ovary
    c   testes
    d   liver
    e   thyroid.

9 The principal mechanism of action of combination oral contraceptive agents is which of the following?
    a   altered oviduct motility
    b   induction of pre-ovulation
    c   inhibition of ovulation
    d   direct inhibitory effect on the ovaries
    e   none of the above.

10 Which of the following is/are true regarding prednisone vs. cortisol?
    a   has shorter duration of action
    b   has greater anti-inflammatory potency
    c   has greater salt-retaining potency
    d   is an endogenous mineralocorticoid
    e   is a precursor of cortisone.

Chapter 10

Chemotherapeutic agents

There have been at least four so-called revolutions in pharmacology. These include (1) the development of vaccines in the nineteenth century; (2) the discovery of antibiotics during the first half of the twentieth century; (3) the therapeutic introduction of psychopharmacological drugs for the treatment of mental disorders during the 1950s; and (4) the development of genetic engineering for drug production during the 1970s and 1980s. This chapter will deal with the discovery and therapeutic principles underlying the use of chemotherapeutic agents, primarily antibiotics and anticancer drugs.

ANTIBIOTICS

Antibiotics (i.e., anti-infective or antimicrobial drugs) may be directed at one of several disease-producing organisms including bacteria, viruses, fungi, helminthes, etc. The vast majority of antibiotics are bacteria fighters; although there are millions of viruses, there are only about half a dozen antiviral drugs. Bacteria are more complex than viruses (while viruses must "live" in a host (us), bacteria can live independently) and so are easier to kill.

The impact of antibiotics on human health is not difficult to assess. The overall death rate from diseases such as pneumonia and tuberculosis has declined from 79.7 per 100,000 in 1900 to 59 per 100,000 in 1996, according to the Centers for Disease Control and Prevention (CDC). As a result, life expectancy during that period increased from 47.3 to 76.1 years. A further correlation between antibiotic introduction and declining death rate can be appreciated by comparing the decline in death rate in the United States with the introduction of antibiotics following World War II (Table 10.1). While the decline in death rate is undoubtedly multifactorial (nutrition, sanitation, etc.), antibiotics have clearly made a great contribution to humanity. Infections such as pneumonia, tuberculosis, and diarrhea/enteritis were the leading causes of death in 1900. Today, the leading causes are heart disease, cancer, and stroke.

HISTORY

In 1546, Girolamo Fracastro of Verona proposed the then remarkable theory that diseases were transmitted by minute particles of living matter with the properties of multiplication and airborne dissemination. He considered that particles with great

Table 10.1 Correlation of antibiotic use with death rate in the United States

Year	Antibiotic	Death rate (per 100,000)
1945	Introduction of penicillin	40
1946	General distribution of penicillin	37
1947	General distribution of streptomycin	34
1951	Introduction of isoniazid	15
1956	Introduction of *para*-aminosalicylic acid	9
1964	Introduction of myambutol	5
1972	Introduction of rifampin	2.5

penetrating power caused diseases such as plague and smallpox. Fracastro's living particles have, of course, been equated with microorganisms, although he did not suggest that they were disease specific. Unfortunately, lack of convincing scientific evidence led to Fracastro's ideas being largely ignored.

Credit for the actual discovery of microorganisms is given to Antony Van Leeuwenhoek in Holland in 1676. Using a microscope of his own invention, he reported seeing "animalcules" in various specimens, including scrapings from his own teeth. Although his discovery was important, it nevertheless did little to counteract the prevailing theory of spontaneous generation.

The concept of spontaneous generation in relation to microorganisms persisted until Louis Pasteur's classical experiments on fermentation in 1861. Pasteur demonstrated that when organisms from the air were excluded from heat-sterilized liquids, such as sugar solutions and urine, fermentation failed to take place. Although the debate regarding spontaneous generation would last into the 1870s, a commission of the Academie des Sciences officially accepted Pasteur's results in 1864. Despite Pasteur's critical demonstrations, and his conceptualization of the "germ theory of disease," Robert Koch did not establish the actual disease role of microorganisms in causing infections, plagues, and epidemics until the late nineteenth century through his work on anthrax, tuberculosis, and cholera.

Robert Koch was a German scientist who is credited with the founding of modern medical microbiology. Koch's first major breakthrough in bacteriology occurred in the 1870s when he demonstrated that the infectious disease anthrax developed in mice only when the disease-bearing material injected into a mouse's bloodstream contained viable rods or spores of *Bacillus anthracis*. Koch's isolation of the anthrax bacillus was a momentous achievement since this was the first time that the causative agent of an infectious disease had been demonstrated beyond a reasonable doubt.

In 1891, the Russian Romanovsky made a significant observation with pharmacological implications when he suggested that quinine cured malaria by damaging the parasite more than the host and suggested that similar situations might also occur with other drugs. The important therapeutic implications of this prediction were most fully developed by Paul Ehrlich (1854–1915), discussed previously, who coined the term chemotherapy. Ehrlich defined chemotherapy as "the use of drugs to injure an invading organism without injury to the host." The essence of chemotherapy is that, ideally, there is some qualitative or quantitative difference between the infecting pathogen and host that can be selectively exploited therapeutically.

Ehrlich's first chemotherapeutic experiments, beginning in 1904, were performed with organic dyes obtained from the prolific German synthetic chemical industry, the most advanced in the world at the time. During 1904, Ehrlich successfully demonstrated the curative properties of the substance trypan red against trypanosome-infected mice, thereby demonstrating the first man-made chemotherapeutic agent. Unfortunately, the drug proved to be inactive in man. For the remainder of his life Ehrlich concentrated his efforts in studying aromatic arsenicals, which had also shown promise in the treatment of trypanosomiasis.

In 1910, Ehrlich made a historic discovery while investigating one of these arsenicals, the antisyphilitic drug arsphenamine. This particular drug, with the laboratory code designation "606," was so effective in laboratory tests that it was announced as a cure for the dreaded disease and was referred to as a "magic bullet". Although the marketed form of the chemical, Salvarsan, ultimately proved to be too toxic for human use, arsphenamine was the opening event in the chemotherapeutic revolution for the treatment of human infections.

Antibiotics are unique in two significant respects. First, they include members of the only class of drugs that actually cure a disease. As indicated previously, most drugs merely provide symptomatic relief while the disease or condition runs its course, or replace an endogenous chemical that is being produced in inadequate amounts. In either case, the drug has not altered the basic etiologic factor that produced the disorder. Antibiotics, on the other hand, can contribute to an authentic cure by eradicating the cause of the disease, namely the pathogen. Second, the utility of antibiotics is intimately related to their ability to produce toxicity, albeit selectively. The selective toxicity of an antibiotic refers to the degree to which the substance is able to perturb the life processes of the pathogen without simultaneously affecting similar functions in the host.

As mentioned earlier, the basis for selective toxicity resides in some uniquely important difference in the biochemistry between host and microbe. Antimicrobial drugs exploit this difference and are able to selectively damage the target cell. For example, the drug may (1) inhibit a reaction vital only to the microbe and not the host. The target reaction may, in fact, have no counterpart in the host. For example, penicillin inhibits the cross-linking of microbial peptidoglycan and thereby prevents microbial cell wall synthesis. Animal cells have membranes of a different composition. Alternatively, the drug may (2) inhibit a reaction that yields a product vital to both microbe and host. However, the host has an alternative mechanism of obtaining the substance. For example, sulfa drugs inhibit intracellular folic acid synthesis by microbes. Human cells can utilize preformed folic acid and are not susceptible to this antimetabolic effect. Also the drug may (3) undergo biochemical activation to a toxic form in the microbe. For example, acyclovir is used to treat herpes infections. In order to be active it must undergo triple phosphorylation before it is able to inhibit herpes virus DNA polymerase. The drug may (4) selectively accumulate in the microbe because of a more active cell membrane transport mechanism. For example, quinine accumulates more readily in the malarial plasmodium cell than in the host cell. Finally, the drug may (5) have a higher affinity for a critical site of action in the microbe. For example, chloramphenicol binds to a fragment of the 70S ribosome of bacterial cells, thereby inhibiting synthesis of bacterial proteins. The drug has a much lower affinity for human ribosomes, which are 80S.

Antibiotics can be either bactericidal or bacteriostatic. That is, they can either kill the pathogen directly or arrest its replication until the body's immune system can be mobilized. Generally, bactericidal drugs are more desirable, especially in the immunocompromised patient. However, when a microbe is killed by a cidal drug and immediately cleared from the body, the antigenic stimulus is greatly reduced. In some cases it is so reduced that no immune response is triggered. Therefore, sometimes it may be more advantageous to use a static drug that will permit the body sufficient time to develop an appropriate immune response. Theoretically, it is not usually a good idea to combine cidal and static antibiotics, since cidal drugs depend upon active bacterial growth in order to be effective. For example, during the 1950s it was found that the human mortality rate for pneumococcal meningitis was higher when chlortetracycline (static) was administered with penicillin (cidal) than penicillin alone.

PENICILLIN

One of the most important events in the history of antibiotics is the discovery and production of penicillin. In 1928, while investigating staphylococcus variants at St Mary's Hospital in London, Alexander Fleming observed that when a particular strain of mold, *Penicillium notatum* (named because the cells were pencil-shaped when viewed under a microscope), contaminated these cultures they underwent lysis. Fleming named the active substance penicillin. Unfortunately, because Fleming was such a poor public speaker, his public presentation of his seminal discovery went unheeded, and it took an additional 12 years before the potential of penicillin was realized.

Fortunately, the production of relatively large quantities of penicillin was achieved by a group of researchers at Oxford University under the direction of Howard Florey, since no pharmaceutical company could be persuaded to take up the challenge. Florey's group experimented with treating both humans and animals during this period. By May 1940, crude preparations were available that were found to produce dramatic therapeutic effects when administered parenterally to mice with experimentally produced streptococcal infections. In 1941 the group accumulated enough material to conduct trials in several patients desperately ill with staphylococcal and streptococcal infections refractive to all other therapy. Their work culminated with publication of a paper in the journal *The Lancet* and concluded with the statement: "Enough evidence, we consider, has now been assembled to show that penicillin is a new and effective type of chemotherapeutic agent, and possesses some properties unknown in any antibacterial substance hitherto described." With classic British understatement the dawn of the antibiotic era had begun.

As an interesting historical footnote, in March 1996 the drug company Pfizer paid $35,160 at auction for a small culture of the original mold used by Fleming. The specimen is one of two that Fleming gave to his laboratory assistant, Dan Stratful, and contains a handwritten inscription ("The mold that makes penicillin." Alexander Fleming). Pfizer was one of the U.S. companies that finally participated in the commercial mass production of penicillin during World War II. The first marketable penicillin cost several dollars per 100,000 units; today, the same dose costs only a few cents. Commercial production results in more than 100 million pounds of penicillin per year.

Several natural penicillins can be produced, depending on the chemical composition of the fermentation medium used to culture penicillium. Penicillin G (benzylpenicillin) has the greatest antimicrobial activity of these natural penicillins and is the only natural penicillin used clinically. However, penicillin G is not stable; it is extremely acid-labile. Only about one-third of an oral dose is absorbed under the most ideal conditions. Therefore, it is generally not given orally but is administered by intramuscular injection. Several newer derivatives of penicillin G have been developed that do have good to excellent oral absorption (e.g., cloxacillin, ampicillin, and amoxicillin).

The selective toxicity of penicillin can be dramatically illustrated by the fact that a person with normal renal function can receive approximately 12.5–15 grams of penicillin per day with no ill effects. However, as little as 0.002 µg/ml may kill some bacteria such as pneumococcus. Therefore, the toxic to therapeutic ratio is extremely high. Unfortunately, this is not always achieved with antibiotics. This can be illustrated with the antifungal drug amphotericin B. For treatment of fungal infections, daily dosages of 0.5–0.6 mg/kg (35–42 mg for a 70-kg person) are needed. However, a dose of 1 mg can cause fever, chills, and low blood pressure in some patients. Chronic use can lead to fatal kidney damage. Therefore, although antibiotics are often associated with a relatively high margin of safety, there are important exceptions.

During the 1930s another significant class of antibiotics was discovered. The sulfa drug Prontosil, with its active metabolite sulfanilamide, was found to be effective against streptococcal infections, first in mice and then in humans. Sulfonamides were in fact the first effective chemotherapeutic agents to be employed systemically for the prevention and cure of bacterial infections in humans, since penicillin was not widely available until the early 1940s. In fact, the individual credited with discovery of this class of drugs, and recipient of the Nobel prize for his work, Gerhard Domagk, allowed it to be administered successfully to his daughter who was suffering from streptococcal septicemia at the time.

MECHANISM OF ACTION OF ANTIBIOTICS

As discussed earlier, there are a number of ways by which an antibiotic can selectively interfere with biochemical processes in a microbe. This part of the chapter deals in more detail with the respective mechanisms. These include the cell wall and membrane, nucleic acid and protein synthesis, and intermediary metabolism.

Penicillins, cephalosporins, and related drugs are known as beta-lactams since they share a four-membered beta-lactam ring. The mechanism of action of beta-lactam type drugs is more complex than originally thought. Penicillin and cephalosporin appear to be analogs of a natural structural unit (D-alanyl-D-alanine) in the cell walls of gram-positive bacteria. These antibiotics become covalently bound to a family of enzymes known as penicillin-binding proteins (PBPs), which are responsible for constructing the peptidoglycan lattice of bacterial cell walls. Failure to achieve adequate synthesis of the cell wall results in increased cell permeability, leakage, and death. Penicillin will not harm any cell wall already made but will interfere with new cell wall formation.

Microbes also have a plasma membrane that resides adjacent to their cell wall. Polymyxins are amphipathic agents (containing both nonpolar, lipophilic and polar, lipophobic groups) that interact with phospholipids in microbial cell membranes. The result is disruption of the membrane and increased permeability. However, because microbial and mammalian cell membranes are not exceedingly dissimilar, polymixins can produce significant toxicity in humans (i.e., they have low selective toxicity). This is also true for the related drug nystatin. This is why these particular antibiotics are not generally used systemically and are usually restricted to topical application.

Some antibiotics are known to interfere with microbial nucleic acid function. Rifampin, for example, inhibits DNA-dependent RNA polymerase, leading to suppression of the initiation of RNA chain formation. Nuclear RNA polymerase from a variety of eukaryotic cells does not bind rifampin, and RNA synthesis is correspondingly unaffected. Drugs belonging to the quinolone group interfere with DNA gyrase, the enzyme responsible for "supercoiling" microbial DNA into a compact form while retaining its functionality. Eukaryotic cells do not contain DNA gyrase (type II DNA topoisomerase is the equivalent and is several orders of magnitude less sensitive).

There are a number of sites within the sequence of protein synthesis where antibiotics can act. These include (1) inhibition of the attachment of mRNA to 30S ribosomes by aminoglycosides; (2) inhibition of tRNA binding to 30S ribosomes by tetracyclines; (3) inhibition of the attachment of mRNA to the 50S ribosome by chloramphenicol; and (4) erythromycin inhibition of the translocation step by binding to 50S ribosomes, thus preventing newly synthesized peptidyl tRNA moving from the acceptor to the donor site.

Finally, sulfonamides can interfere with intermediary metabolism. Because of their structural similarity to *para*-aminobenzoic acid (PABA), they can function as competitive inhibitors for dihydropteroate synthase. The result is interruption of microbial synthesis of folic acid by blocking formation of the folic acid precursor dihydropteroic acid. Sensitive microorganisms are those that must synthesize their own folic acid. Conversely, resistant bacteria and normal mammalian cells are unaffected since they do not synthesize folic acid but use the preformed vitamin.

RESISTANCE TO ANTIMICROBIAL AGENTS

One of the unfortunate realities of antimicrobial therapy has been the sobering realization that pathogens can develop drug resistance. Once on the verge of defeat, thanks to medicine's arsenal of approximately 160 antibiotics, bacteria began a resurgence seveal years ago. With each passing decade, bacteria that defy not only single but also multiple antibiotics—and therefore are extremely difficult to control—have become increasingly common. The emergence of antibacterial resistance in pathogenic strains is a worldwide problem. For example, during the past 50 years the development of penicillin-resistant strains of pneumococci has exceeded 50 percent in isolates from some European countries. In 1997, in three geographically separate patients, a new strain of *Staphylococcus aureus* was encountered. This bacterium, previously resistant to all antibiotics except for vancomycin, now showed resistance to vancomycin. The emergence of vancomycin-resistant organisms has been one of the greatest fears among public health professionals. For many infections, vancomycin is the antibiotic of last resort. *S. aureus* causes 260,000 infections each year in the United States, which, if left untreated, can be fatal. There are now strains of entercocci, pseudomonas, and enterobacters that are resistant to all known drugs.

The remarkable capacity of *S. aureus* to develop resistance to antibiotics is no more clearly illustrated than its recently reported success against linezolid (Zyvox®). Linezoid is the first entirely new type of antibiotic (oxazolidinones) introduced in 35 years. The FDA approved it in April 2000 for the treatment of several infections including resistant strains of *S. aureus*. However, it took only slightly more than a year for resistance to manifest itself. In the summer of 2001, the first report of staph resistance to the new antibiotic was observed in an 85-year-old man undergoing dialysis.

In recent years, strains of multidrug-resistant tuberculosis (TB) have spread around the world, killing thousands. In fact, the death rates for some communicable diseases such as tuberculosis have started to rise in industrialized countries. The number of TB cases worldwide has reached epidemic proportions. The World Health Organization reports that one-third of the world's population is infected, projecting 1 billion new infections and 35 million deaths in the next 20 years. In the United States alone, according to a 1995 report from the former Office of Technology Assessment, 19,000 hospital patients die each year due to hospital-acquired bacterial infections. Until recently, infections caused by *Staphylococcus epidermidis* and *Enterococcus faecium* were treatable with antibiotics. This is no longer the case. Up to 30 percent of the pneumonia found in some areas of the United States no longer responds to penicillin. Heavily used, antibiotics have become an evolutionary force, selecting for and enhancing the survival of bacterial strains that can resist them. According to the CDC, antibiotics are used excessively in 20–50 percent of cases.

The speed with which bacteria "acquire" resistance to antibiotics cautions restraint about prescribing them too frequently. Between 1983 and 1993, the percentage of patients receiving antibiotics rose from 1.4 to 45. During those years, researchers isolated *Eschericia coli* annually from patients, and tested the microbes for resistance to five types of fluroquinolones. Between 1983 and 1990, the antibiotics easily killed all 92 *E. coli* strains tested. However, in the interval from 1991 to 1993, 11 of 40 tested strains (28 percent) were resistant to all five drugs.

While the plea to more closely regulate the clinical use of antibiotics in humans is an obvious admonition to the medical community (humans take an estimated 3 million pounds yearly), there are other sources of concern. For example, the American Medical Association estimates that more than half of the total mass of antibiotics used in the United States is fed to animals, not to cure them of illness, but as growth promoters or to prevent illness. The Animal Health Institute, which represents makers of animal drugs, indicates that more than 20 million pounds of antibiotics are used yearly in the United States. The Union of Concerned Scientists estimates that as little as 2 million pounds go to sick animals. This is exactly the type of profligate usage that promotes the emergence of resistance.

In a study published in 2001, researchers at the University of Maryland collected 200 samples of ground beef, ground chicken, ground turkey, and ground pork from three supermarkets in the Washington, DC area. Twenty percent of the samples were contaminated with salmonella, a bacterium blamed for approximately 1.4 million cases of food poisoning a year in the United States. Of the salmonella strains isolated, 84 percent were resistant to at least one antibiotic, and 53 percent to three or more.

In another study published in the same year, researchers at the CDC found that half of 407 supermarket chickens bought from 26 stores in four states—Georgia, Maryland, Minnesota, and Oregon—carried the sometimes fatal germ *E. faecium* in a form resistant to Synercid®, one of the few drugs of last resort against the infection.

Antibiotics do not usually induce adaptive mutations; instead, they act as fierce agents of selection, killing off all bacteria except a favored few that, by chance, are immune to the antibiotic—a strain that earlier, for other reasons, might not have competed successfully with its fellows. The fact that bacteria quickly evolve resistance to antibiotics reflects the enormous diversity of forms and biochemical capacity at work in the microbial world. In this world there is a continuing conflict of measure and countermeasure, raging between host and parasite—in this case, between the pharmaceutical companies, generating new antibiotics, and the microbes, generating new resistant strains to replace their more vulnerable ancestors.

In order for an antimicrobial agent to be efficacious, it must reach the target pathogen and bind to it in sufficient concentration to express its effect. Bacteria can develop resistance by a number of mechanisms including (1) preventing the drug from reaching the target. For example, the "porin" channel proteins in gram-negative bacteria can become altered, thereby preventing certain antibiotics from gaining entrance. (2) Certain bacteria can increase their ability to metabolize antibiotics. For example, gram-positive bacteria (which do not have an outer cell membrane) such as staphylococci export beta-lactamases into their immediate environment and destroy beta-lactam antibiotics such as penicillins and cephalosporins. This is a major problem with *Haemophilus* and gonococci. In an attempt to circumvent this problem, beta-lactamase inhibitors are sometimes given simultaneously in order to protect the antibiotic. Gram-negative bacteria may also export beta-lactamases as well as having them in their periplasmic space between the inner and outer membrane. (3) Changes can occur at the drug-binding site. For example, a common cause of resistance to protease inhibitors used in the treatment of AIDS is that a phenyl group in the active site "flips" out of reach of the tightly binding inhibitor. This creates a gap where van der Waals contacts once formed by the inhibitor are lost. Finally, (4) some microbes can increase the transport of antibiotics out of the cell.

GENETICS OF BACTERIAL RESISTANCE

Many bacteria possessed resistance genes even before commercial antibiotics came into use. Scientists do not know exactly why these genes evolved and were maintained. One argument is that natural antibiotics were initially elaborated as the result of chance mutations. The bacteria so endowed were more likely to survive and proliferate.

Bacteria can obtain the various types of resistance mechanisms described previously by undergoing modifications in their genetic constitution. Many bacteria simply inherit their resistance genes from their forerunners. In addition, genetic mutations can occur that can confer a new trait. For example, it has been estimated that bacteria undergo spontaneous mutation at a frequency of approximately 1 in 10 cells. These mutations can confer resistant traits to the subsequent progeny. Mutations are believed to be responsible for the development of resistance to streptomycin (ribosomal mutation), quinolones (gyrase gene mutation), and rifampin (RNA polymerase gene mutation). The end result is that the drug does not bind. It is by this vertical, Darwinian process that a few existing members of a heterogeneous population that happen to have a genetic advantage reproduce in the presence of the antimicrobial drug and become the dominant surviving strain. However, although mutation of the microbe's genome can occur, the major mechanism of resistance development in pathogenic bacteria is plasmid mediated.

Plasmids are autonomously replicating pieces of extrachromosomal DNA present in bacteria. They are encoded with subtle, yet vital, changes for the synthesis of important cellular proteins. Because they are relatively large, they can contain information pertaining to several genes. One of these genes codes for beta-lactamase, an enzyme that can hydrolyze the four-member heterocyclic beta-lactam ring present in penicillins and cephalosporins.

There are several mechanisms by which plasmids can serve as the vehicle to transfer resistance determinants to sensitive bacteria. These include transduction, transformation, and conjugation. Resistance that is acquired by this type of horizontal transfer can become rapidly and widely disseminated.

Transduction involves the introduction of new genetic information via a bacteriophage (a virus that infects bacteria). In this situation the bacteriophage contains DNA, which can carry a gene for drug resistance. Transductive transfer of phage DNA is particularly important for the development of resistance among strains of *S. aureus* that become endowed with the ability to synthesize penicillinase.

Transformation is a process whereby fragments of free DNA in the environment of the microbe become incorporated into its own genome. For example, penicillin-resistant pneumococci produce altered PBPs that have low-affinity binding sites for penicillin. Nucleotide sequence analysis of the genes encoding these altered PBPs indicates that the insertion of foreign genetic material has taken place. Presumably, these DNA fragments (transposons) originate in closely related streptococcal strains and become incorporated into resident PBP genes by homologous recombination.

The process by which the passage of genes occurs directly from bacterium to bacterium by direct contact is referred to as *conjugation*. A pilus or tube is temporarily formed that joins the donor and recipient organisms and through which genetic material is passed. The donor must posses two genetic factors in order to participate in conjugation: an R-factor, which codes for the resistance trait, and an RT-factor, which codes for the synthesis of the pilus. Conjugation occurs largely in gram-negative bacteria. The clinical significance of conjugation was first demonstrated in Japan in 1959 after an outbreak of bacillary dysentery. The responsible pathogen, *Shigella flexneri*, was found to be resistant to not just one but four different classes of antibiotics (tetracycline, sulfonamide, streptomycin, and chloramphenicol).

SELECTION OF APPROPRIATE ANTIBIOTIC

Ideally, biological specimens containing the infectious agent would be obtained and identification of the pathogen carried out. In addition, in vitro antimicrobial susceptibility studies might then be determined. In practice this is generally not done, since clinical decisions are often based upon the presentation of patient symptoms. In this manner, therapy can be started immediately with a minimum of expense. The drawback to this expeditious prescribing is that antibiotics are subject to inappropriate use, which has contributed to the development of resistance.

We need only recall the aftermath of the World Trade Center terrorist attack on September 11, 2001, which involved the threat of anthrax infection. Almost all naturally occurring cases of anthrax are cutaneous or gastrointestinal. Blackish sores on the skin characterize cutaneous anthrax. Anthrax was in fact derived from a Greek word that refers to coal or charcoal. Inhalation anthrax is an extremely rare disease that normally results from exposure to contaminated animal hides and hairs, with most transmissions occurring in an industrial setting. Anthrax is a biowarfare threat because its spores can be made into an aerosol form that can resist environmental degradation, and can be milled into an ideal size for reaching the lower respiratory tract (1–6 µm). Although the exact number of inhaled spores required to produce death in humans is unknown, most estimates put the level in the 8000–10,000 range.

As soon as the first case of anthrax was confirmed in Florida, a relatively new drug gained notoriety—Cipro®. This fluoroquinolone (ciprofloxacin) became the mode of therapy for those people exposed to the anthrax bacillus (approved by the FDA for anthrax on July 28, 2000). Despite appeals for restraint in the use of Cipro, pharmacies in Mexican border towns reported being cleaned out of the antibiotic by Americans searching for the readily available and relatively cheap drug. Only time will tell if inappropriate, irrational use of Cipro results in loss of effectiveness in treating anthrax infection. However, the CDC did determine that 19 percent of 490 people in Florida experienced side effects 1–2 weeks after beginning therapy with Cipro.

The use of Cipro to treat anthrax infection emanated from research carried out in 1990 at Fort Detrick, Maryland (see later). The army was concerned that Saddam Hussein could introduce germ warfare in the Gulf War in the form of anthrax. Sixty monkeys were infected with a strain of *Bacillus anthracis* by aerosol and were divided into six groups. One group received a vaccine alone; another received the vaccine and antibiotics; and three groups were treated for 30 days with one of three different classes of antibiotics—penicillin, doxycycline, or Cipro. A control group received saline injections.

By day 8, nine of 10 control monkeys had perished. By day 10, eight of 10 monkeys who received vaccine alone were dead. By contrast, the monkeys treated daily with antibiotics survived into the fourth week. The combination of vaccine and doxycycline performed best. Nevertheless, Pentagon officials recommended using a combination of Cipro and vaccine, since Cipro was a newer drug and presumably more effective against a conceivably genetically engineered anthrax. However, in October 2001 the FDA issued a health advisory update reminding all health professionals that doxycycline is approved for the treatment of anthrax in all its forms (inhalation, cutaneous, and ingested).

BIOTERORRISM

Microorganisms and warfare go back more than two millennia. Scythian archers are known to have dipped their arrowheads in manure and rotting corpses to increase the deadliness of their weapons. In the fourteenth century Tartar forces, in what is now the Ukraine, threw plague-laden bodies over the walls of enemy cities. During the French and Indian War in North America during the eighteenth century, British troops under the command of Sir Jeffrey Amherst gave unfriendly native Americans blankets known to be contaminated with smallpox. In 1797, Napoleon tried to infect residents of a besieged city in Italy with malaria.

During World War I, a German agent grew anthrax and other bacteria in his Washington, DC home. The anthrax was used to infect some 3000 horses and mules destined for allied troops in Europe. Many of the animals died and hundreds of soldiers were infected.

In 1942, the British began testing "anthrax bombs" on Gruinard Island, a 500-acre island off the northwestern coast of Scotland. The Gruinard experiments established the environmental consequences of using anthrax as a weapon of mass destruction—a lesson Soviet scientists would discover for themselves decades later. Instead of the spores dying or being dissipated by the wind, they remained to the point that Gruinard became known as "Anthrax Island."

During World War II, the Japanese dropped fleas infected with plague (*Yersinia pestis*) on Chinese cities, killing hundreds and possibly thousands. Thousands of documents captured from the Japanese following the war further attest to the Japanese use of anthrax, typhoid, and plague on Manchurian towns and cities. This information proved to be a stimulus for the United States to seriously begin to study the area of germ warfare.

By the early 1950s the U.S. government had established its own germ warfare laboratory at an army base located at Fort Detrick, Maryland. Over time, the scientists identified approximately 50 different viruses and rickettsiae that were good candidates for germ warfare, a number that was nearly three times the number of suitable bacteria. Viruses were considered to be particularly ideal agents since they were basically unaffected by antibiotics and they could be selected to primarily debilitate, rather than kill, the victim. Incapacitation ties up more resources of the enemy and is more humane. President Eisenhower was briefed at a National Security Council meeting on February 18, 1960, to the effect that controlled incapacitation promised to "open up a new dimension of warfare."

Despite the allure of incapacitating viruses, the scientists at Fort Detrick continued their research on more virulent viral strains. Among them was an old nemesis—smallpox. Smallpox was an ancient foe, highly contagious, and killed approximately one-third of those infected. It has been estimated that smallpox has killed more people over the ages than any other infectious disease, including the plague. In the twentieth century alone, it has been estimated that smallpox was responsible for the death of half a billion people worldwide, exceeding all of the wars, epidemics, and pandemics combined. Smallpox has been considered an excellent choice for bioterrorism since it has a consistent, long incubation period that allows the operatives responsible for the attacks to leave the country prior to outbreak.

America's participation in germ warfare research took an abrupt turn when, on November 25, 1965, President Richard Nixon proclaimed that "the U.S. shall renounce the use of lethal biological agents and weapons, and all other methods of biological warfare. The U.S. will confine its biological research to defensive measures." In 1972, the United States, the Soviet Union, and more than 100 nations signed the Biological and Toxin Weapons Convention. This document prohibits the possession of deadly biological agents except for research into selective defensive measures. It was the world's first treaty banning an entire class of weapons. Unfortunately, the treaty was filled with loopholes and ambiguities ad nauseum, and, together with a lack of enforcement, therefore achieved virtually nothing.

At the same time that the 1972 treaty was being created, two scientists in Northern California began a collaboration that transformed the world of microbiology. Stanley Cohen and Herbert Boyer applied existing technology to the creation of recombinant life forms that provided the foundation for genetic engineering. The concept was deceptively straightforward; snip a gene from one organism and insert it into another. By using certain enzymes that break DNA at certain points, Cohen and Boyer's team was able to remove the gene for resistance to penicillin from a microbe, for example, splice the gene into plasmid DNA, and allow *E. coli* to take up the plasmid. The result was a new microbe resistant to penicillin. Subsequently, gene expression of other substances, such as insulin and human growth hormone, has created a novel area of drug production. Unfortunately, this technology can also be utilized to convert normally harmless bacteria, such as *E. coli*, to higher levels of pathogenicity, as well as highly pathogenic microbes, such as anthrax, to "superbugs."

Congressional investigations, and inventories, have shown that even after Nixon's ban on offensive germ warfare studies, the Central Intelligence Agency (CIA) had retained a small arsenal (at least 16 pathogens; usually in the milligram to gram range) stored at Fort Detrick. In comparison, the Soviet Union had not only continued to research germ warfare (e.g., the development of "Superplague," and the capacity to produce 300 tons of anthrax spores in 220 days) but had also flagrantly violated the treaty for 20 years. It had produced an industry that created disease by the ton. The Soviet Union's plan for World War III had included hundreds of tons of anthrax bacteria and scores of tons of smallpox and plague viruses. A comparison of germ warfare production between the United States and the Soviet Union during its maximum period of production is shown in Table 10.2.

Table 10.2 Comparison of dry agent production (metric tons per year) in the United States and the Soviet Union

	United States	Soviet Union
Staphylococcal enterotoxin B	1.8	0
Francisella tularensis (tularemia)	1.6	1500
Coxiella burnetii (Q fever)	1.1	0
Bacillus anthracis (anthrax)	0.9	4500
Venezuelan equine encephalitis virus	0.8	150
Botulinum	0.2	0
Yersinia pestis (bubonic plague)	0	1500
Variola virus (smallpox)	0	100
Actinobacillus mallei (glanders)	0	2000
Marburg virus	0	250

Source: J. Miller, S. Engelberg and W. Broad (2001) *Germs: Biological Weapons and America's Secret War.* New York: Simon & Schuster.

According to data collected by the Center for Nonproliferation Studies at the Monterey Institute of International Studies, there have been 285 incidents throughout the world during the past 25 years in which terrorists have used chemical or biological weapons. One of these attacks occurred in the United States almost 17 years to the day prior to the World Trade Center's catastrophe. On September 9, 1984, citizens who had dined in a restaurant in The Dalles, Oregon, began to complain of stomach cramps. Symptoms worsened over the next several days with hospitalization sometimes being necessary. Some customers threatened to sue the local owner for food poisoning. Over the next few days the local health department received complaints regarding two other restaurants.

On September 21, a second wave of reports occurred involving people who had fallen ill at 10 different restaurants in the small town. For the first time in the history of the community's only hospital, all 125 beds were filled. By the end of the outbreak, nearly 1000 people had reported symptoms. The offending agent was identified as *Salmonella typhimurium*. Extensive investigations of employees, water sources, septic-tank malfunctions, as well as suspect food items, did not produce an explanation. In addition, the deputy state epidemiologist proclaimed that there was no evidence to support deliberate contamination. It would take another year before an explanation occurred.

On September 16, 1985, the Bhagwan of the Rajneeshees cult ended a 4-year vow of silence by holding a press conference at his ranch/cult center. The Bhagwan leveled numerous charges at his recently departed personal secretary and the commune's de facto leader. Among the most revealing allegations was that his secretary was responsible for the poisoning. Federal and state police then formed a joint task force to investigate the situation. Analysis of "bactrol discs" revealed that the salmonella in the growth discs was identical to that which had sickened people in The Dalles the previous year. The smoking gun had been found.

The reason for the poisoning of patrons in local diners was related to politics. Since the cult and its followers had arrived in this sparsely populated Oregon area, they had begun to make attempts to take the town over. Numerous strategies had failed. Finally, it was decided that perhaps control of the town could be taken over at the ballot box. In theory, if enough of the locals came down with a sickness during an election, then perhaps the candidates supported by the cult could win. Such was not to be the case. Although little media attention was generated at the time, the incident is still significant since it represents the first large-scale use of bioterrorism on American soil. A comparison of deaths from selected causes is shown in Table 10.3 and can be used to put anthrax fatalities into perspective.

ANTICANCER DRUGS

Cancer involves the uncontrolled proliferation of cells, which can produce the growth of tumors or alter the formation of blood cells. Numerous factors can influence the development of neoplasia but the major causes appear to be environmental and genetic. While most environmental carcinogens appear to be mutagens, normal regulatory control of cell growth in the body can be perturbed by either (1) the expression of oncogenes or (2) the loss of tumor suppressor genes. In a human cell, there are

Table 10.3 Deaths from selected causes in the United States

Cause of death	Number
Smoking-related	23,077
Flu-related	3674
Auto accidents	2448
Alcohol-induced	1101
Murders	971
AIDS	847
Prescription drug errors	404

Sources: American Cancer Society, Institute of Medicine, National Transportation Safety Board, and National Center for Health Statistics.

Note
Deaths are for an average 3-week period not adjusted for seasonal fluctuations.

30–50,000 different genes that can become defective to produce cancer. In any event, the result is malignant transformation.

Therapeutic modalities in cancer treatment may involve surgery, radiation, and/or chemotherapy. The objectives of cancer chemotherapy include (1) cure, (2) reduction in tumor size, and (3) prolongation of life. At the present time, approximately 50 percent of patients with cancer can be cured, with drug treatment estimated to contribute in 17 percent of cases. Cancer chemotherapy can be curative in testicular cancer, diffuse large cell lymphoma, Hodgkin's disease, choriocarcinoma, certain childhood tumors (acute lymphoblastic leukemia, Burkitt's lymphoma, Wilms' tumor, and embryonal rhabdomyosarcoma). Certain cancers are more resistant to chemotherapy than others (e.g., lung and colon).

The objective of cancer chemotherapy is to kill all of the tumor stem cells. This is always a challenge for the attending oncologist. In certain cases of disseminated cancer there may be a total body cell burden of 10^{12} (1 trillion) cancerous cells. Even with a kill percentage of 99.9 percent, there will still be 10^9 cells remaining; the result of a "three log kill." Some of these remaining cells may be resistant or not be accessible to the drug. In comparison, a "three log kill" may be curative for bacterial infections since host resistance factors can eliminate residual disease, unlike the situation in treating cancer. Strategies to maximize the probability of obtaining total cell death with chemotherapy include the following:

• Combination therapy
• Drugs with differing toxicity profiles
• Drugs with differing mechanisms of action
• Drugs with synergistic actions
• Combine with surgical and radiation intervention.

Historically, anticancer drugs have been discovered through large-scale screening of synthetic chemicals and natural products against animal tumor systems. The drugs discovered in the first two decades of cancer chemotherapy (1950–1970) primarily

Table 10.4 Overview of major anticancer drugs

Alkylating agents	Cross-link two strands of DNA leading to impairment of DNA replication and RNA transcription (e.g., cyclophosphamide)
Antimetabolites	Folic acid (e.g., methotrexate), purine (e.g., 2-chlorodeoxyadenosine) and pyrimidine (e.g., 5-fluorouracil) analogs that interfere with synthesis of DNA precursors
Natural products/antibiotics	Anthracyclines (e.g., doxorubicin) damage DNA by intercalating DNA and inhibiting topoisomerase II
Antimitotics	Inhibit microtubule synthesis; inhibit cell division (e.g., paclitaxel)
Hormones	Glucocorticoids, estrogen antagonist (e.g., tamoxifen), and leuteinizing hormone-releasing hormone analogs (e.g., leuprolide)

Table 10.5 Common toxicities of cancer chemotherapeutics

Bone marrow	Suppression of bone marrow function can lead to significant reduction in white blood cells, platelets, anemia, and neutrophils; caused by almost all anticancer drugs.
Gastrointestinal tract	Nausea, vomiting, and diarrhea
Alopecia	Loss of hair (high mitotic index)
Renal damage	(e.g., 2'-Deoxycorformycin)
Pulmonary injury	Pulmonary fibrosis can be produced by bleomycin
Peripheral neuropathy	(e.g., vincristine, binding to tubulin)

Note

Long-term complications such as cardiomyopathy (e.g., doxorubicin), leukemia (i.e., mechlorethamine), and infertility (alkylating agents) can also occur. Amelioration of certain side effects can be achieved with the judicious use of antiemetics and blood transfusions (or erythropoietin).

interacted with DNA or its precursors, inhibiting the synthesis of new genetic material or causing irreparable damage to DNA itself. This strategy was based upon the quantitative difference between tumor cells and most normal cells, that is, a high mitotic index. In other words, because tumor cells divide at a higher rate, their genetic machinery is more prone to be affected by drugs that influence mitosis. Unfortunately, the same can be said for certain normal cells such as hair follicles, explaining why alopecia is a common side effect to drugs that interfere with nucleic acid synthesis. Table 10.4 shows the mechanism of action of major classes of anticancer drugs.

Because anticancer drugs do not affect qualitatively different sites within cancer cells, such as penicillin does in prokaryotic bacteria, they are more prone to produce side effects. As mentioned earlier, organs with active cell division are typically affected. Table 10.5 presents some common side effects of anticancer drugs. It should be noted that certain drugs are associated with certain side effects.

SELECTED BIBLIOGRAPHY

Albert, A. (1979) *Selective Toxicity*. London: Chapman & Hall.
Hardman, J. G., Limbird, L. L. and Gilman, A. G. (eds) (2001) *Goodman and Gilman's: The Pharmacological Basis of Therapeutics*, 10th ed. New York: McGraw-Hill.

Miller, J., Engelberg, S. and Broad, W. (2001) *Germs: Biological Weapons and America's Secret War*. New York: Simon & Schuster.

Moellering, R. C. (1985) *Principles of anti-infective therapy*. In *Mandell, Douglas, and Bennett's Principles and Practice of Infectious Diseases*, 2nd ed. (eds G. L. Mandell, R. G. Douglas, Jr, and J. E. Bennett). New York: John Wiley & Sons.

Pratt, W. B. and Fekety, F. R. (eds) (1986) *The Antimicrobial Drugs*. New York: Oxford University Press.

QUESTIONS

1 Credit for the actual discovery of microorganisms is given to which of the following scientists?
   a Paul Ehrlich
   b Robert Koch
   c Louis Pasteur
   d Alexander Fleming
   e Antonie van Leeuwenhoek.

2 Which of the following is credited with conceptualizing the "germ theory of disease"?
   a Paul Ehrlich
   b Robert Koch
   c Louis Pasteur
   d Alexander Fleming
   e Antonie van Leeuwenhoek.

3 Which of the following is credited with demonstrating the actual disease role of microorganisms?
   a Paul Ehrlich
   b Robert Koch
   c Louis Pasteur
   d Alexander Fleming
   e Antonie van Leeuwenhoek.

4 Which of the following drugs was first referred to as a "magic bullet"?
   a penicillin
   b arsphenamine
   c Cipro
   d sulfanilamide
   e ampicillin.

5 The mechanism of action of penicillin involves which of the following?
   a inhibition of DNA-dependent RNA polymerase
   b inhibition of DNA gyrase
   c inhibition of mRNA attachment to 30S ribosomes
   d inhibition of peptidoglycan formation in cell walls
   e inhibition of mRNA attachment to 50S ribosomes.

6 Microbial resistance to antibiotics can develop by which of the following mechanisms?
   a   uptake of plasmids
   b   inheritance
   c   mutation
   d   all of the above
   e   none of the above.

7 Which of the following is/are true regarding cancer chemotherapy versus microbe chemotherapy?
   a   the therapeutic index is generally lower
   b   the therapeutic index is generally higher
   c   a higher cell "kill rate" is required to effect a cure
   d   cures are virtually never really achieved
   e   a and c.

8 Which of the following is/are not used in cancer chemotherapy?
   a   drugs that cross-link DNA
   b   inhibitors of folic acid synthesis
   c   drugs that damage DNA
   d   drugs that inhibit microtubule synthesis
   e   none of the above.

9 Which of the following is/are true regarding side effects of anticancer drugs?
   a   primarily affect the central nervous system
   b   primarily affect rapidly dividing tissues
   c   are generally unpredictable
   d   gastrointestinal problems are common
   e   b and d.

10 Which of the following is/are most likely to be used to treat side effects from anticancer drugs?
   a   aspirin
   b   antiemetics
   c   emetics
   d   blood transfusion
   e   b and d.

Chapter 11

Drug treatment of symptoms: neuropharmacology and substance abuse

NEUROPHARMACOLOGY

Background

Neuropharmacology is the study and evaluation of the effects of drugs on the nervous system. As mentioned previously, humans have known that chemicals found in plants and animals can cause profound changes in the function of the nervous system and have used natural products such as opium, cannabis, belladonna, and alcohol for thousands of years. As people developed the capacity to extract, purify, and finally synthesize new chemical substances, the number of chemicals that can modify nervous system function has grown rapidly.

To manage the complex tasks involved in behavior, the central nervous system (CNS) employs large numbers of neurons and synapses. Underneath each square millimeter of cortex are some 100,000 neurons, each of which has approximately 6000 synapses. As the surface area of the human brain is of the order of 100,000 square millimeters, a single brain will contain 10 billion neurons interconnected by 60 trillion synapses. It is because of this complexity, and because of the inherent function of the nervous system, that ample sites for drug action exist. Although some drugs can provide physiological replacement, and others can actually cure a disease state, the majority of drugs are taken to relieve symptoms often relating to nervous system function/ dysfunction. Because of the significant role that neuropharmacological agents play in our lives, a significant amount of space is devoted to them in this chapter.

The methods by which the neuropharmacological effects of drugs can be studied are numerous. The surest, but the most dangerous, method is to study the effects directly in the human population. Obviously, this is normally only done under highly regulated circumstances, as discussed in Chapter 14. Unfortunately, however, there do occur periodic unregulated episodes within the general population that do provide significant neuropharmacological information. For example, such an event occurred during the 1980s in northern California with a substance known as 1-methyl-4-phenyl-1,2,3,5-tetrahydropyridine (MPTP).

MPTP is a chemical widely employed in various organic synthesis reactions. However, the general public is not normally exposed to it. Nevertheless, its potential for neurotoxicity was sensationalized after a number of young individuals began to appear in California clinics in 1982 with symptoms of advanced Parkinson's disease. These individuals exhibited the characteristic symptoms of Parkinson's disease, including an inability to walk, a mask-like facial expression, impairment of speech and skilled acts such as writing and eating, and in the most severe cases, a rigid immobility that was life-threatening. Because Parkinson's disease is usually a progressive disease that develops in older people, its sudden, full-blown development in young adults was immediately recognized as a highly unusual situation. Questioning soon revealed that the affected people had taken an illicit street "designer" drug that had properties similar to heroin. The drug, unfortunately, contained a small amount of MPTP as a contaminant introduced during its clandestine synthesis. The mechanism whereby MPTP produced its deleterious effect is described later in this chapter since it has contributed to our understanding of neurochemistry.

Animal testing is the traditional, more controlled means of discovering both desired neuropharmacological effects and undesired neurotoxicity. Fortunately, neurons and basic neuronal circuitry are very similar between mammalian species. Neurons from rats, cats, dogs, and humans share similar critical macromolecules with high conservation of structure and function through evolution. The enhanced intellectual capacity of humans results more from quantitative than from qualitative differences in the structure and function of neurons. It is the increase in size and complexity of the nervous system in humans that accounts for this, not the presence of a new type of neuron or other cellular element. For this reason, neuropharmacological responses in humans and animals are usually quite similar. Thus, animals can serve as valid models for most, though not all, neuropharmacological responses in humans.

As mentioned earlier, there are several reasons why the nervous system is frequently involved in response to drugs and chemical substances. Despite the existence of a blood–brain barrier, the morphological and biochemical complexity of the nervous system makes it a sensitive and selective target for drug attack. For example, the weight of the average adult human brain is approximately 2 percent of the whole body, yet the blood flow to the adult brain is about 20 percent of the cardiac output. The adult human brain relies almost entirely on the metabolism of glucose to meet its energy demands, and most (> 90 percent) of this carbohydrate is oxidized to carbon dioxide. Very little brain glucose (a few percent) is normally converted to lactate and released to the venous blood. The very high capacity of the brain to oxidize glucose suggests that this organ may be vulnerable to oxidative stress from drugs, toxins, and ischemia.

Another point of interest is that the brain expresses more of the total genetic information in its DNA than does any other organ, perhaps 10–20 times as much. Thus, in addition to the metabolic and maintenance machinery shared by most cell types, neurons contain many unique macromolecules, including enzymes, ion channels, neurotransmitters, and receptors that are not found in other cells. Drugs that target these sites produce selective changes in nervous system activities that are directly related to altered behavior. In some cases the effect is desired while in others this is obviously not the case.

With exposures to drugs severe enough to kill nerve cells or parts of cells, long-term, often permanent, deficits in sensory processes, motor function, behavior, learning capacity, and memory can occur. Since neurons do not reproduce, recovery of lost function occurs only if the remaining nervous system can "take over" the functions of the cells that were killed. Less severe exposures will modify function, often profoundly, until the drug is eliminated from the body. In most cases, normal behavior returns, and there may be no evidence of chronic consequences. With repeated exposures to some substances, however, the consequences may take on an irreversible quality.

A brief history of neuropharmacology

Man's earliest notions with regard to the nervous system were that nerves contained ethereal and nonquantifiable spirits. It was the Frenchman René Descartes, in the 1600s, who suggested that the spirits were, in fact, composed of minute physical entities. The key discoveries during the first half of the twentieth century include the demonstration that the vagus nerve liberates a chemical (i.e., acetylcholine) that controls heart rate (neurotransmission) and that nerve action potentials could be recorded and analyzed using the squid giant axon as a model.

In 1920, the Austrian scientist Otto Loewi discovered the first neurotransmitter. In his classic experiment (which came to him in a dream), he used two frog hearts. One heart (heart #1) was placed in a chamber that was filled with saline. This chamber was connected to a second chamber that contained heart #2. Fluid from chamber #1 was allowed to flow into chamber #2. Electrical stimulation of the vagus nerve (which was attached to heart #1) caused the heart rate of heart #1 to slow down. Loewi also observed that after a delay, heart #2 also slowed down. From this experiment Loewi hypothesized that electrical stimulation of the vagus nerve released a chemical into the fluid of chamber #1 that flowed into chamber #2. He called this chemical "Vagusstoff." We now know this chemical as the neurotransmitter acetylcholine. A diagram of Loewi's classic experiment is shown in Figure 11.1.

It was also during this period that Henry Dale assigned a variety of names to characterize different classes of pharmacological agents based upon their action on receptors. Thus, receptors at the postganglionic nerve endings of parasympathetic nerves (which were stimulated by muscarine, and acetylcholine, and blocked by atropine) were classified as "muscarinic." Those agents that blocked the responses of muscarine, thereby resembling atropine, were designated as antimuscarinic or atropine-like. In contrast to the muscarinic sites, the sites stimulated by small doses of nicotine (and acetylcholine) and blocked by large doses of nicotine were called "nicotinic." Otto Loewi and Sir Henry Dale shared the Nobel prize for medicine in 1936 for their discoveries regarding chemical transmission of nerve impulses.

In the 1950s and 1960s, a model was developed for the ionic basis of the "action potential," largely based on the work of Sir John Eccles in England. The model defined the voltage dependence and time course of activation for the sodium and potassium currents that underlie the sudden reversal of membrane potential (going from −70 mV resting to +30 mV). During this same time frame, the synapse was visualized by utilizing the electron microscope, and calcium ions were demonstrated to be essential for neurotransmitter release at the neuromuscular junction.

During the 1970s, electron micrographs of active zones from freeze-fractured neuromuscular junctions confirmed earlier electrophysiological evidence that vesicles fuse to the presynaptic membrane to release neurotransmitter into the synaptic cleft. In addition, acetylcholine-generated electrophysiological "noise" was correlated with opening and closing of acetylcholine-activated ion channels and successful recordings were made from single acetylcholine receptor–channel complexes.

These collective data led to a general view of neurotransmission. The transmission of messages from one nerve cell to another takes place in several steps. Packages of a neurotransmitter held in special vesicles are moved up to an active zone in the sending—or presynaptic—cell and dock at their release sites. Then, when an electrical signal arrives at the synapse, some of the vesicles fuse to the membrane, burst,

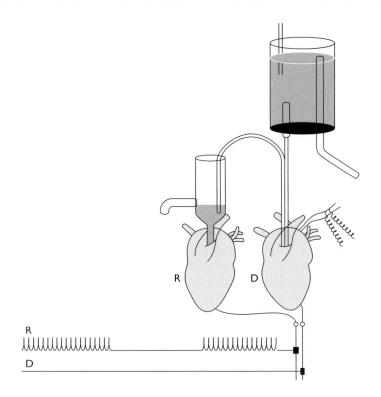

Figure 11.1 Loewi's demonstration of the chemical nature of neurotransmission. Heart D (donor) represents heart #1 while heart R (recipient) represents heart #2. Tracings R and D represent the respective heart beats of the two hearts. When fluid from the stimulated donor heart was allowed to interact with the recipient heart (middle of tracing R), heart rate was obviously abbreviated.

and release their neurotransmitter. The chemical messenger diffuses across the gap to the receiving cell, attaches to receptors on the postsynaptic neuron, and, depending on the nature of the neurotransmitter, stimulates or inhibits electrical activity in this second neuron. Changes in synaptic strength are largely attributed to changes in the probability of any vesicle fusing and releasing its contents.

During the 1980s and 1990s, sequencing of individual subunits of receptor proteins (e.g., nicotinic) was achieved, as well as their cloning. Researchers have identified more than 20 classes of proteins that function in synaptic-vesicle fusion and recycling at the presynaptic membrane.

ANATOMY OF THE NERVOUS SYSTEM

During the course of evolution an efficient system has evolved that enables the functions of individual organs to be orchestrated in increasingly complex life forms and permits rapid adaptation to alterations in a changing environment. This regulatory system is composed of a number of major anatomical divisions. These include the

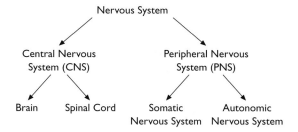

Figure 11.2 Subdivisions of the nervous system.

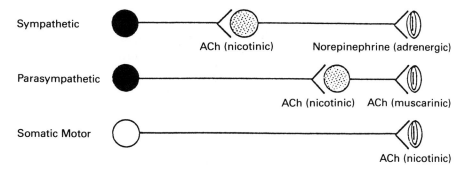

Figure 11.3 Diagram of autonomic and somatic motor neurons. Presynaptic neurons are depicted with solid cell bodies. Postsynaptic neurons are speckled. The neurotransmitter released by the presynaptic neuron and the type of receptor it activates are listed below each synapse.

CNS—brain and spinal cord—and two separate pathways within the peripheral nervous system (PNS) for two-way communication with the peripheral organs. The PNS subdivisions are the somatic and autonomic nervous systems (Figure 11.2). The latter is further divided into sympathetic and parasympathetic divisions (Figure 11.3).

The somatic nervous system is composed of sensory afferents and motor efferents and serves to perceive external states and to modulate appropriate body responses. The autonomic nervous system (ANS), together with the endocrine system, controls the milieu interieur. It adjusts internal organ functions to the changing needs of the organism. The ANS operates largely autonomously, beyond voluntary control, at the subconscious level. Its central components reside in the hypothalamus, brain stem, and spinal cord. The ANS has sympathetic and parasympathetic branches. Both are made up of afferent, mainly in the vagus nerve, and efferent fibers.

The sympathetic and parasympathetic branches usually work in opposition to each other. In simplistic terms, activation of the sympathetic division can be considered a means by which the body achieves a state of maximal work capacity as required in "fight or flight" situations. For example, blood flow to skeletal muscle is increased (for running or fighting) and cardiac rate and contractility are enhanced (to provide more oxygen for muscle exertion). Parasympathetic nerves regulate processes connected with energy assimilation (food intake, digestion, and absorption) and storage. These processes become quiescent when the sympathetic system becomes activated, and operate when the body is at rest, allowing decreased respiration and cardiac activity and enhanced peristaltic activity.

The various components of the nervous system can be further differentiated into three basic cellular elements: (1) neurons, (2) interstitial cells, and (3) connective tissue, blood vessels, and microglia. The neuron is the only cell type in the nervous system involved in information processing. Each neuron is, in its own right, a receiver, an integrator, and a transmitter of information. Neurons are always in contact with other neurons so that they create simple or complex channels through which many different responses can be transmitted. All behavior, no matter how complex, results from the interactive function of the billions of neurons.

Neurons

Neurons vary tremendously in form and size, but they all share the ability to respond to stimuli and to create new stimuli to affect other cells. Regardless of their structural diversity, all neurons are bounded by a plasma membrane and possess a cell body (soma), one or more axons, and, with very few exceptions, dendrites (Figure 11.4).

The bounding membrane of the neuron is typical of all cells. It is a continuous lipid bilayer sheet of thickness about 60–80 angstroms. Embedded in it, or passing through it, are numerous proteins and glycoproteins, many of which are found only in nerve cells. These have many functions. Some provide structural support to the membrane, but most form ion channels and receptor sites that are essential to nerve function.

The membrane of the neuron is differentially specialized. The membrane of the soma and dendrites is designed to react to chemical stimuli and contains both neurotransmitter-gated ion channels and neurotransmitter-gated receptors associated

Figure 11.4 Structural components of nerve cells.

Source: T. M. Brody, J. Larner, K. P. Minneman and H. C. Neu (eds) (1994), *Human Pharmacology: Molecular to Clinical*, 2nd ed. St Louis, MO: Mosby. Reprinted with permission.

with various G proteins. The former evoke rapid changes in the cell's membrane potential, while the latter initiate slower, more persisting changes in neuronal excitability via the second messengers cyclic adenosine monophosphate (cAMP) and inositol triphosphate (IP$_3$).

The axon is specialized to react to changes in membrane potential. When the cell's membrane potential reaches a certain "threshold" the axon responds with an action potential that rapidly transmits an electrical signal from the cell body to its terminals. Finally, the nerve terminal is specialized to convert the electrical signal of the action potential back into a chemical signal. It responds to depolarization by releasing a neurotransmitter that acts either upon the soma or dendritic membranes of the next neuron or, in the PNS, on an effector site (Figure 11.5). The specialized membrane is essential to the electrochemical properties of neurons.

The cell body contains many structures of importance. The nucleus is usually located in the center of the cell body. It contains widely dispersed, fine chromatin material. The chromatin is composed of deoxyribonucleic acid (DNA) and its associated histone proteins. The nucleolus contains the specific portion of DNA encoding the ribonucleic acid (RNA) of future ribosomes.

In the neuroplasm of the neuron are located mitochondria, Nissl substance, and the Golgi apparatus. Mitochondria contain their own DNA and function as the major oxidative organelles, providing energy through the production of adenosine triphosphate (ATP). The Nissl substance, which is absent from the axon, represents the nodal points of the endoplasmic reticulum that exists throughout the soma. The endoplasmic reticulum is the major protein-synthesizing organelle and manufactures in 1–3 days an

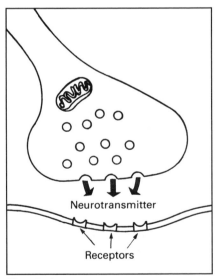

Chemical synapse

Figure 11.5 Simplified representation of the relationship between a nerve terminal and its effector site.

Source: T. M. Brody, J. Larner, K. P. Minneman and H. C. Neu (eds) (1994), *Human Pharmacology: Molecular to Clinical*, 2nd ed. St Louis, MO: Mosby. Reprinted with permission.

amount of protein equal to the total protein content of the cell. The Golgi apparatus is primarily responsible for synthesis of the membrane and the incorporation of membrane-bound proteins into it. It pinches off the membrane with its associated proteins as "vesicles." Some of these vesicles contain protein needed to maintain the neurolemma, while others become secretory vesicles destined to contain neurotransmitter.

The dendrites represent all the processes of the cell body except for the specialized axonal process (axon). They are usually numerous and serve to increase the surface area of the neuron available for receiving synaptic input. Neurons will have one or more main dendrites that successively branch and arborize to form many smaller processes.

The axon of the typical neuron arises from a cone-shaped region of the cell body, the axon hillock. The initial segment of the axon is both the smallest region in diameter and the region with the lowest threshold to electrical activation. Distal to the initial segment the axonal diameter enlarges and the diameter remains constant out to the terminal ending or until the axon branches. Myelinated neurons have their axons ensheathed by myelin segments, each segment provided by an oligodendrocyte or a neurolemma cell. Between segments the axonal membrane is exposed. These regions are termed the "nodes of Ranvier." Unmyelinated axons do not possess such a segmented sheath. Rather, they tend to collect in bundles that are loosely enclosed in troughs formed by neurolemmal cells or oligodendrocytes. The terminal end of an axon most often is profusely branching, each branch ultimately terminating in a synaptic ending.

Transport mechanisms are available within the neuron that allow the passage of substances from the soma to axon terminal and vice versa. Most of the vesicles formed by the Golgi apparatus are transported through the axon to the nerve terminal by fast anterograde transport. Within the terminal the secretory vesicles recycle many times, binding and fusing with the terminal membrane, then being "pinched off" via endocytosis and returned to the vesicle pool. The terminal membrane is continually being replaced by newly arriving vesicles. Old membrane and proteins are returned to the cell body for degradation by way of a fast retrograde transport system.

Fast anterograde transport can reach rates as high as 400 mm/day. It is dependent upon microtubules that provide a track along which the vesicles move. The movement is energy dependent and is mediated by a specific "motor" protein, kinesin. A similar process is responsible for fast retrograde transport. A second motor protein, dynein, is needed for movement in that direction. A third type of transport process is termed slow axoplasmic transport. It ranges from 0.2 to 5 mm/day and is responsible for the transport of cytoskeletal proteins, the neurofilaments, and microtubules, as well as an assortment of cytoplasmic proteins.

Glial cells

There are three types of glial cells in the CNS: astroglia (astrocytes), oligodendroglia (oligodendrocytes), and microglia. There are corresponding neurolemma cells (Schwann cells) in the PNS. Glial cells in the CNS perform a wide variety of "support" functions; while these cells are absolutely integral to neuronal function, they do play more of a support and modulatory than an information transmission role. For example, astrocytes are known to function in the removal of degenerative debris as well as in maintaining ion homeostasis and in metabolism of putative and acknowledged neurotransmitters. In response to virtually any form of neural insult, astrocytes become hypertrophic, displaying a response that includes enlargement of the cell body and increases in both the number and length of astrocytic processes. These are the cells, in fact, that form glial scars after brain or spinal cord injury. Astrocytes also contribute importantly to the blood–brain barrier by forming an additional layer of cells around brain capillary endothelial cells.

Oligodendroglia provide the insulating myelin sheath for many CNS axons and are responsible for maintaining this sheath, as well as for control of the local ionic environment of the axon. In addition, oligodendroglia provide a loose covering through which unmyelinated fibers course. The functions of microglia are not well understood but are believed to be of mesodermal origin and related to macrophage/monocyte lineage. Some microglia are resident within the brain, while additional cells of this class may be attracted to the brain during periods of inflammation following either microbial infection or other postinjury inflammatory reactions. They are phagocytic and remove debris throughout the CNS.

In addition to neurons and glial cells, the nervous system contains blood vessels, fibroblasts, and other connective tissue elements. In the PNS, processes from Schwann cells that form the multilayered myelin sheaths characteristic of peripheral myelinated nerves surround most neuronal elements.

Morphological considerations

Neurons assume a vast array of forms in accordance with the functions they serve. In most neurons the cell body and dendrites are separated from the axonal terminal by a very long tube, the axon. This creates problems unique to nerve cells. In the motor neurons that innervate hands and feet, for example, more than 90 percent of the mass of the neuron is in the cell processes. An often given example of this relationship is that if the cell body of a motor neuron were enlarged to the size of a baseball, the corresponding axon would be about 1 mile long, and the dendrites and their branches would arborize throughout a large amphitheater.

The neuron is put at a metabolic disadvantage because of this relatively large size. The cell body is the only part of the neuron that can synthesize proteins, but it may make up less than 5 percent of the total cell mass. Because of this, very high rates of protein synthesis are required. As all proteins are synthesized in the cell body, most have to be transported long distances to their eventual target. For proteins destined for the distal portions of the axon and for the axon terminal, the specialized transport systems mentioned earlier must function continuously to get them to their targets in a reasonable length of time. These systems require a large, complex cytoskeleton to maintain them. Anything that compromises protein synthesis, axonal transport, or cytoskeletal integrity may reduce new functional and structural protein arrival to a point where structure and function of the neuron have been damaged. Neurotoxicity associated with the anticancer drug vincristine, for example, may be related to such a site of action since this alkaloid is known to damage microtubules.

Nutritional and biochemical aspects

As mentioned previously, the CNS is protected from certain drug effects by the blood–brain barrier. This barrier is primarily created by (1) the tight junctions that occur in brain capillaries between neighboring endothelial cells and (2) the supporting glial cells. Nonpolar, lipid-soluble compounds can penetrate the barrier readily by passing directly through the endothelial cells. However, highly polar, non-lipid-soluble compounds do not penetrate well, if at all. Active transport mechanisms to maintain the blood–brain barrier require significant energy expenditure. Erosion of the blood–brain barrier is of special concern because increased permeability permits the entry into the brain of blood-borne toxic or infectious agents.

Because the blood–brain barrier is less well developed in immature brains, children are more susceptible to CNS toxicity from certain toxic substances, such as lead salts, than are adults. The patency of the blood–brain barrier may also become increased under conditions of disease and dehydration. Although the CNS is generally well protected from certain drugs by the blood–brain barrier, the PNS does not have a comparable structure. Therefore, it is possible to have drug effects restricted to peripheral structures only, if their entry into the CNS is excluded.

The metabolic requirements of neurons often make them more susceptible than other types of cells to drug actions. Neurons are highly active metabolically in order to support their unusual demands, and are very sensitive to drug actions that interfere with normal nutrient utilization. The high metabolic activity results in part from the high rates of protein synthesis needed to maintain the specialized nerve cell and from the fact that a neuron constantly generates action potentials as part of its information-processing function. Each action potential, in turn, erodes the ionic gradients existing across the nerve cell membrane. Large amounts of energy are expended by the nerve cell in restoring and maintaining these gradients, which are critical to normal function. This requires the continuous formation of large amounts of ATP, which requires aerobic metabolism.

It should also be remembered that even neurons "at rest" are highly electrically charged by virtue of uneven distributions of ions across the cellular membrane. Ionic pumps and carriers are continually maintaining the ionic gradients with the expenditure of energy. Therefore, given an adequate supply of energy, the concentrations of Na^+, K^+, Cl^-, Ca^{2+}, HCO^-, and H^+ ions are maintained inside the cells at levels to support the metabolic processes of the cell. It follows that even at rest the nerve cells are in a state of dynamic homeostasis, which is essential for life. The homeostasis is self-adjusting; that is, enzymes that produce energy and pump the ions require an appropriate ionic milieu to function. A brief disruption of this steady-state situation can be tolerated by nerve cells because of an elaborate system of "buffers" that can temporarily compensate for disruption, such as change in concentration of an ion, but in the long term there is a limit beyond which the homeostasis cannot be perturbed without fatal results.

As mentioned earlier, neurons are almost entirely dependent upon glucose as an energy supply. The neuron has little capacity for anaerobic metabolism, and is therefore highly susceptible to a lack of oxygen or glucose. The oxygen consumption of neurons is nearly 10 times higher than adjacent glial cells, and therefore neurons are more often damaged by anoxic or hypoglycemic conditions. Certain large neurons, such as pyramidal cells in the cerebral cortex, cerebellum, and hippocampus or motor neurons in the spinal cord, have a particularly high metabolic rate. Damage is often seen first at these sites when oxygen or glucose levels are not sufficiently maintained.

Neuronal damage can start within minutes and becomes irreversible within 5–6 minutes after oxygen or glucose delivery is stopped.

Role of myelin

Schwann cells differentiate to form the protective myelin sheath that surrounds the nerve axon and promotes long-distance propagation of the action potential in the autonomic nervous system. The myelin sheath is a greatly extended and modified plasma membrane that is wrapped around the nerve axon in a spiral fashion. Each myelin-generating cell furnishes myelin for only one segment of any given axon. The axon and its myelin sheath are important to each other metabolically as well as functionally. Axons direct the formation of myelin and can provide a mitogenic stimulus for Schwann cell or oligodendrocyte cell proliferation. The myelin-forming cells can influence axonal diameter and play a role in determining the composition of the axonal membrane.

Although in nonmyelinated fibers sodium and potassium channels are distributed uniformly across the axonal membrane, in myelinated fibers sodium channels are concentrated at the nodes of Ranvier and potassium channels in the internodal regions. This greatly improves the efficiency of action potential propagation. A nerve signal can travel from your spinal cord to the tip of your toe in less than 25 ms. Such rapid nerve transmission is only possible because the axons have very good insulation. Layers of glial cells (astrocytes) wrap axons much like gauze wrapped around an injured finger, forming an insulating myelin sheath.

As an example of the advantages imparted by myelin, we can compare two different nerve fibers, one myelinated and the other nonmyelinated, that both conduct action potentials at 25 m/s. In the case of a nonmyelinated axon (e.g., squid giant axon) a diameter of 500 μm is required, while a corresponding myelinated human axon would only be 12 μm in diameter. The nonmyelinated axon requires 5000 times as much energy to conduct an action potential, and occupies approximately 1500 times as much space. If the human spinal cord contained only nonmyelinated axons, it would need to be as large as a good-sized tree trunk to conduct action potentials at the same speed as it does at present.

When myelin is lost, axonal function is rapidly affected. Conduction velocity slows in proportion to the degree of demyelination and, in extreme situations, conduction can be blocked. Loss of the myelin may also lead to loss of the axon. Axons can generally survive some demyelination, but extensive loss of myelin can result in axonal degeneration. Because myelin-forming cells can proliferate, they generally reestablish a myelin sheath around an axon once the demyelinating stimulus is removed.

The synapse

The synapse is a critical structure in the nervous system and serves as the communication link between neurons (Figure 11.5). Synapses in the mammalian CNS are chemical in nature. They possess three components: (1) a presynaptic element, (2) a postsynaptic element, and (3) a synaptic cleft. At a typical synapse, neurotransmission requires four steps: (1) synthesis and storage of neurotransmitter, (2) transmitter release, (3) receptor activation, and (4) transmitter inactivation.

Most neurotransmitters are synthesized within the presynaptic terminal by enzymes made in the cell body and transported to the ending by axoplasmic transport. They are subsequently stored in vesicles in the terminal. These vesicles, as well as the presynaptic terminal membrane, contain specific proteins that play essential roles in the docking and fusing of vesicles to the membrane during the process of neurotransmitter release. The release of neurotransmitter is triggered by a sequence of events that begins with the propagation of an action potential that ultimately arrives at the terminal region.

The depolarization that accompanies the action potential induces an increase in membrane permeability to calcium ions. A large inward electrochemical gradient exists for calcium and it moves into the terminal. The calcium that enters the terminal activates enzymes that cause the attachment of some of the vesicles to releasing sites on the terminal membrane, membrane fusion, and the release of the vesicular contents into the synaptic cleft. Transmitter release is terminated by the removal of calcium from the terminal cytoplasm, either via a calcium pump, which pumps it out of the cell, or by uptake into the endoplasmic reticulum or into mitochondria.

Once the neurotransmitter is released from the presynaptic terminal it diffuses across the synaptic cleft. On the postsynaptic side it complexes with a membrane-bound macromolecule, its receptor. In synapses that have to generate action potentials within microseconds of neurotransmitter release, the receptors must be clustered in the postsynaptic membrane at high density, close to where the neurotransmitter is released. Such a synapse exists at the neuromuscular junction, where acetylcholine is the neurotransmitter. Acetylcholine is released from the presynaptic nerve terminal within 50 nm of the postsynaptic muscle membrane that contains densely arrayed acetylcholine receptors ($\sim$ 10,000 acetylcholine receptors/μm^2). There is a steady turnover of receptors, with newly synthesized receptors replacing those that are periodically degraded or not being utilized.

Binding leads to one of two consequences. If the receptor is coupled to an ion channel, the channel is opened, ions move down electrochemical gradients, and the membrane potential is changed. If the receptor is linked to a G protein, the binding initiates a sequence of biochemical events that result in the production of a second messenger such as cAMP or IP_3. These evoke long-term changes that alter excitability of the postsynaptic cell. The complexation process is usually rapidly reversible with an occupancy half-life of 1–20 ms.

Action of the neurotransmitter is terminated by several means. For many neurotransmitters, the bulk is recycled back into the presynaptic terminal via an active uptake process to be reused. Alternatively, some of the neurotransmitter may simply diffuse away and be enzymatically destroyed elsewhere. In other cases enzymes may be located on the postsynaptic side of the cleft, in the vicinity of the receptor, which serves to rapidly break the transmitter down into inactive metabolites.

Clearly, there are many components involved in the process of neurotransmission. These can be the targets of useful drugs as well as neurotoxicants. Examples include the local anesthetics, which target sodium channels in nerve axons, neuromuscular blocking drugs, which target the nicotinic receptor at the motor end-plates, and some tranquilizers, such as diazepam, which target the GABA receptor on neurons in the CNS (see later discussion).

Table 11.1 Representative receptors and their actions

Receptor type	Location, effect, and mechanism of action
Cholinergic	
Muscarinic	Postsynaptic and presynaptic, variable effects, some increase IP_3, others inhibit adenylate cyclase
Nicotinic	Postsynaptic, excitatory, opens an Na^+,K^+-selective ion channel
Adrenergic	
Alpha$_1$	Postsynaptic, excitatory, linked to formation of IP_3
Alpha$_2$	Presynaptic, reduce transmitter release, reduce calcium entry
	Postsynaptic, depressive, ?
Beta$_1$	Postsynaptic, excitatory, activates adenylate cyclase
Beta$_2$	Postsynaptic, depressive, activates adenylate cyclase
Dopaminergic	
D$_1$ family (D$_1$, D$_5$)	Postsynaptic, variable effects, stimulates adenylate cyclase
D$_2$ family (D$_2$, D$_3$, and D$_4$)	Postsynaptic and presynaptic, variable effects, inhibits adenylate cyclase
GABAergic	
GABA$_A$	Postsynaptic, inhibitory, opens a Cl^--selective ion channel
GABA$_B$	Presynaptic, inhibitory, reduces calcium entry
	Postsynaptic, inhibitory, increases K^+ conductance
Glycinergic	Postsynaptic, inhibitory, opens a Cl^--selective ion channel
Glutamatergic	
AMPA	Postsynaptic, excitatory, opens an Na^+,K^+-selective ion channel
Kainate	Postsynaptic, excitatory, opens an Na^+,K^+-selective ion channel
NMDA	Postsynaptic, excitatory, opens an Na^+,K^+,Ca^{2+}-selective ion channel

SPECIFIC NEUROTRANSMITTER SYSTEMS

Certain neurotransmitter systems are more frequently involved in neuropharmacological and toxicological responses than others. We have briefly discussed the importance of the dopaminergic system previously with regard to Parkinson's disease. Additional systems for drug targeting include the cholinergic, adrenergic, glutamatergic, GABAergic, and glycinergic neurotransmitter systems (Table 11.1). To understand their significance, a more comprehensive description of their function is now given.

Acetylcholine

Acetylcholine was the first identified neurotransmitter. It is the neurotransmitter released by the motor neurons that innervate skeletal muscle, all preganglionic and many postganglionic autonomic neurons in the PNS, which innervate smooth muscle, cardiac muscle, and glands, and many neurons within the CNS. Extensive loss of cholinergic neurons in the CNS has been found in patients with Alzheimer's disease. The structure of acetylcholine is shown in Figure 11.6.

$$
\overset{+}{(CH_2)_2}NCH_2CH_2O\overset{O}{\overset{\|}{C}}CH_2
$$

Figure 11.6 Structure of acetylcholine.

Two distinct receptor groups have been identified for acetylcholine, the nicotinic and the muscarinic groups (Table 11.1). Furthermore, there are at least four subtypes of nicotinic and five subtypes of muscarinic receptors. Nicotinic receptors are ubiquitous and exist at the neuromuscular junctions of skeletal muscles and on ganglion cells in the autonomic nervous system. Nicotinic receptors located on cation-specific ion channels, when opened, evoke fast, transient depolarizations of the recipient cell. Muscarinic receptors are found in smooth muscle receiving parasympathetic innervation and elsewhere, and can be blocked by atropine. Muscarinic receptors are coupled indirectly to slow and fast ion channels via G proteins.

Acetylcholine is synthesized from acetyl coenzyme A (acetyl-CoA) and choline within the presynaptic terminal by the enzyme choline acetylase. The acetylcholine formed is stored in small, lightly staining synaptic vesicles that are concentrated around the synaptic contact area. The release of acetylcholine is calcium dependent. The entire content of a synaptic vesicle is released into the cleft in an all-or-none manner, where it interacts with its receptors and then is rapidly destroyed by acetylcholinesterase. Under normal circumstances, the half-life for acetylcholine in the synaptic cleft is about 1 ms. The acetylcholine is hydrolyzed to choline and acetate, and the choline is actively pumped back into the presynaptic terminal to be used to synthesize more acetylcholine.

Glutamate

Glutamate is the primary excitatory neurotransmitter in the brain. Glutamate is formed by the Krebs cycle and is found free and stored in vesicles in synaptic terminals. Its release is calcium dependent, and an uptake system exists in presynaptic terminals and in glia to terminate its action after release. It is possible that glia metabolize glutamate to glutamine and return it to the neuron for reuse. An excessive release of glutamate can be lethal to cells in the immediate vicinity.

Three subtypes of glutamate receptors are known (Table 11.1). Two of these, the AMPA and kainate receptors, are part of a cation-selective ion channel that is permeable to sodium and potassium. These channels are responsible for the fast, transient excitatory postsynaptic potentials (EPSPs) evoked by glutamate release. The third, the *N*-methyl-D-aspartate (NMDA) receptor, is part of a cation channel permeable to sodium, potassium, and calcium. Activation of this channel leads to calcium entry into the cell, which can act as a second messenger in its own right to modulate cellular processes. This receptor is critical to the development of neuronal plasticity in experimental model systems and is thought to be essential to higher processes of the brain, including memory and learning.

Inhibitory modulation of neurotransmission in the CNS is carried out by two substances, gamma-aminobutyric acid (GABA) and glycine. They are differentially distributed, GABA being found primarily in the brain and glycine primarily in the spinal cord.

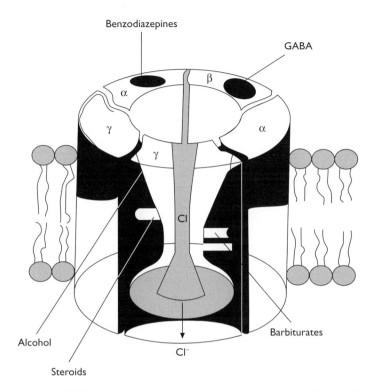

Figure 11.7 Schematic three-dimensional representation of the GABA$_A$ receptor complex with the recognition sites for GABA, benzodiazepines, alcohol, steroids, and barbiturates.

Source: G. Zernig, A. Saria, M. Kurtz and S. S. O'Malley (eds) (2000), *Handbook of Alcoholism.* Boca Raton, FL: CRC Press. Reprinted with permission.

GABA

GABA is formed from glutamate, which is derived from the Krebs cycle, by the enzyme glutamic acid dehydrogenase. In GABAergic neurons about 10 percent of glutamate is converted to GABA rather than being processed further by the Krebs cycle enzymes. Synthesis occurs in the terminal cytoplasm, and GABA is found free and bound in vesicles. Once released, GABA is taken up into the presynaptic terminal via a high-affinity, sodium-dependent transport system. It is also rapidly taken up by a similar process into glia, where it is metabolized.

Two major subtypes of GABA receptors are known: GABA$_A$ and GABA$_B$. The GABA$_A$ receptor is part of a chloride channel. It mediates postsynaptic inhibition and gives rise to fast transient inhibitory postsynaptic potentials (IPSPs). GABA$_B$ receptors are found both pre- and postsynaptically. Presynaptically they act via a G protein to reduce calcium entry. Postsynaptically they act via a G protein to increase potassium conductance. In either case they mediate inhibition. A representation of the GABA$_A$ receptor is shown in Figure 11.7.

Glycine

Glycine is an important inhibitory transmitter in the spinal cord. The postsynaptic receptor for glycine is very similar to the $GABA_A$ receptor and forms part of a chloride channel complex. When it is activated by glycine, the channel opens transiently to produce IPSPs in spinal neurons. Both gaseous anesthetics and alcohol are believed to activate glycine receptors. Strychnine reversibly antagonizes the effects of glycine on spinal neurons, and this is thought to be responsible for its convulsant properties.

MECHANISM OF ACTION OF SELECTED NEUROPHARMACOLOGICAL AGENTS

As mentioned previously, there are many potential targets available in nerve cells for interaction with a drug. Some targets are general to all nerve cells, and drugs that affect them will produce widely dispersed effects. Other targets are found only in a subset of nerve cells, and in these cases drug effects will be restricted to them. The most common reason specific interactions occur is that neurons differ in the transmitter system they possess.

In the first part of this chapter, the unfortunate experience of young adults with MPTP was discussed briefly. It might be instructive at this point to complete the story. As soon as it was recognized that MPTP was the neurotoxicant, a number of laboratories began to investigate its mechanism of action. It was eventually demonstrated that MPTP readily diffused into neurons and glial cells and that it served as a substrate for the "B" isozyme of monoamine oxidase (MAO) found predominantly in astrocytes. In the glial cell, the MPTP was oxidized to the primary neurotoxicant, the pyridium ion, MPP^+. Because of its structural similarity to dopamine, the MPP^+ was selectively taken up by dopaminergic neurons of the substantia nigra via the dopamine uptake system. Within these dopaminergic cells, the MPP^+ acted as a general cellular poison, ultimately blocking oxidative phosphorylation and killing the neuron (Figure 11.8).

A chilling follow-up to this acute development of Parkinson's disease/syndrome was subsequently found. Some of the individuals who had taken small amounts

Figure 11.8 Conversion of MTPT to MPP^+.

of the illicit street drug, and therefore small amounts of MPTP, did not develop Parkinsonism within the short term following its ingestion. It was observed subsequently, however, that some of these individuals began to show delayed, early signs of the disease years after the drug's ingestion. The basis for this delayed effect is not known with certainty, but it is likely that the initial exposure killed too few dopaminergic cells to result immediately in Parkinson's disease. However, the progression of the disease via natural degeneration of the dopaminergic cells may have been accelerated by MPTP exposure. In excess of 200 people who used MPTP one or more times, under the impression that it was a synthetic heroin, were subsequently identified.

We now know that the appearance of MPTP in the northern California drug market was part of the advent of "designer drugs." The term was coined to reflect the increasing sophistication of street-drug suppliers, who were beginning to tailor their products to individual preferences regarding the nature and duration of the drug effect. By slightly changing the molecular structure of a drug, its potency, length of action, euphoric effects, and toxicity can be modified.

Designer drugs

A designer drug is an analog, a chemical compound that is similar in structure and effect to another drug of abuse but differs slightly in structure. Designer drugs are produced in clandestine laboratories to mimic the psychoactive effects of controlled drugs. The most commonly known types of synthetic analog drugs available through the illicit drug market include analogs of fentanyl and meperidine (both synthetic opioids) phencyclidine, and amphetamine and methamphetamine (which have hallucinogenic and stimulant properties).

Designer drugs came into vogue to circumvent the Controlled Substances Act of 1970. Many designer drugs when introduced in the 1970s in the United States were initially legal, but the Federal Drug Enforcement Administration quickly invoked its emergency authority to place an immediate ban on them by declaring them federally scheduled drugs under the Comprehensive Crime Control Act of 1984. Subsequent federal legislation (1986) has prohibited the illicit manufacture of all forms of designer drugs.

The first designer drug that rapidly became part of the drug scene was methylenedioxymethamphetamine (MDMA), known by the street names of "Ecstacy," "Adam," and "Essence." MDMA is synthesized from molecular components of methamphetamine or from safrole. Users describe its effect as similar to hallucinogens produced by other psychedelics (e.g., mescaline), but its subdued effects leave them feeling "more emphatic, more insightful, and more aware." The ease with which drugs can be modified is illustrated by the identification of at least 35 variants or analogs that have been synthesized from phencyclidine (PCP, "Angel dust"); several dozen analogs of methamphetamine have also been produced. Such drugs proved to be exceptionally potent and presented significant health hazards.

This situation became particularly acute with respect to the development of illicit analogs of fentanyl to derive heroin substitutes. Fentanyl is a synthetic opioid, a μ-receptor agonist, and is about 100–200 times more potent than morphine as an analgesic. As with other narcotic analgesics, respiratory depression is the most significant acute toxic effect of the fentanyl derivatives. Fentanyl analogs can be 80–1000 times more potent than heroin in causing respiratory depression. Fentanyl analogs are responsible for more than 150 of the overdose deaths in the United States.

One of the relatively new designer drugs was identified in 1994, when U.S. Drug Enforcement Agents reported that a very potent drug, methacathinone ("cat"), was introduced to the streets as a cocaine-like drug whose effects could last up to 5–7 days. At least three deaths have been associated with the drug.

Alcohol

Ethyl alcohol is one of the most widely consumed drugs in the world. It is a good example of a drug that is a general CNS depressant. Ingestion of even small amounts diminishes performance, particularly performance dependent on training and previous experience. Mood is affected and can range from euphoria to deep depression. Memory, concentration, insight, and motor function are impaired in a dose-dependent fashion. With large ingestions, a state similar to general anesthesia develops. The doses that produce death are not much higher than those inducing anesthesia.

For many years it was thought that alcohol and other lipophilic solvents exerted their depressant effects on the CNS by virtue of "nonspecific" membrane-fluidizing properties causing neuronal swelling. This swelling was believed to be responsible for perturbing the functions of key macromolecules embedded in the membrane, including the ion channels and various receptors. However, the discovery that alcohol acts on receptor-gated ion channels ($GABA_A$, NMDA, and $5HT_3$) in a saturable and specific manner has now led to the belief that the behavioral and neurochemical properties of alcohol are the consequence of a number of specific receptor interactions of this chemical in the brain.

An important finding relating to alcohol's mechanism of action is that ethanol interacts with the $GABA_A$ receptor–channel complex in the CNS, and augments $GABA_A$-mediated synaptic inhibition. This occurs at concentrations that do not produce comparable effects on other types of neurotransmitter receptors. Normally, activation of the $GABA_A$ receptor–channel complex increases the permeability of the nerve cell to chloride ions for approximately 10–20 ms. Inebriating amounts of ethanol prolong the time that the channel remains open, by two- to threefold, when alcohol binds to the receptor. At higher concentrations neurotransmitter release is reduced from all nerve terminals, probably due to reductions in calcium entry.

The effects of alcohol on the $GABA_A$ receptor may be important to the development of tolerance and physical dependence that occurs to individuals who drink large amounts of alcohol on a chronic basis. There is evidence that chronic alcohol ingestion leads to a reduction in the number of $GABA_A$ receptors in the brain as a compensatory response to the continual presence of the drug (i.e., downregulation). After this process occurs, when alcohol levels in the CNS fall, and its potentiating effect on $GABA_A$ receptors is lost, the brain becomes hyperexcitable and the dependent individual experiences anxiety, general malaise, and tremors. This acts as a powerful stimulus for the alcoholic to ingest more. During a prolonged withdrawal, the lack of alcohol to potentiate inhibition causes increasing hyperexcitability and frank signs of withdrawal including tremors, hyperreflexia, and convulsions.

Many important pharmaceutical agents produce CNS depression and have been studied extensively to determine their mechanism of action. One group of drugs, exemplified by the barbiturates, affects the nervous system much like alcohol does, whereas members of a second group, the benzodiazepines, are remarkably selective potentiators of $GABA_A$-mediated inhibition. Since they are commonly found in the home and are responsible for a number of suicides and alcohol-related deaths, they merit consideration.

Barbiturates

The barbiturates (e.g., phenobarbital) were at one time extensively used as sleeping pills and as sedative agents to reduce stress and anxiety in people. They, like alcohol, produce a spectrum of depressant effects that are dose dependent. Small doses promote tiredness and sleep, while higher doses can produce a general anesthetic state and death. The barbiturates can also produce tolerance and physical dependence after chronic ingestion of high doses. The withdrawal complications are very similar to those seen with alcohol. Although not prescribed to a great extent today, barbiturates continue to be readily available on the street.

Barbiturates probably interact more specifically with hydrophobic domains of membrane proteins than does alcohol. Interestingly, they produce opposite effects on the $GABA_A$ receptor-mediating inhibition in the CNS and the glutamate receptors that mediate excitation. Barbiturates enhance $GABA_A$ receptor-mediated inhibition by binding to a site within the chloride channel part of the complex. Barbiturates are more effective channel stabilizers than alcohol and can maintain the channel in its open state 2–10 times longer than normal. The same levels of barbiturates depress excitatory transmission mediated by glutamate. Why the function of one receptor complex should be enhanced while another is attenuated remains unknown.

Benzodiazepines

The benzodiazepines, of which valium is a prototype, are very selective drugs that target only the $GABA_A$ receptor–chloride channel complex. First discovered in the 1960s, this class of drugs was soon observed to produce marked changes in animal behavior and aggressiveness and eventually was marketed for use in humans. Most produce modest sedation and quite effectively alleviate anxiety resulting from any cause. Some produce a greater degree of sedation (e.g., halcion) and have become the modern "sleeping pills." The benzodiazepines are remarkably good at what they do, and they are among the most widely prescribed drugs in medicine today.

The advantages benzodiazepines possess over barbiturates are due to their relatively selective interaction with the $GABA_A$ receptor. They bind to a location on the receptor complex distinct from the binding site for the neurotransmitter GABA (an allosteric site). When they bind, they alter the structure in a way that increases the affinity of the GABA binding site for GABA. This increase in affinity for GABA results in a potentiation of GABA's effects when it is released from GABAergic nerve terminals. The benzodiazepines do not affect the $GABA_B$ receptor, any other receptor, or transmitter release. Figure 11.9 illustrates the major difference in the dose–response properties of barbiturates and benzodiazepines. For drugs with a dose-dependent plateau, such as the benzodiazepines, this translates into a significant improvement in safety profile.

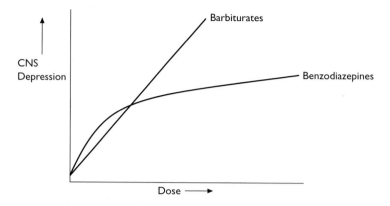

Figure 11.9 Comparison of dose–response curves in producing CNS depression.

Cannabinoids

Marijuana (Δ^9-tetrahydrocannibinol, THC) is unusual among drugs of abuse in that there is little evidence that it serves as a reinforcer in animal models of self-administration. It has also been difficult to demonstrate physical dependence.

During the 1990s, the brain receptors for THC in brain GB[1] and immune system GB[2] were isolated and cloned. The cannabinoid receptors belong to the G-protein-coupled superfamily of receptors. Since the discovery of a brain receptor implies an endogenous ligand for that binding site, the search for such a compound began immediately thereafter. In 1992 a compound that occurs naturally in the brain, called arachidonylethanolamide, belonging to the class of endogenous compounds known as eicosanoids, was shown to bind to the THC receptor and to produce pharmacological effects similar to those of THC itself. The compound has been given the name anandamide by its Hebrew discoverers, after the Sanskrit word *ananda*, meaning bliss. Interestingly, chocolate contains three compounds related to anandamide that may be related to chocolate craving. A second endogenous ligand is 2-arachidonoyl glycerol (2-AG). 2-AG is capable of binding to and activating both receptor types, whereas anandamide only activates the GB[1] receptor.

Cannabinoids may share at least some common neuronal mechanisms with opioid compounds. Studies of intracellular events associated with ligand binding to either cannabinoid or opiate receptors indicate that these receptors are linked via G proteins to the production of cAMP. Certain studies have also indicated that there may be some interaction between cannabinoid binding sites and opiate receptors in the reward pathway. In addition, there is increasing evidence that cannabinoids interact with opiate systems involved in the perception of pain. In fact, cannabinoids clearly produce analgesic effects in both experimental animals and humans, and of all the potential clinical uses of cannabinoids, the mediation of analgesia has received the most attention. Some evidence also indicates that the cannabinoid receptor system is an analgesic system.

Partly because of THC's analgesic property, efforts have been made to facilitate the availability of THC to the public. Several states have passed initiatives to decriminalize the use of "medicinal" marijuana. In 1985 THC was made available as a pill sold under the brand name Marinol®. The drug was found to be useful in relieving glaucoma and pain, nausea and vomiting in cancer patients, and in enhancing appetite and inducing weight gain in AIDS and cancer patients. In July 1999 Marinol was reclassified as a Schedule III drug. Unfortunately, Marinol lacks one of the main advantages of smoking: quick onset of effect. So the debate goes on with no clear resolution in sight.

Cocaine

Cocaine is a natural product originally isolated from a bushy shrub, *Erythroxylon coca*, that grows in the Andes mountains of Peru. Cocaine's potential for addiction was known and used with sinister intent by South American Indian chiefs hundreds of years ago. The chiefs maintained a messenger system along the spine of the Andes to control their thinly populated kingdoms, which stretched for thousands of miles along the mountains and were isolated from each other by rugged terrain. The messengers had to run at high altitude and needed stimulants for this exhausting task. Their wealthy employers provided the runners with coca leaves along their routes for this purpose and enslaved them further by paying them with more coca leaves, thus maintaining the addiction for which the runners were willing to continue their jobs. When coca leaves reached Europe with the Spanish conquistadors, their introduction led to one of the first European waves of psychoactive drug use.

Cocaine enjoyed a short popularity in human medicine as a local anesthetic, but the primary concern today is that cocaine's CNS effects appeal to many people, and cocaine is presently a major drug of abuse. Its popularity boomed in the 1980s when "free base" cocaine, known as "crack," became available. The ability to achieve rapid, high brain levels of cocaine by smoking crack has greatly increased its abuse potential and also its toxicity.

Although cocaine can function as a local anesthetic, most of its actions relate to a second mechanism. Cocaine increases synaptic concentrations of catecholamines (i.e., dopamine and norepinephrine) in the brain by blocking their reuptake mechanisms. Normally, when these transmitters are released from nerve terminals, they are rapidly removed from the synaptic cleft by specific energy-dependent "transporter" proteins that carry them back into the terminal. By blocking these transporter systems, cocaine prolongs the time the catecholamines remain in the synapse and intensifies their actions. This increase in dopamine concentration in the CNS appears to be the basis for the various euphoric and related changes that occur in people who use cocaine. A similar mechanism has been suggested for methamphetamine.

Interestingly, the breeding of a strain of "knockout" mice devoid of the gene for synthesis of the dopamine transporter protein results in hyperactive animals. This is probably because their neurons cannot remove released dopamine from synapses and consequently dopamine remains in the synapse 100 times longer. The animals attempt to compensate for this defect in their brain by "downregulating" the entire dopamine system, including (1) decreased synthesis of dopamine within the neurons and (2) reducing the number of postsynaptic receptor sites. Eventually, because of the absence of the dopamine transporter protein in these animals, they lose their sensitivity to cocaine.

Cocaine also blocks the reuptake of norepinephrine in the PNS; the combination of central and peripheral actions leads to a high probability of toxicity. The cardiovascular system is particularly sensitive to the actions of cocaine, and cardiac arrhythmias, marked increases in blood pressure, cerebral hemorrhage, myocardial ischemia, and outright heart failure are not uncommon with cocaine use. Even young, otherwise healthy individuals with normal coronary and cerebral arteries have died suddenly after cocaine use from cerebral hemorrhage or ventricular fibrillation. There have been several deaths of famous athletes attributed to cocaine cardiotoxicity. These cardiotoxic effects may be related to increased intracellular calcium levels and involve both cardiac and vascular actions of the drug.

The cardiovascular complications of cocaine abuse now account for a major fraction of drug-related emergency room visits and deaths. In 1986, for example, cocaine use was the third highest drug-related cause for an emergency room visit, ranking behind only opioids and alcohol in drug-induced death. Approximately 1700 cocaine-related deaths were reported to the National Institute of Drug Abuse in 1987.

ANESTHETICS AND ANALGESICS

Pain—the ultimate, universal symptom. It is virtually impossible to comprehend the collective pain and distress that members of our species, as well as others, have endured through the millennia. Broken bones, impacted wisdom teeth, infections, animal bites, amputations, and childbirth, to name just a few. Prior to 1846, attempts to provide comfort during surgical operations were minimally effective, at best, and the development of surgery was necessarily limited. From the earliest days of medicine, surgeons had tried all manner of primitive techniques to ease their patients' pain. The Egyptians, for example, used diluted narcotics (probably the best method). Other surgeons made their patients drunk with alcohol and then tied them to wooden benches that served as operating tables. In Europe, some surgeons choked their patients unconscious before operating. Still others applied pressure to a nerve (sensory) or artery (depriving the distal area of oxygenation) to make an area "fall asleep." In the sixteenth century, the French surgeon (and barber) Ambroise Pare devised a novel expedient. He put a wooden bowl over the head of a patient and pounded a hammer against it to knock him/her unconscious (much like heavy-metal "music"). Today, the two principal areas of pain management with pharmacological agents include anesthetics and analgesics.

Although the analgesic properties of both nitrous oxide (NO) and diethyl ether (ether) had been known since the late 1700s (NO was synthesized by Priestley in 1776), these agents were not used for medicinal purposes at the time. However, because of their effects on the CNS, these drugs were used in carnival exhibitions to entertain the audience, by producing "highs," as well as in social gathering ("ether frolics") to entertain the participants. It remained for the emergence of two dentists in the mid-1840s to usher in one of the most significant advances in the history of medicine: the successful achievement of reversible general anesthesia.

Dentists were instrumental in the introduction of gaseous anesthetics because they came in daily contact with persons suffering from excruciating pain, often of their own making. It was during a theatrical production that Horace Wells, a dentist,

Table 11.2 Gaseous anesthetics after 1846

1847	Chloroform; pleasant odor, nonflammability, hepatotoxin, cardiovascular depressant
1863	Nitrous oxide reintroduced
1868	Nitrous oxide with oxygen described
1920	Four stages of anesthesia described[a]
1929	Cyclopropane discovered
1956	Halothane introduced, noninflammable

Note
a   The somewhat arbitrary division is as follows: I, stage of analgesia; II, stage of delerium; III, stage of surgical anesthesia; IV, stage of medularry depression.

observed that one of the participants became injured during his performance yet felt no pain while under the influence of nitrous oxide. Wells was so impressed with the effect that he had one of his own teeth extracted the next day while breathing the gas. Unfortunately, Well's attempt to publicly demonstrate this remarkable effect in 1845 was a failure (the patient cried out during the operation).

In 1846, William T. G. Morton, a former associate of Wells, performed a demonstration using ether on a patient named Gilbert Abbot. Both Wells and Abbot must truly be considered heroes in this regard. In a scene reminiscent of Hollywood, Morton arrived late to the proceedings just as the surgeon was about to begin. After administering the ether Morton turned over responsibility of the event to the surgeon. When the surgery was complete, with the absence of consciousness and pain, the surgeon declared to the audience, "Gentlemen, this is no humbug." Unfortunately, the subsequent lives of Wells and Morton were humbug. Wells died insane while Morton failed in his attempt to patent the use of ether and died an embittered man. The subsequent development of major general anesthetic agents is shown in Table 11.2.

Special factors govern the transport of gaseous anesthetic molecules from inspired gas through the lungs to blood and then to the brain, including (1) concentration of the anesthetic agent in inspired gas; (2) pulmonary ventilation rate delivering the anesthetic to the lungs; (3) transfer of the gas from the alveoli to the blood flowing through the lungs; and (4) transfer of the agent from the arterial blood to all the tissues of the body. The steady-state concentration in the brain is, of course, of greatest importance. Because the brain is well perfused, anesthetic partial pressure in brain becomes equal to the partial pressure in alveolar gas (and in blood) over the course of just several minutes.

One of the troublesome aspects of the inhalation anesthetics is their relatively low margin of safety. They have therapeutic indices in the range of 2–4, making them among the most dangerous drugs in clinical use. The toxicity of these drugs is largely a function of their side effects, and each has a unique side-effect profile. Therefore, the selection of a particular agent is often based on matching a patient's pathophysiology with drug–effect profiles.

Although inhalation anesthetic agents have an analgesic component (stage I), in that the response to noxious stimuli can be blunted, the analgesic effect is mild at low doses and is only satisfactory at dangerously high doses. Therefore, the use of most general anesthetics is accompanied with some type of analgesic adjunct. Nonsteroidal anti-inflammatory drugs, such as cyclooxygenase-2 inhibitors or acetaminophen

Table 11.3 Chemical classes producing anesthesia

Inert gases	(xenon, argon, and krypton)
Diatomic gases	(hydrogen and nitrogen)
Simple organic compounds	(chloroform, cyclopropane)
Ether and halogenated ether	(isoflurane, enflurane, methoxyflurane, desflurane, sevoflurane, and fluroxene)
Polyhalogenated alkane	(halothane)

(Chapter 13), sometimes provide adequate analgesia for minor surgical procedures. However, because of the rapid and profound analgesia produced, opioids (e.g., fentanyl and its derivatives, as well as morphine, etc.) are the primary analgesics used during the perioperative period. The primary analgesic activity of each of these drugs is produced by agonist activity at μ-opioid receptors.

General anesthetics are rarely given alone. In addition to the analgesic agents just mentioned, benzodiazepines (midazolam, Versed®; diazepam, Valium®) are commonly used as adjuncts for the relief of anxiety, amnesia, and sedation prior to induction of anesthesia. Neuromuscular blockers (e.g., succinylcholine or pancuronium) can also be administered during the induction of anesthesia to relax skeletal muscles.

How do gaseous anesthetics produce their effects?

Perhaps the most unusual aspect regarding the structure of gaseous anesthetics is the lack of a basic chemical structure that can produce anesthesia. Table 11.3 compares the diversity of chemical classes that can produce anesthesia.

The first chemical clue relating the structure of anesthetics to their potency was discovered in 1899 by a pharmacologist, Hans Horst Meyer, and an anesthetist, Charles Ernst Overton. Working independently, Meyer and Overton noted a strong correlation between the polarity of a compound and its potency as an anesthetic. They expressed polarity as the oil/gas partition coefficient, while anesthetic potency was expressed as the partial pressure in atmospheres. Figure 11.10 is a Meyer–Overton correlation for 18 anesthetics used on mice. Note that olive oil is used, and it has become the most commonly used reference solvent.

The slope of the regression line implies that the MAC (minimal alveolar concentration effective in 50 percent of animals) is inversely proportional to partition coefficient or potency is directly proportional to partition coefficient. The Meyer–Overton correlation suggests that the site at which anesthetics bind is primarily a hydrophobic environment. Although a wide variety of compounds lie on the Meyer–Overton correlation line, there are many compounds that do not. This suggests that the chemical properties of the anesthetic site differ from those of olive oil.

The prevailing debate among investigators in the field of volatile anesthetics with regard to the mechanism of action is the lipid/protein controversy. The center of the debate is whether lipids or proteins are the primary targets for general anesthetics. In the fluid mosaic model of the cell membrane, proteins have been envisioned as having active functions while lipids have played a passive, supporting function. Recent advances in cell physiology, however, question a simple dichotomy between lipids and protein. Therefore, the divisions in the lipid/protein controversy have become less clear.

Figure 11.10 Meyer–Overton correlation for volatile general anesthetics in mice. The slope of the regression line is −1.02 and the correlation coefficient, $r^2 = 0.997$. CTF, carbon tetrafluoride; NIT, nitrogen; ARG, argon; PFE, perfluoroethane; SHF, sulfur hexafluoride; KRY, krypton; NO2, nitrous oxide; ETH, ethylene; XEN, xenon; DDM, dichlorodifluoromethane; CYC, cyclopropane; FLU, fluroxene; DEE, diethylether; ENF, enflurane; ISO, isoflurane; HAL, halothane; CHL, chloroform; MOF, methoxyflurane.

Source: E. Moody and P. Skolnick (eds) (2001), *Molecular Basis of Anesthesia*. Boca Raton, FL: CRC Press. Reprinted with permission.

Interesting calculations have been carried out by others dealing with the interaction of anesthetic molecules on lipids and proteins. For example, at the MAC, the concentration of anesthetic molecules in the hydrophobic phase is approximately 50 mM. Assuming that the anesthetic molecules are uniformly distributed throughout the lipid bilayer of a cell membrane of thickness 50 Å, there would be only one anesthetic molecule for every 60 lipid molecules (i.e., 1.5 percent of the molecules in the membrane and only 0.5 percent of the membrane volume). Under these circumstances, the anesthetic molecules would be distributed too diffusely to have a significant effect on membrane status. If, however, anesthetic molecules became preferentially located adjacent to a protein, then a local effect on protein function might occur.

A similar argument has been made for anesthetic–protein interactions. Halothane, for example, has a molecular weight of 197. The GABA$_A$ receptor channel (a putative receptor site for volatile anesthetics) has a molecular weight of approximately 250,000. Is it possible that a single molecule of halothane could significantly affect the function of such a large protein? Some proteins are designed to undergo allosteric changes upon the binding of small molecules. GABA, for example, the neurotransmitter that permits the GABA$_A$ receptor channel to undergo the closed-to-open channel transition, has a molecular weight of 103.

The GABA$_A$ receptor

The GABA$_A$ receptor is a ligand-gated chloride channel that underlies synaptic inhibition in the brain. When the endogenous neurotransmitter, GABA, binds to the receptor the anion channel opens and chloride enters the cell. This sequence of events hyperpolarizes the neuron, rendering further depolarization or transmission of impulses less likely.

The $GABA_A$ receptor has been recognized for many years as the target of alcohol, barbiturates, and benzodiazepines. More recently, it has been recognized that other drugs such as volatile anesthetics act at these receptors as well (e.g., the concentration at which these drugs enhance $GABA_A$ function correlates well with their anesthetic potencies). The suggestion that increased inhibition of the CNS might be expected to produce "anesthesia" has resulted in the identification of this receptor as a significant anesthetic target.

Studies using synaptoneurosomes (produced by homogenizing brain tissue and recovered by differential ultracentrifugation) have demonstrated that volatile anesthetics can enhance the uptake of chloride ion in a stereoselective manner. The results of these neurochemical studies have been found to correlate reasonably well with data obtained using electrophysiological techniques. Although the $GABA_A$ receptor has received the most recent attention regarding the mechanism of action of volatile anesthetics, it still appears premature to totally disregard excitatory amino acid receptors (NMDA, AMPA, or kainite), as well as calcium and potassium channels; glutamate receptors apparently can be eliminated.

Parenteral anesthetics

In addition to gaseous anesthetics, there are several drugs that can achieve anesthesia when given parenterally. Parenteral anesthetics are small, hydrophobic, substituted aromatic or heterocyclic compounds. Lipophilicity is the key factor governing the pharmacokinetics of these drugs. After a single intravenous bolus, these drugs preferentially partition into the highly perfused and lipophilic brain and spinal cord tissue where they produce anesthesia within a single circulation time. Termination of anesthesia after a single bolus dose is primarily by redistribution out of the nervous system rather than by metabolism.

The two principal parenteral anesthetic drugs used clinically are thiopental (an old prototype) and propofol (a relatively new drug). Thiopental is a derivative of barbituric acid, while propofol is a substituted propylphenol. Onset and duration of anesthetic effect for the two drugs are similar. However, recovery is more rapid following infusion with propofol (a desirable feature). The relatively rapid clearance of propofol explains its less severe hangover in patients compared to thiopental and may allow for a more accelerated discharge from the recovery room.

Local anesthetics

The development of local anesthetics and their structure–activity relationship are described in Chapter 13 in the drug screening section. Suffice it to say that the development of these drugs has opened up an entirely new era in relieving pain in the conscious patient. When applied locally to nerve tissue in appropriate concentrations, local anesthetics reversibly block the action potentials responsible for nerve conduction. They act on any part of the nervous system and on every type of nerve fiber. Their action is reversible at clinically relevant concentrations and nerve function recovers

Table 11.4 Various types of local anesthesia techniques

Infiltration anesthesia	The injection of local anesthetic directly into tissue without taking into consideration the course of cutaneous nerves; duration can be extended with the addition of epinephrine (vasoconstrictor)
Field block anesthesia	Produced by subcutaneous injection in such a manner as to anesthetize the region distal to the injection site
Nerve block	Injection of anesthetic into or about individual peripheral nerves or nerve plexuses; produces area of anesthesia greater than with the above techniques
Spinal anesthesia	Injection of local anesthetic into the cerebrospinal fluid in the lumbar space. In most adults, the spinal cord terminates above the second lumbar vertebra. Therefore, in this region there is a relatively large space to accommodate injected drug. Various specific gravity preparations can be used to manage the height up the spinal cord that the drug will travel

with no evidence of damage to nerve fibers or cells. The first local anesthetic, cocaine, was accidentally discovered to have anesthetic properties in the late nineteenth century.

Cocaine was first isolated in 1860 by a chemist named Albert Niemann. Like most organic chemists before and after, Niemann had the habit of tasting compounds that he isolated. On this particular occasion Niemann noted that it caused a numbing of the tongue. Carl Köller, who used it as a topical anesthetic for ophthalmological surgery, first introduced cocaine into clinical practice in 1884. Subsequently, cocaine became popular for its use in infiltration and conduction block anesthesia.

Local anesthetics block nerve conduction by decreasing or preventing the large transient increase in the permeability of excitable membranes to Na^+, which is normally produced by depolarization of the nerve cell membrane. This effect is due to their direct interaction with voltage-gated Na^+ channels. As the anesthetic action progressively takes effect, the threshold for electrical excitability correspondingly increases, the rate of rise of the action potential declines, and impulse conduction slows. These factors decrease the probability of propagation of the action potential, and nerve conduction eventually fails. Examples of different types of local anesthesia are shown in Table 11.4.

Analgesics

Unfortunately, to feel pain is an essential condition for survival. Pain-initiated avoidance behavior protects the individual. Morphine, obtained from opium, from the juice of the opium poppy (*Papaver somniferum*), has been known for millennia to alleviate pain. As mentioned in Chapter 5, endogenous opioids have also been identified. The word "opioid" is now used to refer to all drugs with morphine-like actions. The structure of morphine is shown in Figure 11.11. Diacetylmorphine (heroin) is made by acetylation at the 3 and 6 positions.

In human beings, morphine-like drugs produce analgesia, drowsiness, changes in mood, and mental clouding. A significant feature of the analgesia is that it occurs without loss of consciousness. When therapeutic doses of morphine are given to

Figure 11.11 Structure of morphine.

patients in pain, they describe the pain as being less intense, less discomforting, or entirely dissipated; drowsiness can occur. An additional component can be the experience of euphoria.

Opioid analgesics function as agonists at opioid receptors widely distributed in both spinal cord and brain to produce a decrease in the perception of pain (particularly slow pain). It is well established that the analgesic effects of opioids arise from their ability to inhibit directly the ascending transmission of nociceptive information from the spinal cord dorsal horn and to activate pain control circuits that descend from the midbrain. Opioid receptors in the spinal cord may mediate various analgesic reflexes, and agonists acting at these sites produce significant analgesic responses. These receptors are most concentrated in the limbic system, which regulates emotional behavior, as well as in areas such as the medial thalamus and periaqueductal gray, which mediate pain perception. A preponderance of evidence indicates that analgesic effects of opioids are mediated predominantly by μ receptors.

Botulinum toxin

Although not normally considered a drug, botulinum toxin has proved to be a useful tool in understanding neuronal function. In addition, it has recently found a therapeutic use in treating prolonged muscle spasm. In one study, 185 children with cerebral palsy were prescribed botulinum toxin type A (BTX-A) to treat leg and ankle muscle contractions. A small amount of the toxin is injected directly into the muscle fiber to cause that muscle to relax. After 1 year, 46 percent reported improved walking after receiving injections of BTX-A into the calf muscle once every 3 months. After 2 years, up to 58 percent had maintained improvements in their walking ability. The toxin acts to reduce muscle contractions by inhibiting acetylcholine release at all cholinergic synapses, including the CNS, as discussed later. At the skeletal muscle motor end-plate, reduced acetylcholine release leads to weakened muscles, decreased spasticity, and less discomfort. BTX-A has also been used to treat severe muscle spasms in stroke patients and cosmetically to reduce the appearance of wrinkles.

Botulinum toxin is produced by the bacterium *Clostridium botulinum*. It is among the most lethal substances known, and it has been estimated that 1–2 ounces of the pure toxin could kill the entire population of the United States. Poisoning of man and animals occurs when food containing the toxin is ingested. The most common source is improperly prepared canned fruits and vegetables or fish products. Although only about 100 cases are reported in the United States per year, botulinum poisoning is still a world problem, particularly in Asia where thousands of cases occur yearly. The lethality rate is 15–40 percent. Clinical symptoms usually develop 18–36 hours after ingestion. Most are due to cholinergic blockade and include weakness, blurred vision, difficulty in swallowing and speaking, progressive weakness of skeletal muscles, and eventually respiratory paralysis. Sensation and consciousness are left unaffected.

There are seven distinct botulinum neurotoxins that differ somewhat in structure and potency. All are polypeptides of molecular weight about 150 kDa. Their amino acid homology is generally high. The mechanism of action of botulinum toxin is now well understood. The toxin is synthesized as a single polypeptide chain that is proteolytically cleaved by the bacteria to form two peptides held together by a disulfide bond. One, the heavy chain, is approximately 100 kDa in size and the other, the light chain, is approximately 50 kDa in size. When the toxin is ingested, it is absorbed from the gastrointestinal tract and distributed via the bloodstream to nerve terminals in the periphery. The toxin binds to a site on cholinergic nerve terminals and is subsequently internalized by endocytosis.

The endocytotic vesicles are processed to form endosomes, which normally ferry their contents to lysosomes for destruction. As part of their function, the endosomes contain enzymes that progressively render their contents more and more acidic. At a pH of approximately 4, the heavy chain of botulinum toxin undergoes a conformational change that leads to its insertion into the endosomal membrane. This insertion creates a large channel through which monovalent cations can move and through which the light chain likely leaves the endosome to gain access to the nerve terminal cytoplasm.

The light chain, when separated from the heavy chain, behaves as an enzyme that selectively cleaves a peptide associated with synaptic vesicles. This peptide, synaptobrevin, is required for docking and fusion of the vesicle during acetylcholine release. By enzymatically cleaving it, botulinum toxin renders vesicle docking and fusion impossible, and cholinergic neurotransmission comes to a halt. Because the light chain has enzymatic activity, just a few molecules can catalyze the destruction of synaptobrevin on thousands of vesicles. In this way, extreme potency is achieved via amplification of the process.

Nicotine

Nicotine is an alkaloid derived from the tobacco plant *Nicotiana tabacum*. It is a liquid at room temperature and acquires a brown appearance with a characteristic odor when exposed to air. It is widely available in tobacco products and in certain pesticides. Tobacco products can contain 0.2–5 percent nicotine and if ingested, particularly by children, can be very toxic. Only a small amount of nicotine found in tobacco is volatilized and absorbed during smoking. However, the nicotine that is absorbed is done so quite rapidly through the alveoli and is detectable in the brain only 8 seconds after the first inhalation. Nicotine is believed to be the major component of tobacco associated with its addictive potential, or its abuse liability.

The actions of nicotine relate to its ability to activate one of the two groups of cholinergic receptors, the nicotinic receptors. Nicotine and a second substance, muscarine, a mushroom toxin, were known long before acetylcholine was identified as a neurotransmitter, and the receptors in the PNS were initially distinguished by whether they responded to nicotine or to muscarine. Thus, the nomenclature of nicotinic and muscarinic cholinergic neurons was established.

Nicotinic receptors are located in autonomic ganglia, at neuromuscular junctions (Figure 11.3), and within the CNS. Activation of the latter is involved in the psychoactive and addictive properties of nicotine. Like most addictive drugs, nicotine can cause dopamine to be released in a specific brain region known as the shell of the nucleus accumbens. The shell links the amygdala and the core of the nucleus accumbens. Stimulation of peripheral ganglia leads to acceleration in heart rate, increase in blood pressure, and constriction of blood vessels, particularly in the skin. At high concentrations a pronounced tremor develops and convulsions are possible. Even higher exposure promotes a "depolarization block" of ganglionic and neuromuscular function. Under these conditions heart rate drops precipitously, blood pressure plummets, and skeletal muscle paralysis can develop.

Cholinesterase inhibitors

As mentioned in Part 2, there are drugs that can interfere with the inactivation of neurotransmitters. In that particular case the reversible cholinesterase inhibitor neostigmine was discussed within the context of treating myasthenia gravis. Excessive blockade of acetylcholinesterase at both muscarinic and nicotinic synapses results in a sustained excess of acetylcholine, which persistently activates the effector they innervate. Muscarinic stimulation results in excessive salivation, lacrimation, bronchiolar secretions, and bronchoconstriction. Nicotinic stimulation produces effects such as those described earlier for nicotine.

Reversible cholinesterase inhibitors find their greatest clinical use in the treatment of open-angle glaucoma. Relief is achieved by enhancing the contraction of the ciliary muscle and the iris sphincter. This contracture pulls the iris off the lens and facilitates fluid movement through the canal of Schlemm. The result is decreased pressure with reduced distortion of the lens and increased movement of aqueous humor out of the anterior chamber of the eye.

There is another class of cholinesterase inhibitors known as irreversible organophosphates. Their mechanism of action involves phosphorylation of serine residues in the esteratic site via covalent bonds. These compounds are highly toxic and are not used clinically. Human exposure occurs through the use of pesticides or nerve gases. An example of a nerve gas is the infamous sarin, which was used in the terrorist attacks in Japan during the mid-1990s. Nerve gases are among the most potent synthetic toxic agents known; they are lethal to laboratory animals in submilligram doses. Antidotal treatment in cases of this type of poisoning includes (1) general supportive measures, as well as (2) management with atropine for the treatment of muscarinic symptoms and pralidoxime (2-PAM) for the regeneration of the enzyme. 2-PAM exerts a nucleophilic attack on the phosphorus; the oxime phosphate is then split off, leaving the regenerated enzyme. However, this is not a rapid process.

Schizophrenia/antipsychotic drugs (neuroleptics)

Schizophrenia is a complex psychotic disorder affecting multiple functional modalities and is one of the two most common psychotic emotional disturbances (the other

Phenothiazines

Chlorpromazines (THORAZINE)
R1: —(CH$_2$)$_2$—N(CH$_3$)$_2$
R2: —Cl

Figure 11.12 Chemical structure of the prototypic phenothiazine antipsychotic.

being manic-depressive illness). One percent of the world's population is affected by classic schizophrenia. Records show that in 1955 a patient with schizophrenia occupied one out of every four hospital beds in the United States. The symptoms of schizophrenia include virtually the complete range of abnormal phenomena that afflict the human mind. The symptoms most characteristic of schizophrenia include delusions, hallucinations, formal thought disorder, inappropriate affect, blunted affect, impoverished thought, and diminished volition.

Antipsychotic drugs (neuroleptics) may be defined as medications effective in the palliative treatments of psychotic disorders, most notably schizophrenia, although not exclusively. Phenothiazines are the oldest and largest class of antipsychotic drugs. They include the prototypical antipsychotic chlorpromazine, which in the mid-1950s initiated the present era of pharmacological treatment of psychiatric disorders. Soon after chlorpromazine was introduced in the United States, the population of the state mental hospitals—which until then had been increasing by 10–15 percent yearly—began to plummet. The drugs belonging to this class are three-ring heterocyclic compounds in which two aromatic rings are linked by a third ring containing sulfur and nitrogen atoms (Figure 11.12).

The antagonism of central dopamine receptors by antipsychotic drugs has been postulated as a critical determinant of the therapeutic efficacy of this class of drugs and forms a core of the "dopamine hypothesis." In essence, this hypothesis postulates that schizophrenia is a manifestation of hyperdopaminergic activity in the CNS. In support of this theory are the facts that: (1) all widely used antipsychotic drugs have a profound affinity for binding to dopamine D$_2$ receptors; (2) the clinical potencies of antipsychotic drugs are directly related to their affinities for the dopamine D$_2$ receptor; and (3) the therapeutic concentrations of antipsychotic drugs in the plasma or the spinal fluid exactly match the antipsychotic dissociation constants at the dopamine D$_2$ receptor.

The words "neuroleptic" and receptor "occupancy" have similar semantic connotations. The term neuroleptic originates from the Greek *leptikos*, which means "to seize" and implies that the drug seizes the neurons. The term occupancy, of course, evokes a similar meaning at a receptor level through its roots in the Latin *occupare*, which also means to seize. Research has shown that the fraction of brain dopamine D$_2$ receptors occupied by antipsychotic drugs is consistently on the order of 75 percent, as calculated from the therapeutic concentration and the antipsychotic dissociation constant. The clinical potencies of neuroleptics and their blockade of dopamine receptors correlate while there is a lack of correlation with serotonin, alpha adrenergic, and histamine receptors. Additional support for the dopamine hypothesis comes from the finding that the density of dopamine D_2 receptors is elevated in postmortem brain tissue from schizophrenic patients. Furthermore, positron emission tomography reveals elevated dopamine D_2 receptors in brains of schizophrenics.

Despite the preponderance of data correlating the dopamine D_2 receptor with schizophrenia, alternative sites in the brain (serotonergic, adrenergic, glutamatergic, and GABAergic) are also being investigated to explain the actions of "atypical" neuroleptics.

Antidepressant drugs

Depressive illness constitutes one of the most frequently seen mental disorders. The morbidity and mortality associated with alteration of mood is one of the major problems facing behavioral health professionals, with the U.S. National Comorbidity Study of 1994 showing a lifetime prevalence of major depression of 12.7 percent in males and 21.3 percent in females. Most mood disorders are chronic and require long-term management. Pharmacotherapy continues to be a mainstay treatment of depression. Because depressant mood disorders are so prevalent in our society, antidepressant drugs are among the most frequently prescribed medications.

The discovery of the antidepressant effect of medications was coincidental to their use for other disorders. Initial work published in 1952 reported that iproniazid (originally used for the treatment of tuberculosis) could elevate mood. Although the use of iproniazid was discontinued due to toxicity, many other additional medications have been tested and approved for the treatment of depression. These include monoamine oxidase inhibitors, tricyclics, selective serotonin reuptake inhibitors, and a heterogeneous class of atypical drugs.

The principal groups of antidepressants available today are all presumed to exert their action via alteration of brain monoamine metabolism. These amines include norepinephrine, dopamine, and serotonin. The involvement of catecholamines in the pathogenesis of depression was invoked as early as 1965. A deficiency in brain serotonin was theorized in 1967, while a role for dopamine in depression was formally proposed in 1975. The drugs that are used to treat depression basically act to increase neurotransmitter concentration in the synaptic cleft either by (1) decreasing neurotransmitter degradation or (2) inhibiting neurotransmitter reuptake.

An example of a class of drugs that interrupt neurotransmitter degradation is the monoamine oxidase (MAO) inhibitors. MAO is a mitochondrial enzyme that exists in two forms (A and B). Its major role is to oxidize monoamines such as norepinephrine, serotonin, and dopamine by removing the amine grouping from the neurotransmitters. Under normal circumstances, MAO acts as a "safety valve" to degrade any excess transmitter molecules that may spill out of synaptic vesicles when the neuron is in a resting state. MAO inhibitors prevent this inactivation. In their presence, any neurotransmitter molecules that leak out of the synaptic vesicles survive to enter the synapse intact. Receptors are thus exposed to a greater amount of the neurotransmitter.

Several clinically utilized MAO inhibitors such as phenylzine and tranylcypromine are irreversible inhibitors of both MAO-A and MAO-B (presumably via covalent binding). The irreversible inhibition of MAO means that neurons so affected must synthesize new enzyme before normal biological activity is reestablished. Research indicates that the antidepressant effect of these drugs is primarily due to inhibition of MAO-A. Relatively new MAO inhibitors are of the reversible type and include moclobemide.

MAO inhibitors were the first widely used antidepressants, but because of various undesirable side effects they are employed today in only a more limited number of cases. People who are treated with MAO inhibitors, for example, must be careful of their diet. They should not eat food rich in tyramine or other biologically active amines. These foods include cheese, beer, and red wine. Individuals on MAO inhibitors are unable to inactivate tyramine present in the food. Because tyramine causes the release of endogenous norepinephrine, patients are susceptible to increased blood pressure (e.g., potential lethal cerebral hemorrhages) and cardiac arrhythmias.

Fortunately, another group of antidepressant drugs was developed to take the place of MAO inhibiters. These drugs are called tricyclics, because all have chemical structures resembling a three-ring chain. Imipramine was the first of the tricyclic antidepressants (TCAs), synthesized as a "me-too" follow-up to chlorpromazine. All TCAs inhibit the presynaptic reuptake of the monoamine neurotransmitters norepinephrine and serotonin. By inhibiting reuptake more neurotransmitter is left in the synaptic cleft, thus potentiating their effects. The relative effect on serotonin or norepinephrine reuptake inhibition varies from one TCA to another. In addition to the blockade of neurotransmitter uptake, most TCAs have direct affinities for several heterogeneous receptors.

As scientists improved their techniques for detecting low levels of amines, they began to measure the amine concentrations in postmortem human brains. Several researchers measured levels of serotonin and norepinephrine in the brains of people who had committed suicide as a result of depression and compared the levels to individuals of the same age who had been killed in accidents. The suicides' brains had lower levels of serotonin. Subsequent studies also revealed that certain depressed patients had lower levels of serotonin metabolites in their cerebrospinal fluid. These findings accelerated the effort to develop drugs that would be effective on serotonergic neurons.

This new class of antidepressants, with relatively few side effects, is the selective serotonin reuptake inhibitors (SSRIs). This group of compounds has a selective effect on the presynaptic reuptake of serotonin and has assumed the role of first-line anti-depressant agents in the management of depression. Most SSRIs have only modest clinically relevant effects on other brain systems. As such, their clinical profile is primarily a reflection of their effect in enhancing the synaptic availability of serotonin. The prototypic drug in this class is prozac, which has received considerable publicity since its entry into the market. Fortunately, initial concerns relating to increased suicide risk have not been confirmed with larger clinical trials. As the name of this class of drugs implies, the mechanism by which they work to alleviate depression is by selectively blocking the reuptake of serotonin.

Mania

While neuroleptics can effectively treat the depression present in bipolar disorder, the metal ion lithium exerts a therapeutic effect on the other aspect; it relieves the symptoms of mania. For many years the only treatment for mania was sedation. Before the advent of neuroleptics, manic patients typically received large doses of barbiturates that simply rendered them unconscious. When they woke up, their manic behavior would take up where it had left off. Later, psychiatrists preferred to prescribe sedating neuroleptics, such as chlorpromazine, for their manic cases because those drugs did not put the patients to sleep, but while chlorpromazine effectively hampers a maniac's activity it does not affect the underlying disorder.

In contrast to neuroleptics, the simple metal lithium, introduced to psychiatry in the mid-1960s, truly aborts the manic condition. Unlike the neuroleptics, lithium does not cause sedation, nor does it transform mania into depression. Instead, it appears to restore the patient to a normal state of mind. The calming effect of lithium was discovered by accident in a flawed experiment during the 1940s. While investigating whether urine from manic patients contained some toxic nitrogenous substances (uric acid), John Cade, an Australian psychiatrist, mixed uric acid with a number of metals to increase solubility. When lithium urate was administered to guinea pigs they appeared to be calmed. Cade then tested lithium in another salt, lithium carbonate, to determine whether the key factor in the "calming effect" was the uric acid or the lithium. This lithium also "calmed" the guinea pigs. Impressed with these results he proceeded with experiments to administer lithium salts to manic patients in the clinic.

We now know that there is nothing abnormal about the urine of manic patients. In all probability, lithium appears to calm guinea pigs only because it makes them sick. Nevertheless, his clinical results were sufficiently positive that Cade published the results in an obscure Australian journal in 1949. In 1954, a Danish psychiatrist confirmed Cade's findings and the use of lithium began to spread in Europe. It was not until the mid-1960s, however, that lithium was marketed commercially in the United States, but it was not used for the treatment of mania until 1970.

The precise mechanism of action of lithium remains unknown.

Methylphenidate (Ritalin®)

One of the most controversial CNS-acting drugs in contemporary society is methylphenidate (Ritalin®). This drug is structurally related to amphetamine and is a "mild" stimulant that has abuse potential similar to amphetamine. Methylphenidate is classified as a Schedule II controlled substance. It is effective in the treatment of narcolepsy and attention-deficit hyperactivity disorder (ADHD). Its use in ADHD has caused the greatest controversy.

ADHD is a frequently diagnosed disorder particularly among juveniles, boys being diagnosed at three to four times the rate of girls. Symptoms are generally thought to include inappropriate levels of attention and concentration, inappropriate levels of distractibility and impulsivity of some sort, and a combination of both of these. A psychologist, psychiatrist, or pediatrician typically diagnoses the condition but diagnostic methods remain controversial.

Since 1990, the number of American children taking Ritalin has more than doubled to between 1.5 million and 2.5 million. Defenders of the drug give testament to the profound effect it can have in turning problem adolescents into model students.

Proponents point to studies showing that 75 percent of children on Ritalin experience positive effects. Opponents label the drug as "kiddie cocaine" and assert that the current state of ADHD diagnosis and treatment is tenuous at best. Undoubtedly, the truth lies somewhere in between, with the proper diagnosis being the key. It is a diagnosis that really did not exist prior to the late 1970s to early 1980s. A correct diagnosis is basically ratified when the medication works.

One of the unfortunate realities of Ritalin use has been its propensity for abuse. A number of studies have revealed that grade-schoolers have obtained the drug from their peers who are undergoing therapy for ADHD. In one study published in 2001, 651 students aged 11–18 from Wisconsin and Minnesota were focused on. The researchers found that more than a third of the students who took ADHD medication said they had been asked to sell or trade their drugs. Users have crushed the pills and snorted the powder in order to get a "cocaine-like" rush. It is hoped that newer-generation products, e.g., time-release medications, will be less prone to this abuse since their formulation makes them more difficult to crush.

Curare

Curare is a natural product isolated from trees and bushes of the *Strychnos* and *Chondodendron* geni. The active principle (*d*-tubocurarine) is a water-soluble and heat-stable alkaloid that can be extracted, heated, and concentrated to produce a pasty residue containing a high concentration of curare. This extract has been used for centuries in South America as an "arrow poison." Curare is not absorbed from the gastrointestinal tract, nor can it penetrate the blood–brain barrier. In order for curare to produce its effects, it must be "injected" into the body.

The effects of curare develop rapidly after it enters the body. Victims develop rapid weakness of voluntary muscles followed by paralysis, respiratory failure, and death. The cause is a blockade of nicotinic cholinergic receptors at the neuromuscular junctions in skeletal muscle. Unlike botulinum toxin, release of acetylcholine by the cholinergic nerve terminals is not affected. When curare is present, however, the acetylcholine that is released cannot bind to the receptors because they are reversibly occupied by the curare. As a consequence, nerve–muscle communication fails and paralysis ensues.

It is critical to the use of curare by hunters as an arrow poison that it is not absorbed from the gastrointestinal tract. Animals killed by curare-tipped arrows can contain many lethal doses of curare in their carcasses around the point of arrow penetration. Because curare is heat stable, it is not destroyed by cooking and is normally ingested by the hunters. If it were absorbed from the gastrointestinal tract to an appreciable degree they would become paralyzed and die from systemic toxicity.

Curare has no effect on sensation, consciousness, or pain and it does not enter the CNS (see Chapter 15). Victims injected with many lethal doses of curare will survive with no apparent damage if adequate respiration can be provided for them. Because of this, curare and derivatives of it are used in medicine to produce paralysis during delicate surgical procedures where involuntary or reflexive movement would be disastrous. The anesthetist provides artificial respiration for the patient until curare is eliminated from the body.

Table 11.5 Main types of abused drugs

Class	Example(s)
Opiates	Morphine
CNS stimulants	Cocaine, amphetamines
CNS depressants	Barbiturates, benzodiazepines, alcohol
Hallucinogens	LSD, mescaline
Miscellaneous	Marijuana, nicotine, caffeine

SUBSTANCE ABUSE

Background

One of the unique aspects of the CNS is that it is the driving force behind the myriad of factors relating to substance abuse. Man has been "abusing" chemicals possessing pharmacological effects on the CNS for millennia. It is the specific quality of certain drugs for influencing CNS function that makes them candidates for abuse. If one examines the main types of abused drugs (Table 11.5) there is considerable diversity in chemical structure. However, they all share the single common feature of affecting brain function to the extent that certain elements of "reality," or consciousness, are altered. Within this context, they are typically taken for religious experiences, to "explore" the subconscious, or to suppress anxiety in social settings. Conversely, drugs that do not affect brain function do not represent societal drug abuse problems. For example, one does not hear of insulin or penicillin "junkies."

There are numerous theories as to what the underlying factors are in drug abuse, be they psychologically or biochemically based. In essence, psychological factors driving drug abuse are believed to be based upon either some "positive effect" or some "negative avoidance." Biochemical factors appear to be somewhat more complicated, since our understanding of the relevant processes are not as clearly understood. However, we do have a reasonably good understanding of a very important component of drug abuse, namely the "reward pathway."

Reward pathway

Various experimental paradigms have, over the years, indicated that specific limbic structures in the brain (nucleus accumbens and the amygdala) appear to be consistently associated with what has become to be considered as a common reward pathway through the brain. At present, the reinforcing or rewarding properties of drugs, modulated by specific discriminative cues and concurrent aversive properties, are considered essential in determining the addictive potential or abuse liability of these compounds. The neuropharmacological correlates of reward are considered to be the key to our scientific understanding of drug addiction, and these neuronal mechanisms are the targets of research efforts to elucidate effective pharmacological adjuncts to drug addiction treatment programs.

Natural reward centers have developed over the course of evolution to reinforce useful behaviors (e.g., pleasure, sexual satisfaction, eating, and drinking). These reward centers are innervated by dopaminergic neurons. Highly addicting drugs such as cocaine and methamphetamine substitute for natural neurotransmitters to produce an artificial state of reward (euphoria) and a compulsion to sustain that state. We now know that cocaine and methamphetamine can increase the level of dopamine in the synapses of dopaminergic fibers by blocking dopamine reuptake transporter proteins.

Tolerance

Tolerance is characterized by a diminishing drug effect following repeated administration. The result is a requirement for higher doses with subsequent use to produce the same effect. The term does not give any indication of the mechanism, however. We have already considered one type of tolerance, pharmacokinetic tolerance, when discussing phenobarbital. This barbiturate has the capacity to stimulate hepatic microsomal enzymes. Since many other drugs are metabolized by the same enzymes, they too are metabolized more quickly. In other situations, pharmacodynamic tolerance can occur in which there are alterations at the receptor level. This is believed to be the case with opiates such as morphine and its receptor, while barbiturates can apparently decrease the number of $GABA_A$ receptors in the brain.

There are several important aspects of the tolerance phenomenon. For some drugs, tolerance will develop to one effect of the drug and not to other effects. For example, with the opiates, tolerance to the euphoric and analgesic effects is routine following chronic use, but less tolerance develops to the respiratory depression that opiates can produce. This has obvious toxicological implications since the opiate abuser is placed in greater jeopardy as the dose required to achieve euphoria becomes elevated, and the margin of safety for inhibition of the respiratory center decreases. Cross-tolerance infers that individuals tolerant to one drug will be tolerant to other drugs in the same class, but not to drugs in other classes. For example, a person tolerant to the sedative effects of one barbiturate will be tolerant to this effect of all barbiturates. However, that individual will not be tolerant to the sedative effects of opiates. A schematic representation of tolerance is shown in Figure 11.13.

Drug dependence

Drug dependence can manifest itself as physiological and/or psychological dependence. Physiological dependence is characterized by a syndrome of signs and symptoms manifested upon withdrawal of the drug. Dependence on drugs of abuse develops only when the drug is administered in sufficiently large doses, at a high enough frequency, and over a long enough period of time. It is believed that excessive bombardment of relevant receptors under these circumstances causes long-lived molecular adaptations in the signaling properties of neurons. Physical dependence is more marked with the opiates and barbiturates than with cocaine or methamphetamine.

The mechanism of addiction and physical dependence formation is probably best understood for the opiate class of drugs. A single dose of opiate is believed to inhibit the firing of neurons in the locus ceruleus (LC) by interacting with their μ-receptors. Long-term opiate administration causes a decrease in μ-opiate receptor signaling in the LC (tolerance) without causing a decrease in the number or affinity of these receptors—thus implicating postreceptor signal transduction mechanisms as the site

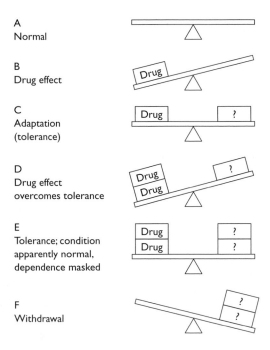

Figure 11.13 Representation of the body's response to an addicting drug that develops tolerance.

of adaptation. The adaptation may involve upregulation of a cAMP cascade leading to increased phosphorylation of a "slow" depolarizing Na^+ channel, producing increased neuronal excitability. This hyperactive state does not become manifested until either the drug is withdrawn or an antagonist is given. The factor believed to be responsible for inducing the hyperexcitable state is cyclicAMP-responsive element-binding protein (CREB).

The withdrawal syndrome for drugs within a pharmacological class is similar, but differs between various drug classes. For example, barbiturate withdrawal is different from opiate withdrawal. A withdrawal syndrome can be precipitated by abrupt cessation of drug use or the administration of a specific antagonist (e.g., nalorphine with morphine). Withdrawal syndromes vary in intensity depending upon the drug class. For example, opiate withdrawal rarely constitutes a medical emergency and is considered far less dangerous than withdrawal from alcohol and barbiturates (i.e., possible death). As drugs within a certain class can produce cross-tolerance, they can also generally support physical dependence produced by other drugs in the same class (i.e., cross-dependence).

Caffeine

The "drug of choice" for most Americans is caffeine. In fact, caffeine is the most widely used psychoactive drug in the world. Many of caffeine's effects are believed to occur because of competitive antagonism at adenosine receptors. Adenosine is a neuromodulator that influences a number of functions in the CNS. The mild sedating

Table 11.6 Approximate amount of caffeine (mg) in a 12-ounce serving

Coffee (200)
Jolt (72)
Josta (59)
Pepsi Kona (56)
Surge (53)
Mountain Dew (52)
Coca-Cola (47)
Pepsi (38)

effects that occur when adenosine activates particular adenosine receptor subtypes can be antagonized by caffeine. Caffeine's stimulant effect in relatively normal doses (100–500 mg) is an arousal of the cerebral cortex, resulting in greater wakefulness, mental alertness, and improved psychomotor functioning.

Caffeine qualifies as an addicting drug because it presents qualities of reinforcement and its withdrawal induces a syndrome of symptoms. These include headache, drowsiness, fatigue, decreased performance, depression, and occasionally nausea and vomiting. Symptoms appear within 12–24 hours of last caffeine use, peak at 20–48 hours, and last about 1 week. Although withdrawal symptoms are more common in moderate to heavy users of caffeine (in excess of three cups of coffee a day), it can also occur with low to moderate intake (235 mg/day, equivalent to 2.5 cups of coffee).

Coffee is not the only source of large doses of caffeine. Chocolate bars, for example, contain approximately 30 mg of caffeine. In addition, over the past 10–15 years soft-drink manufacturers have produced a number of caffeinated beverages including orange juice and water. However, colas remain the principal vehicle to "Feed the Rush." A comparison of caffeine content of various colas is shown in Table 11.6.

Methadone maintenance

One of the unique aspects of physical dependence on heroin is the legal availability of free methadone (a structurally related opiate agonist) through clinics. Methadone is a highly effective analgesic after oral administration. Its use is based on the principle of replacing the addict's heroin with an orally active agonist with a long duration of action. This reduces drug craving in the addict and prevents withdrawal. Methadone is usually supplied on a maintenance basis (chronic use of the same dose) or on a withdrawal basis (gradually reducing the dose over 1–6 months). Because of the inherent difficulties in the withdrawal program most recipients of methadone are in the maintenance program.

The primary objectives of the methadone maintenance programs are the prevention of progressive health deterioration and to keep in touch with drug users. This makes continuous medical supervision more possible. This is particularly important regarding the prevention of a further spread of infectious diseases such as AIDS and hepatitis. Supplying methadone may also enable addicts to live a structured life, which in turn may increase their chances of successful social integration and, possibly, in the long run a drug-free existence.

The United States pioneered the use of methadone in the 1960s and 1970s, but now lags behind much of Europe and Australia in making methadone accessible and effective. Methadone is the best available treatment in terms of reducing illicit heroin use and associated crime, disease, and death. In the early 1990s the National Academy of Sciences Institute of Medicine stated that of all forms of drug treatment, "methadone maintenance has been the most rigorously studied modality and has yielded the most incontrovertibly positive results . . . Consumption of all illicit drugs, especially heroin, declines. Crime is reduced, fewer individuals become HIV positive, and individual functioning is improved."

Popular misconceptions and prejudice, however, have all but prevented any expansion of methadone treatment in the United States. The 115,000 Americans receiving methadone today represent only a small increase over the number receiving treatment 20 years ago. For every 10 heroin addicts, there are only one or two methadone slots available. Efforts to make methadone more available in the United States run up against the many Americans who dismiss methadone treatment as substituting one addictive drug for another and are wary of any treatment that does not fulfill the single-minded, quixotic goal of leaving the patient "drug free."

In 1994, the Swiss carried out an interesting nationwide study to determine whether prescribing heroin, morphine, or injectable methadone could reduce crime, disease, and other drug-related ills. Some 1000 heroin addicts took part in the study. Not surprisingly, the trial quickly determined that virtually all participants preferred heroin, which was subsequently prescribed to them. In the summer of 1997 early data were reported. Criminal offenses and the number of criminal offenders declined by 60 percent, the percentage of income from illegal and semilegal activities fell from 69 to 10 percent, illegal heroin and cocaine use decreased dramatically, stable employment increased from 14 to 32 percent, and physical health improved significantly. There were no deaths from drug overdoses, and no prescription drugs were diverted to the black market. A cost benefit analysis of the program found a net economic benefit of $30 per patient per day (primarily due to reduced criminal justice and health care costs). The results of the Swiss study imply that given relatively unlimited availability, heroin users will voluntarily stabilize or reduce their dosage and some will even choose abstinence, and that long-addicted users can lead relatively normal, stable lives if provided legal access to their drug of choice.

Because of the success achieved with methadone maintenance facilities, similar strategies are being sought to treat other forms of drug dependence. As described later, cocaine has an extremely high addiction liability. Cocaine is basically available in two forms: water-soluble cocaine hydrochloride, which can be given orally, intravenously, or by nasal insufflation, and cocaine free base, which is water insoluble and is usually administered by smoking. The free base is referred to as "crack" cocaine because of the popping sound it makes when the crystals are heated. Crack cocaine is highly desirable to the user because CNS effects are achieved within 1–2 minutes, while "snorting" requires 30–60 minutes to achieve peak effect.

The search for an agent to treat cocaine addiction, one that would not produce euphoria but would still prevent withdrawal, is currently under way. Unfortunately, to date, cocaine dependence has proved to be highly resistant to therapy, primarily because of its powerful reinforcing potency. Recently, however, animal studies have produced what may be a new direction in treating cocaine addiction. As described previously, cocaine activates the mesolimbic dopamine system by preventing the neuronal reuptake of dopamine. Dopamine acts at two general classes of dopamine receptors, termed D_1 and D_2. Studies in the rat indicate that selective agonists for the two receptor sites can produce different effects. Of particular interest is the observation that D_1-like receptor agonists prevent cocaine-seeking behavior while D_2 agonists do the opposite. Further evaluation of this lead may produce a possible pharmacotherapy for cocaine addiction.

An alternative strategy for the treatment of cocaine addiction involves the use of an anticocaine vaccine. Experiments in rats have demonstrated reduced desire for the drug as well as reduced uptake of cocaine into the brain. The vaccine consists of a synthetic cocaine derivative attached to proteins that trigger immune responses to cocaine. The cocaine derivative is not addictive and brain levels of free cocaine were reduced by 40–60 percent in the study. There are approximately 400,000 cocaine abusers in drug-treatment programs in the United States.

Addiction liability

Drugs vary in their propensity to produce dependence. One way to experimentally assess this quality is to expose animals to a behavior paradigm within which the animal can self-administer a drug by pressing a lever attached to a drug delivery system (see Figure 11.14). When exposed to a variety of drugs, one can quantify that a rat or monkey prefers to self-administer certain drugs more than others by recording the number of lever presses over time. Not surprisingly, both the rat and monkey,

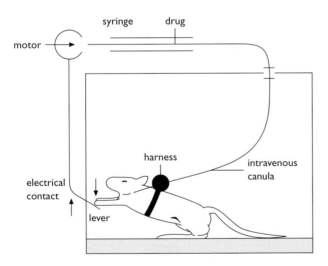

Figure 11.14 Apparatus for self-injection of drugs by laboratory animals. The diagram shows a rat pressing a lever to receive an intravenous injection of the drug contained in the syringe above the cage. Rats and other laboratory animals in this situation will readily self-inject most of the drugs that humans regard as pleasurable, though exceptions include hallucinogens such as lysergic acid diethylamide (LSD). Because there is good agreement between animal and human data, tests such as this can be used to assess the likely "abuse potential" for new drugs.

Table 11.7 Addiction risk of major psychoactive drugs

Drug	Liability index
Cocaine, amphetamine	1
Nicotine	2
Opiates (e.g., morphine, heroin)	2
CNS depressants (e.g., alcohol, barbiturates, benzodiazepines)	3
Cannabis	4
Caffeine	5
Hallucinogens (e.g., LSD, PCP)	5

like humans, prefer psychoactive drugs. The degree to which animals will go to self-administer drugs is illustrated by the fact that, in some cases, monkeys will self-administer cocaine until death. If the drug concentration in the administered solution is reduced, the animals will try to compensate by increasing the frequency of lever presses. Similarly, the animals will lever press more frequently if they begin to go into withdrawal. A comparison of psychoactive drugs assessed in this type of situation is shown in Table 11.7 (a liability index of 1 is the highest).

What drives addictive behavior? There are many laboratories pursuing this question, with the attendant expenditure of significant resources. The rationale is that if we can understand the neurobiological factors driving this type of deleterious behavior, the scientific community may be able to develop efficacious pharmacological agents to combat the problem. At the present time, a popular model revolves around certain "reward pathway centers" (mentioned previously) in the brain. These are, basically, dopaminergic neurons in the ventral tegmental area projecting into the nucleus accumbens in the forebrain and onto the prefrontal cortex, an area involved in learning. New data indicate that dopamine release within the brain highlights, or draws attention to, certain significant or surprising events. These include not only those the organism finds rewarding, such as consuming a tasty morsel of food, but also events that predict rewards. By underscoring such events the dopamine signal helps the animal learn to recognize them.

These natural reward centers have developed over the course of evolution to reinforce useful behaviors (e.g., pleasure, sexual satisfaction, eating, and drinking). It is believed that drugs such as cocaine and amphetamine directly stimulate these centers, while opiates free the pathways from inhibitory control. Nicotine, on the other hand, reaches the brain in as little as 10–20 seconds, where it stimulates nicotine receptors to cause dopaminergic neurons to release large quantities of dopamine. After a few hours, dopamine levels decline, causing withdrawal symptoms to readily appear (e.g., anxiety, irritability, and inattentiveness). When cigarette smokers say they need a smoke to steady their nerves, what they really mean is that they have to contend with nicotine withdrawal.

The development of pharmacological strategies to deal with addiction is not limited to those described above. In 1996, the FDA approved a nicotine nasal spray as a treatment for adults trying to quit smoking. The efficacy of the nicotine nasal spray is comparable to other smoking cessation products such as nicotine gum or patches (which are now available OTC). It is recommended that patients use the nasal spray

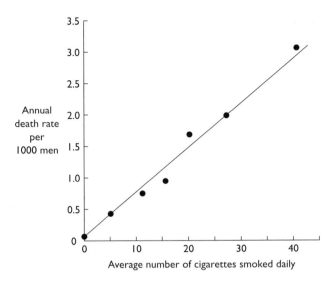

Figure 11.15 Number of cigarettes smoked daily and death rate from lung cancer.
Source: R. Doll and A. B. Hill (1964), *British Medical Journal* 1: 1399–1410.

for 3 months. Because nicotine is highly addictive, it is possible to become addicted to the nasal spray. Patients' chances of becoming dependent on the nasal spray increase if they use it longer than 6 months (its recommended maximum duration of usage). Nor surprisingly, most people using the spray experience nasal or sinus irritation. Approximately $500 million is spent annually in the United States on nicotine replacement patches and gum, yet these quitting aids do not work for most smokers. For example, about 80 percent return to smoking after removing the patch.

In the late 1990s, a new approach to nicotine addiction was introduced. It involves the use of an antidepressant known by its generic name as bupropion. Bupropion is believed to act like nicotine in that it apparently can boost brain levels of dopamine as well as norepinephrine. Some patients have successfully terminated drug therapy after a few months with no ill effects.

According to 1997 figures, 25 percent of the adult population in the United States cannot or will not give up the habit of smoking cigarettes, despite the knowledge that smoking causes cancer, heart disease, and numerous other health problems. Quite a testament to the addictive liability of nicotine. The financial cost that drug addition extracts from society is, of course, very high. For cigarettes alone, it has been estimated that the average annual excess medical costs incurred per smoker compared to non-smoker is approaching $1000; total annual value of lost productivity and disability time related to smoking is approximately $50 billion; total deaths in the United States per year attributed to smoking in excess of 400,000. The relationship of cigarette consumption to mortality rate in males has been known for years and is shown in Figure 11.15.

Addiction has been defined by some as a chronic, relapsing disease of the brain. If this is an accurate portrayal, then there are numerous implications for society, including altering our criminal justice strategies as well as medical treatment. If we know that criminals are drug addicted, it may no longer be reasonable to simply incarcerate them. If they have a brain disease, imprisoning them without treatment would appear to be a futile expedient. Understanding addiction as a brain disease can also affect how society approaches and deals with addicted individuals. Society has learned to deal with people in different brain states such as schizophrenia and Alzheimer's disease. As recently as the beginning of this century, individuals with schizophrenia were institutionalized in prison-like asylums. If, in fact, the brain were the core of the addiction problem, then it would appear reasonable to approach the brain's needs as a central part of the solution.

WAR ON DRUGS

A predictable consequence of the illicit use of psychoactive drugs is the imposition of societal "guidelines" as to what constitutes their licit or illicit use. In this context, a more accurate title for this section might read "War on Some Drugs." Those drugs that are licit in our society, such as alcohol and tobacco, which have arguably more undesirable qualities than many illicit drugs, have, of course, enjoyed a somewhat exempt status historically. While alcohol use can certainly involve legal sanctions, its use has basically been decriminalized with an emphasis placed on restriction of use. Tobacco has enjoyed even less governmental regulation of use (although this has been changing; see Appendix). If you are "legally of age," you can buy the drug unsupervised from a vending machine. In both cases, sale of the drug occurs despite governmental health warnings either on the package itself or in close proximity to the site of purchase and/or consumption.

If there is to be a war, of any kind, one would presume that it could be justified on some rational basis. Perhaps the three main historical reasons typically cited to justify wars are a perceived threat, some driving "moral principle," or the desire for more geographical territory. Obviously, the latter factor is not involved in our country's war on drugs. Therefore, the energy for our government's position probably emanates from the first two and it might be instructive to examine some of the relevant issues. For example, how successful has the war on drugs been? In 1988 Congress passed a resolution proclaiming its goal of "a drug-free America by 1995." Despite this obviously absurd declaration, as subsequent history has shown, the beat goes on. Politicians refuse to deal with the reality of illicit drug use as a disease for fear of being labeled "soft" on drugs, and continue to increase the "Drug Czars'" budget to ludicrous proportions, all to appease the well-intentioned conservative members of society.

So, how many people actually use illegal drugs? Obviously, this is a very difficult question to answer with certainty. Because of this, there are disparate figures in the literature. All of them are subject to a certain degree of skepticism. For example, the federal government's Household Survey on Drug Abuse, conducted annually, is probably the most commonly cited set of statistics (including that by the Drug Enforcement Agency) on the prevalence of drug use. According to the 1994 survey, there were approximately 12.6 million people who indicated they had used some illegal drug in the past month and perhaps 30–40 million who had used some illegal drug within the past year. Of the 12.6 million who used an illegal drug within the

Table 11.8 Number of yearly drug-related deaths in the United States

Drug	Deaths
Tobacco	400,000
Alcohol	80,000
Cocaine	2200
Heroin	2000
Aspirin	2000

Source: NIDA research monographs.

Note
No reported deaths due to marijuana.

past month, approximately 10 million were presumed to be casual drug users, and approximately 2.6 million classified as addicts.

It should be appreciated that these data are generated by making random phone calls to the public. Therefore, only people who have phones and answer them are included in the study. In addition, the respondents are essentially being asked if they have committed a felony. Other surveys of drug use have put the number at twice as high. Obviously, there are no highly precise, accurate data available on this important question. This lack of hard data is one of the problems associated with attempting to establish an appropriate drug policy.

While the question of prevalence is an important criterion, it would also be helpful if there were some statistics relating to the dangers of illicit drug use. We mentioned previously that there are some addiction data relating to animal research models as well as rating scales devised by experts in the field. These generally result in a drug profile characterized by the following sequence, in order of decreasing addiction liability, of some common drugs: heroin, cocaine, alcohol, nicotine, caffeine, and marijuana.

The ultimate undesirable property of a drug is its propensity to take human life. Interestingly, if we look at data published by the National Institute of Drug Abuse (Table 11.8), we see that tobacco and alcohol are by far associated with death with the highest frequency. It is also interesting to note that all illegal drugs combined are responsible for approximately 1 percent of the total number killed by alcohol and tobacco. It has been estimated that tobacco is responsible for killing more people each year than all of the people killed by all of the illegal drugs in the last century.

Often, before people die, it is necessary that they spend a considerable amount of time in the hospital with all of the attendant costs. Both alcohol and tobacco play significant roles in this regard. In fact, a series of lawsuits were generated in the 1990s by several states with this in mind. It is the states' contention that tobacco companies should be held liable for health costs caused by their products, and they should be required to compensate the states for this expense (see Appendix). The city of San Francisco has also taken this position.

How effective has the war on drugs been? Three important criteria addressing this question have to do with illicit drug availability, the prevalence of their use, and the incarceration rate of violators. With regard to availability, the Rand Corporation's

Table 11.9 Average price and purity of cocaine in the United States, 1981–1996

	Price per pure gram ($)	Purity (%)
1981	275.12	47.53
1985	212.50	55.00
1989	105.09	76.75
1993	110.45	72.01
1996	94.52	68.61

Source: *System To Retrieve Information From Drug Evidence*, DEA, 1981–1996.

Table 11.10 Average price and purity of heroin in the United States, 1981–1996

	Price per pure gram ($)	Purity (%)
1981	3374.40	6.73
1985	2652.71	14.16
1989	1457.89	30.31
1993	1404.20	37.20
1996	1126.57	41.48

Source: *System to Retrieve Information From Drug Evidence*, DEA, 1981–1996.

1988 analysis of drug interdiction effectiveness at the border and the General Accounting Office's 1991 report on cocaine flow indicate that the answer is, virtually no effect at all. This is further substantiated by the government's 1994 survey of illicit drug use, which actually demonstrates an increase. According to a 1997 General Accounting Office study, over the 7 years that began in 1988, "farmers planted new coca [plants] faster than existing crops were eradicated." Despite costing billions of dollars and half a dozen lives over 7 years, international drug eradication efforts have not reduced the supply of illegal drugs. In fact, cost has gone down while availability has gone up (Tables 11.9 and 11.10). Obviously, if drug availability were significantly curtailed, this negative correlation would not be expected. Despite this information, government expenditures on various aspects of interdiction continue to increase.

One statistic that might be referred to as indicating "success" of the war on drugs is the number of drug-related incarcerated prisoners in the United States. Between 1926 and 1970, according to the Department of Justice, the total prison population (state and federal) remained quite consistent at approximately 200,000 per year. However, in the 20-year period between 1974 and 1994 the corresponding prison population increased approximately sevenfold to 1.4 million, according to Uniform Crime Reports of the Federal Bureau of Investigation. This era coincided with the successive administrations of Presidents Nixon, Reagan, and Bush, all proponents of the war on drugs theme. One can, of course, also conclude that these data indicate exactly the opposite; that is, because of greater market demand and availability, the number of "users" and "sellers" in their respective pools increased in a corresponding manner.

Carrying out a war is always expensive. In 1980 the federal budget for drug control was approximately $1 billion, and state and local budgets were approximately two or three times that. By 1997, the federal budget had ballooned to $16 billion, two-thirds of it for law enforcement agencies, and state and local funding to at least that. On any day in 1980, approximately 50,000 people were behind bars for violating a drug law. By 1997, the number had increased to approximately 400,000.

According to a Justice Department study, 30,099 people were charged with federal drug offenses in 1999, more than double the number 15 years earlier, and, significantly, most of those convicted were drug traffickers. The study reported that only 4 percent were convicted of simple possession. It also found that drug offenders are serving longer sentences. The average prison stay rose to 5.5 years in 1999 from 2.5 years in 1986. Drug prosecutions made up 32 percent of the federal criminal caseload in 1999 compared with 18 percent in 1984.

The above data are mirrored in the experience of the state of California. During the 1980s, California achieved the highest incarceration rate in the world, exceeding South Africa and the Soviet Union. In 1980 there were 23,726 inmates in California prisons. By 1992, the prison populations jumped to 102,554 (approximately 32 percent for drug law violators) as 18 new prisons were built. A corresponding effect was an increase in the total number of employees working in the Department of Corrections to 30,800, or approximately one for every three inmates. At that time, the average total yearly custodial expense to maintain an inmate was $22,000.

Drug War theory holds that harsh punishments can make inner-city high-school students graduate and accept minimum wages rather than drop out and clear $1500 a week selling drugs. It assumes Columbians can be forced to give up $500 an acre for producing coca leaves and accept $5 for growing coffee beans. For the smuggler, the profits are even more attractive. One kilogram of heroin is worth $11,000 in Columbia. In Miami, heroin sells for between $50,000 and $70,000—three times as much as a kilogram of cocaine. Drug War theory proposes that enlarging prisons and filling them to overflowing will crush a very profitable industry. Capitalism theory and the Drug War theory are mutually exclusive. One may be true and the other false, or they may both be false, but they cannot possibly both be true.

In 1936, August Vollmer, a leading expert on American policing, spoke on drugs: "Repression has driven this vice underground and produced the narcotic smugglers and supply agents who have grown wealthy . . . Drug addiction is not a police problem: it never has and never can be solved by policemen. It is first and last a medical problem." In June 1995 the European Parliament issued a report acknowledging that "there will always be demand for drugs in our societies . . . the policies followed so far have not been able to prevent illegal drug trade from flourishing."

In closing, the following should be pointed out. In February 2002, President Bush announced two important new aspects of his drug policy. First, instead of making an absurd, unrealistic date to win the war on drugs, his goal is to reduce illegal drug use by 10 percent in 2 years. This appears more realistic. Second, instead of the "Just Say No" campaign of the 1980s, the Bush administration is pushing a policy that in essence reads, "Please get help." This represents a significant alteration in emphasis from punishment to assistance. As part of the $19.2 billion to fight illegal drugs in the fiscal year 2002–2003, budgetary increases will go toward drug treatment and research. As part of Bush's historic announcement, he declared: "We must aggressively promote drug treatment because a nation that is tough on drugs must also be compassionate to those addicted to drugs." Serious and welcome words indeed.

Decriminalization

The United States is not the only country in the world with a drug "problem." How have other countries dealt with the situation and is there anything instructive we can gain from their experience? Probably the most interesting current situation involves the Netherlands. Like many other European countries, the Netherlands is a signatory of the Frankfurt Accord, which adopts decriminalization as the primary approach to drugs. The primary objective of Dutch drug policy has always been health protection rather than incarceration. Therefore, drug legislation in the Netherlands is quite different than in the United States.

Although the harm done to society is taken into consideration, a great effort is made by the Dutch to prevent criminal prosecution from being more damaging to the individual drug user than the drug itself. Since 1976 (the Baan Commission), the goal of Dutch policy is to maintain a distinction between the market for "soft" drugs (i.e., cannabis products such as hashish and marijuana) and the market for "harder" substances such as heroin and cocaine. Criminal penalties for and police efforts against heroin trafficking were increased while those against cannabis were relaxed. The Dutch approach is part of a long tradition of "gedoogbeleid"—the formal, systematic application of discretion.

The Dutch goal is achieved by allowing some limited freedom of movement for the retail trade and possession of small quantities of soft drugs for personal use. However, possession of even soft drugs for commercial purposes outside of regulated outlets is considered a serious offense. For example, for soft drugs the maximum penalty for possession, selling, or production of approximately 1 ounce is detention for 1 month and/or a fine of approximately $3125. In comparison, the maximum penalty for hard drugs varies from 1 year imprisonment (and/or a $6250 fine), for the possession of "consumer amounts," to 12 years imprisonment (and/or a $62,500 fine) for import and export. The maximum penalties may be increased by one-third if the crime has been committed more than once.

Over the years, Dutch flexibility regarding drug regulations has led to the establishment of so-called "coffee shops" where the commercial sale of soft drugs is not prosecuted if certain regulations are observed. These rules of operation include no advertising, no sales to individuals under 16 years of age, no "hard" drugs in or near the premises, and no breach of "decorum," and they are permitted only in certain specified sections of the community. Interestingly, the fact that cannabis is relatively easy to obtain in the coffee shops has not resulted in a larger consumption increase than in other countries. In fact the opposite occurs. For example, in the Netherlands, the teenagers are less likely to sample marijuana than their American peers; from 1992 to 1994 only 7.2 percent of Dutch youths between the ages of 12 and 15 reported having tried marijuana, compared to 13.5 percent of Americans in the same age range.

According to Dutch police estimates, there were between 1200 and 1500 coffee shops in the Netherlands in 1991. Most of these coffee shops offer a wide range of hashish and marijuana products from various countries and of varying quality. Prices in 1995 ranged from 10 to 15 Dutch guilders per gram (approximately $175 to $270 per ounce) compared with a street price of approximately $400 per ounce in the United States.

The trend toward decriminalization of cannabis has accelerated in Europe. Across much of Western Europe, possession and even minor sales of the drug are effectively decriminalized. Spain decriminalized private use of cannabis in 1983. In Germany, the Federal Constitutional Court effectively sanctioned a cautious liberalization of cannabis in a 1994 decision. In Australia, cannabis has been decriminalized in several states. By contrast, in 1996 in the United States, 641,642 people were arrested for marijuana, 85 percent of them for possession, not sale, of the drug. Add to this the discrepancy in sentences for crack use and for powdered cocaine use. In the United States, a person caught with just 5 grams of crack gets a mandatory prison sentence of 5 years, with no chance of parole. It takes 500 grams of powder-cocaine to trigger the same response. Is a 100 to 1 ratio the result of rational thinking or discretion?

The United State's "drug-free" mentality can also be seen in its myopic approach to needle exchange *vis-à-vis* the Europeans. The spread of HIV among people who inject drugs illegally was what prompted governments in Europe to experiment with harm-reduction policies. During the 1980s health officials realized that infected users were spreading HIV by sharing needles. Having already experienced a hepatitis epidemic attributed to the same mode of transmission, the Dutch were the first to tell drug users about the risks of needle sharing and to make sterile syringes available and collect dirty needles through pharmacies and other facilities. Governments elsewhere in Europe soon followed suit. Local authorities in Germany, Switzerland, and other countries authorized needle exchange machines to ensure 24-hour access. In some European cities, addicts can exchange used syringes for clean ones at local police stations without fear of prosecution or harassment.

Despite the logic of the needle exchange program the United States has refused to adopt it; this even though AIDS was the leading killer of Americans aged 25 to 44 for most of the 1990s. In 1991 the National AIDS Commission appointed by President Bush called the lack of federal support for such programs "bewildering and tragic." In 1993 a CDC-sponsored review of research on needle exchange recommended federal funding, but officials in the Clinton administration de-emphasized a favorable evaluation of the report within the Department of Health and Human Services. In July 1996 President Clinton's Advisory Council on HIV/AIDS criticized the administration for its failure to heed the National Academy of Sciences' recommendation that it authorize the use of federal money to support needle exchange programs. An independent panel convened by the National Institute of Health reached the same conclusion in 1997. In 1998 the American Medical Association, the American Bar Association, the World Bank, and the U.S. Conference of Mayors endorsed the concept of needle exchange. The United State's failure to adopt needle exchange programs as national policy has resulted in the infection of an estimated 10,000 people with AIDS.

DRUGS IN SPORTS

Background

In addition to the "recreational" use of illegal drugs, one of the more "creative" uses of drugs is to improve athletic performance. While the use of performance-enhancing drugs in the world of sports is not really drug abuse in the common use of the term, it does involve the illicit use of "banned" substances. Therefore, it is appropriate to include a discussion of this topical subject in this particular section. It is an issue that constantly appears in the headlines.

Viewed objectively, we seem to have a somewhat schizophrenic attitude toward the various components that can make up an athletic event. Let's examine the situation. Basically, an athletic event is composed of athlete + equipment + conditions = performance. Humans have constantly striven to improve athletic performance. Which of the factors have people attempted to modify in order to improve athletic performance? First, how about conditions? One of the most significant developments in the history of sprinting is the rubberized track. Ask any runner if their times are faster on a rubberized track and he/she will laugh. Why was the rubber track developed? How about equipment? The world record in the pole vault increased 9 inches the year the fiberglass pole was introduced. You either used the fiberglass pole or you were finished in the pole vault event. No amount of training by human pole-vaulters could have achieved the same unprecedented increase in height. Was there an outcry from purists? There are other numerous examples of equipment changes including starting blocks, lighter shoes with sharper spikes, electrical timing, and the use of "rabbits." One of the few physiological factors that some athletes are able to legally utilize is training or performing at high altitude (Bob Beamon's long-jump record set in Mexico City in 1968 lasted for approximately 25 years, an unprecedented duration). Creatine monohydrate is routinely taken as an athletic performance enhancer because it is believed to restore muscle function. "Carbohydrate loading" is also practiced in order to increase the amount of glycogen stored in the muscles, thereby increasing endurance. Why not use drugs?

History

Among the earliest reported uses of drugs to enhance performance is by the ancient Scandinavian warriors called the Berserkers. The Berserkers were reputed to be invulnerable, of enormous strength, and filled with a wild frenzy in battle. These qualities were ascribed to the consumption of mushrooms containing muscarine and other psychoactive alkaloids before battle. The use of drugs in the Olympics is not new and dates back to before Christ when Greek Olympians attempted to elevate their performance levels by eating bread soaked in opium. As mentioned previously, Peruvian Indians have chewed coca leaves for centuries in order to sustain strenuous work and athletic ability.

After amphetamine, strychnine, and ephedrine became commercially available in the 1800s, there shortly followed reports of their abuse by canal swimmers and cyclists in Europe and the United States. In 1886 a French cyclist became the first known athlete to die from performance-enhancing drugs (in this case cocaine plus heroin). In the 1904 Olympic Games marathon in St Louis, an American reportedly sped to victory aided by a preparation of egg whites, brandy, and strychnine. One might wonder why an individual would use a component now used in rat poison to increase performance. At that time, however, strychnine was used because of its crude excitatory effect on the CNS, which we now know is due to blocking inhibitory glycinergic fibers in the spinal cord. Despite strychnine's crude pharmacological properties, it still appears to be used to a certain extent. As recently as 1992, the presence of strychnine metabolites in the urine of a Confederation of Independent States athlete caused her disqualification from the Olympic Games marathon.

Stimulant abuse escalated until the mid-1960s when more rigid antidoping and drug testing laws were introduced. In 1968, the International Olympic Committee (IOC) introduced drug testing for the first time at the Winter Games in Grenoble, France. In the same year, the Kentucky Derby winner, Dancer's Image, was disqualified for having received the anti-inflammatory drug phenylbutazone. During the early 1970s, the "Sunday Syndrome" was described in the United States, referring to the use of amphetamine and anabolic steroids in the National Football League (NFL). The NFL banned the use of amphetamine in 1971.

The term doping is believed to have evolved from the Dutch word *doop* that denotes viscous opium juice. The word became modified to become dope, referring to any stupefying substance, while today it has a more general meaning. The IOC's Medical Commission (established in 1967) defines its doping policy as consisting of two parts: (1) a ban on the administration of substances belonging to selected classes of pharmacological agents; and (2) a ban on the use of various doping methods. The original concept was to ban only substances that clearly enhanced performance. When reports appeared that certain drugs could seriously impair performance and render competitors vulnerable to injury (e.g., narcotics), medical safety became a rationale. In 1998 Juan Antonio Samaranch, then president of the IOC, rocked the sports world when he stated that if a drug only improved performance and was not deleterious to health it was *not* doping. When some organizations added marijuana to their lists, social acceptability became a rationale. Although not explicitly banned by the IOC, the National Collegiate Athletics Association (NCAA) and various national governing bodies ban marijuana. Marijuana has no performance-enhancing potential and, in fact, it has been shown that performance skills can be impaired for as long as 24–36 hours after marijuana usage. The IOC's list of banned substances has now reached approximately 150.

The doping classes include stimulants, narcotics, anabolic agents, diuretics, and peptide and glycopeptide hormones and analogs. Because the banning of drugs is by class, no substances belonging to the banned classes may be used even if they are not specifically listed. For this reason, the term "and related substances" is also used. With only two exceptions (caffeine and testosterone) the mere detection of the substance is grounds for disciplinary action. In the case of caffeine, the definition of a "positive" is if the concentration in the urine exceeds 12 µg/ml. Present technology allows routine detection of drugs at the picogram level (10^{-12} g).

Stimulants

As indicated earlier, amphetamine, cocaine, and strychnine dominated early doping incidents until the introduction of testing. Amphetamines were initially commercially available for OTC use as a nasal decongestant. During World War II, amphetamines were used as a means of delaying the onset of fatigue and increasing alertness in soldiers. Subsequently, amphetamines became prominent as an appetite suppressant and as a drug to ward off sleepiness.

The first dope-testing program at a major sporting event, a cycle race in France, revealed positive urinalysis tests in over 20 percent of the competitors. Not surprisingly, experience has shown that runners, swimmers, speed skaters, and cyclists account for most of the problems with stimulants. The efficacy of stimulants as ergogenic agents in these athletes is undoubtedly due to their ability to delay the onset of fatigue, primarily via CNS effects. For example, cyclists receiving 250 mg of amphetamine before and during monitored cycling achieved a 7 percent increase in work productivity while reporting that they were not working harder. Unfortunately, this beneficial effect does not come without a potential price. For example, the death of a Danish cyclist in 1960 is believed to be due to the peripheral vasoconstrictor effect of amphetamine (i.e., decreased heat loss leading to "sunstroke"). With regard to cocaine, the few studies that exist suggest that little to no performance gains are incurred from cocaine. In 1985, 17 percent of NCAA student-athletes reported having used cocaine; by 1997, that figure was down to 1.5 percent. Unlike amphetamine, cocaine is readily metabolized in the body to its major metabolite, benzoylecgonine. In fact, it is benzoylecgonine that is tested for in urine.

Successful detection of the "old-guard" drugs inevitably led to the use of alternative stimulant drugs such as caffeine, phenylpropanolamine, and ephedrine. Because these drugs are commonly found in OTC medications, this obviously presents a problem for the competitor who is taking the medication for legitimate health reasons. This conundrum still represents one of the most complicated aspects of regulating drug use among athletes. Therefore, athletes are warned not to use this type of preparation without first checking with a pharmacist or medical doctor that their medications do not contain any of the banned stimulants.

One of the most tragic episodes relating to the use of "stimulants" during the Olympics is that of Rick DeMont. In 1972, as a 16-year-old, DeMont won the 400-meter freestyle in Munich. However, a urinalysis revealed the presence of ephedrine that DeMont had been taking as an asthma medication. DeMont was required to return his gold medal (his father mailed the medal to IOC headquarters paying the postage himself) and was prohibited from swimming in the 1500-meter freestyle, his best event. Should he have been disqualified? According to IOC rules, yes. However, what about pharmacological rules?

The amount of ephedrine that DeMont had taken was equivalent to 10 mg of amphetamine. Studies during the 1950s, supported by the American Medical Association, had indicated that as much as 20 mg of amphetamine failed to improve swimming performance of 440-yard swimmers (the equivalent of 400 meters). One report concluded that the "findings do not prove that athletes performing in intercollegiate meets would be helped by amphetamine." Even if DeMont had gained some pharmacological effect (i.e., ergogenic) from the ephedrine, the presence of an additional component normally present in the medication (hydroxyzine) would have been expected to produce a sedative effect, thus operating in the opposite direction.

The recurrence of a similar situation was avoided in 1996. An 18-year-old American swimmer about to compete in the qualifying meet for the Olympic team realized that he had taken a dose of his asthma medication (prednisone) too close to the event. Knowing that it would be detected, he chose to withdraw from the meet, saying he would wait another 4 years.

Among the stimulant class of drugs are a group of drugs known as beta-2 agonists. These are drugs commonly taken to treat asthma (they are bronchodilators). Two such drugs are salbutamol and terbutaline. These drugs are permitted to be used by athletes by inhaler only and their use must be declared to the appropriate medical authority. Presumably, the use of aerosol administration is permitted because less of the drug will be administered and it will be localized in the airways.

Narcotics

This class of drugs, of which morphine is the prototype, includes many powerful analgesics and is mainly used medically for the management of severe pain. There is evidence that such drugs have been abused in sports, creating a false sense of prowess beyond the athlete's inherent ability, particularly if injured. The IOC has banned them entirely, even their legitimate use as painkillers. A range of alternative painkillers exists, although less efficacious, including aspirin and ibuprofen. Athletes are also cautioned against some OTC preparations, including certain cough and cold remedies, which include banned substances such as the antitussive drug dextromethorphan.

Anabolic agents

Stimulant and anabolic agents are the two classes of drugs most frequently used in the sports world to enhance performance. The principal group of anabolic drugs is the anabolic androgenic steroids (AASs). The AAS class includes the natural male hormone testosterone and structural derivatives of it. More than 40 synthetic derivatives have been developed that can be taken orally or parenterally. The derivatives have been developed for legitimate medical purposes to increase their anabolic/androgenic ratio for the treatment of such disorders as bone marrow failure and certain anemias. In addition, they can induce significant increases in skeletal muscle mass and strength. In a well-controlled (diet, exercise), 10-week double-blind study, published in 1996, moderately high doses of testosterone enanthate resulted in an average gain of 13 pounds of virtually pure muscle in men who could bench press an extra 48 pounds.

One of the problems with this group of drugs is that they all retain some androgenic activity, which is largely responsible for their side effects. For example, in males AASs decrease the size of the testes, diminish sperm production, and produce impotence. Females experience masculinization, loss of breast tissue, clitoral hypertrophy, hirsutism, deepening of the voice, and diminished menstruation. In 1972 when the dominant East German women's swimming coach was asked about his swimmers' low voices he replied that he was concerned with swimming, not singing. To counteract these side effects, scientists manufactured steroids that retain their anabolic effects but have much lower androgenic effects (e.g., androstenedione and nandrolone).

The East German swimmers used androstenedione in the 1980s to improve their performances. It was banned by the IOC in 1997, but is permitted by some sporting bodies such as Major League Baseball (Mark McGuire admitted using the drug in 1999 when he broke Roger Maris' home run record). Nandrolone was allegedly detected in a urine sample provided by British sprinter and Olympic gold medallist Linford Christie in 1999.

In addition to the East Germans, perhaps the widest use of AASs in swimming has been by the Chinese. During the early 1990s, their female swimmers produced remarkable results including domination of the 1992 Olympics. This continued at the World Championships in Rome in 1994 when they won 12 of 16 gold medals.

However, in 1994 seven Chinese swimmers tested positive for steroid use. As a result of this, China was excluded from the Pan Pacific Games in 1995. Their overall weak performance in the sprints at the 1996 Games in Atlanta suggests that the use of AASs was eliminated.

The use of AASs by teenagers can stunt growth. This is particularly significant since surveys indicate that 5–12 percent of high-school boys reportedly use AASs in the United States. One of the youngest athletes to fail a drug test was the 14-year-old South African runner Lisa de Villiers. She tested positive for the AAS nandrolone. In addition to the side effects listed above, AASs have been reported to be associated with a significant increase in aggressiveness both in men and women. In men, this is sometimes referred to as "roid rage." However, in the 1996 study alluded to above, psychological tests and questioning of the men's spouses found no evidence that steroids made them angrier or more aggressive. It should be noted that the duration of that study was only 10 weeks, however.

Although banned by the IOC in 1974, AASs have been continued to be used. Among the more notable examples is the disqualification of Ben Johnson at the 1988 Seoul Olympic Games. Johnson, whose urine contained metabolites of the anabolic steroid stanazalol, had won the 100-meter dash gold medal in world record time. He was disqualified and his medal returned. Johnson was subsequently banned for life following another positive test, of another nature (discussed later), in 1993.

In addition to being disqualified for having an AAS detected, an athlete can also be disqualified for having alterations in hormonal balances. For example, the presence of a testosterone to epitestosterone ratio (T:E) greater than 6 to 1 in the urine of a competitor constitutes a *prima facie* violation (unless there is evidence that the ratio is due to a physiological or pathological condition—the likelihood of which appears to be < 1.0 percent). The use of this particular test is based upon the following biochemistry. Epitestosterone is a nonmetabolite, stereoisomer of testosterone with no known physiological function normally produced in a fixed ratio to testosterone. Therefore, an elevated ratio above 6 indicates exogenous administration of an AAS. It was this parameter that led to Johnson's lifetime ban, not simply detection of an AAS per se. In order to circumvent this testing procedure, athletes have learned to take the "epi" form in carefully calibrated doses to maintain a "normal" ratio.

The use of AASs involves high doses that exceed the medical replacement dose by 10–100-fold depending upon the sport (swimmers use lower doses while weight and power lifters use the most). Simultaneous use of several AASs is common. Most users begin with one oral drug and then add others either orally or by injection. This regimen, known as "stacking," can include as many as 14 drugs or more. Another strategy involves "cycling," when the drugs are taken for 14–18 weeks followed by a break. The former East Germans were the acknowledged experts on the use of AASs and actually developed a testosterone nasal spray under their state plan 14.25. Unlike earlier oil-based injectable forms of testosterone, newer water-soluble oral AASs can wash out of an athlete's system in days, making detection more problematic.

Another type of drug classified as an anabolic agent is actually a beta-2 agonist (the same type of drug used to treat asthma discussed above). Clenbuterol is the prototypic drug. Its use by athletes emanates from use of the drug in the livestock industry to promote growth. Its efficacy in humans is highly questionable. However, the innocent consumption of clenbuterol-treated meat could conceivably lead to disqualification, if detected, since it is banned. This is a conceivable situation since one study has shown that the urine of four of eight men who consumed chicken injected with an AAS tested positive 24 hours later. In a somewhat more domestic situation, a Russian weightlifter, Aleksey Petrov, won the 1995 World Championship but tested positive for a banned substance and received a lifetime suspension. Fortunately, a former girlfriend later confessed in writing that she had slipped the substance into his food. Petrov was reinstated and won a gold medal in Atlanta.

Although not within the AAS class, female hormones have also been used to feminize males so they can compete in women's events. A "female" gold medal sprinter in the 1964 Olympics was shown by chromosome testing to be a male; she/he was required to return the medal. Cyproterone, an antiandrogenic agent, is suspected of having been used to delay puberty in females. This is particularly important in female gymnastics since puberty shifts the center of gravity lower in the body and changes body proportions. The top three Soviet gymnasts in international competition in 1978 were 17 or 18 years old but their height and weight were 53 inches, 63 pounds; 60 inches, 92 pounds; and 57 inches, 79 pounds.

Diuretics

Drugs in this class have been creatively used by athletes for two reasons. First, they promote rapid urine excretion, thus increasing the urinary clearance of drugs primarily eliminated via this mechanism. In this way, they can be used in an attempt to conceal evidence of the misuse of other drugs in subsequent urinalysis tests. Second, diuretics can be used to achieve rapid weight loss. In sports in which competitions are in weight classes, such as boxing and wrestling, this can give an unfair advantage if taken before weigh-in. For this reason, the IOC reserves the right to take urine samples from competitors in these sports at the time of weigh-in.

Other drugs affecting renal function are also banned. For example, "masking agents" such as probenecid have been used to prevent the tubular secretion of AASs in order to minimize their urinary detection. On February 17, 1998, an Australian National Swimming Team member tested positive for probenecid. He had received the drug 3 days previously to prolong the action of penicillin for the treatment of a respiratory infection. Probenecid was a banned substance because it had been used in the past to prolong the effects of AASs. Neither the swimmer nor the physician involved knew the drug was banned. After an Australian Swimming Inc. Disciplinary Committee hearing on March 28, 1998, it was decided that the swimmer had taken probenecid inadvertently and solely for therapeutic purposes. Nevertheless, on May 5, 1998, the Australian Olympic Committee remarkably imposed its own ban of 3 months and a fine of $6500. This in a country with a relatively rational view of drugs.

Because the original use of probenecid by athletes was in amounts that far exceeded therapeutic doses it was extremely easy to detect. Because of its ease of detection dishonest athletes no longer use it. Detected small amounts, as occurred with the Australian swimmer, only indicates therapeutic use. Once again the pharmacological voice of reason was muted.

Another substance classified as a masking agent is epitestosterone (mentioned earlier). Once athletes and/or their trainers realized that a T:E ratio in excess of 6 could be grounds for disqualification, they attacked the problem in a straightforward manner by simply administering more epitestosterone. The counterresponse of the regulatory agencies to this cat-and-mouse game has been to consider an absolute epitestosterone level of greater than 200 ng/ml grounds for further investigation.

Miscellaneous drugs

It has been mentioned previously that certain types of beta agonists have been taken to enhance performance. Beta blockers were originally developed to reduce blood pressure and heart rate in cardiac patients (see Chapter 12). They have been widely used clinically to control hypertension, cardiac arrhymias, and angina. Some competitors in sports have also used beta blockers where physical activity is of little or no importance. For example, they have found use in shooting and archery where their calming effect can be advantageous. Even a slight reduction in heart rate can be beneficial in maintaining a bead on a target. Although they are unlikely to be of benefit to athletes in sports where physical exertion and endurance are required, the IOC reserves the right to test for these substances in those events it deems appropriate. However, beta blockers would be expected to limit performance in aerobic endurance events.

It is well known that the administration to males of human chorionic gonadotropin and other compounds with related activity leads to an increased production of endogenous androgenic steroids and is considered equivalent to the exogenous administration of testosterone. Corticotropin (the adrenal stimulatory trophic hormone) has been misused in an attempt to increase the blood level of endogenous corticosteroids in order to achieve their euphoric effect. The utilization of corticotropin is considered to be equivalent to the oral, intramuscular, or intravenous administration of corticosteroids. According to the Council for Prevention of Drug Use, 45 percent of riders in the 2000 Tour De France tested positive for drug use. Of the positive tests 28 were for corticosteroids.

The misuse of human growth hormone (hGH) in sport is unethical and dangerous because of various adverse effects. For example, cardiomyopathy, hypertension, diabetes mellitus, and acromegaly can occur when hGH is given in high doses for a long period of time. In addition, whether or not hGH can enhance athletic performance is highly speculative. Substances that act as releasing factors for corticotropin and hGH are also banned. In 1996 the IOC launched a $2 million effort with European drug firms to develop a test for hGH in time for the Sydney Olympics.

The list of proscribed drugs is constantly growing as more performance-enhancing substances come into use and the analytical methods to detect them are developed or improved. At the Lillehamer Winter Olympics in 1994, competitors were, for the first time, tested for erythropoietin (EPO). This naturally occurring hormone is produced by the kidney and regulates red blood cell production and, hence, the oxygen-carrying capacity of the blood. This is useful for athletes, since red blood cells shuttle oxygen to the cells, including muscle cells, enabling them to operate aerobically. Assay for EPO requires, for the first time, the taking of blood samples from athletes. Disqualification can occur not only for its presence in the body but also simply for its mere possession. For example, in 1998 the Festina-sponsored bicycle team was disqualified from the Tour De France after being caught with large quantities of EPO. Synthetic EPO is currently available and has been demonstrated to induce changes similar to a procedure known as "blood doping."

Blood doping

An efficient way to increase the oxygen-carrying capacity of the blood is the technique of "blood doping." This process basically consists of withdrawing approximately 1 liter of an athlete's blood and storing it under frozen conditions for 9–12 weeks. During this period of time the individual's hemoglobin levels will return to normal by compensatory erythropoiesis. The withdrawn blood is then reintroduced into the athlete just before competition. In this way, a higher hemoglobin level is achieved. Blood doping is difficult to detect because of normal variations in hemoglobin levels or the effect of training at high altitude.

Regardless of what type of doping, the U.S. Olympic Committee created a stiff antidoping program prior to the Atlanta games. The drug program mandated a no-notice, out-of-competition testing for steroids and other performance boosters for all 41 Olympic and Pan American Games sports in the United States. One drug that is not presently banned is creatine, an endogenous compound involved in the production of ATP by muscle. It is normally infused just before an event with the hope of increasing energy production.

Herbal and nutritional supplements

Vitamin and mineral supplements, herbal preparations, and homeopathic remedies are becoming increasingly popular and are being used more and more by athletes. Competitors are continually striving to achieve an edge over their opponents; many look to these alternatives to gain the advantage. A great number of manufacturers sell their products to the sporting community as a way of gaining increased performance. The marketing of these types of products often relies on personal endorsements by well-known athletes or on anecdotal evidence, neither of which may be based on scientific studies or reliable evidence. These types of products are not licensed. Unlicensed products are not subject to the strict regulatory requirements regarding the manufacturing and labeling of constituent substances that licensed pharmaceutical products are. Therefore, it is very difficult to determine the purity of the product or whether the manufacturer has varied the constituents without notice. Some unlicensed products have been found to contain prohibited substances, such as ephedrine and caffeine, although neither item appeared on the label.

There are more than 20 different varieties of ginseng plants. Some of them have a stimulant effect in that they reduce tiredness. It is also claimed that the root of the plant improves concentration and has antiaging properties as well. However, there has never been any scientific support for these claims or the alleged enhancement of sporting performance. Pure ginseng is not a banned substance but frequently products claiming to be "Pure Ginseng" include banned substances such as ephedrine, pseudoephedrine, and steroids. A related product known as Chinese ephedra or Ma huang is converted into ephedrine.

Creatine is an amino acid found in meat and fish. It is also produced in the human body by the liver, kidneys, and pancreas. Most of it is stored in skeletal muscle. Of the creatine stored, more than half of it is stored as creatine phosphate, which is involved in the production of energy (by cleavage of the high-energy phosphate bond) for high-intensity activity. It is the lack of creatine phosphate that causes fatigue during high-intensity activity. Additional creatine is taken by competitors in an attempt to increase the body's natural store of the phosphate form in the belief that it will ultimately improve performance. It is thought that this supplementation will assist sporting performance by speeding up the resynthesis of intermediary substances to provide energy for short, high-intensity activity and offset lactic acid production. Lactic acid contributes to muscle fatigue in such activity. Although there have been many studies about the effects of creatine, published papers from large-scale, well-controlled studies are noticeable by their absence.

There is little information on the short- or long-term side effects on the safety of creatine supplementation. However, there have been reports of some athletes suffering side effects with the alleged overdosing of creatine (e.g, the natural production of creatine being curtailed in the athlete's body). The European Commission's Scientific Committee on Food (September 7, 2000) has concluded that high doses of creatine supplementation should be avoided (i.e., > 3 grams per day).

Chromium picolonate is alleged to improve muscle gain. This enhancement has yet to be proven scientifically and there is considered to be a very real potential of serious side effects if chromium is taken in large doses over a period of time.

SELECTED BIBLIOGRAPHY

Baskys, A. and Remington, G. (eds) (1996) *Brain Mechanisms and Psychotropic Drugs*. Boca Raton, FL: CRC Press.

Brody, T. M., Larner, J., Minneman, K. P. and Neu, H. C. (eds) (1994) *Human Pharmacology: Molecular to Clinical,* 2nd ed. St Louis, MO: Mosby.

Goldberg, R. (1994) *Drugs Across the Spectrum*. Minneapolis, MN: West Publishing Co.

Goldstein, A. (1994) *Addiction from Biology to Drug Policy*. New York: W.H. Freeman and Co.

Hardman, J. G., Limbird, L. E. and Gilman, A. G. (eds) (2001) *Goodman and Gilman's The Pharmacological Basis of Therapeutics,* 10th ed. New York: McGraw-Hill.

Karch, S. (1993) *The Pathology of Drug Abuse*. Boca Raton, FL: CRC Press.

Lidow, M. S. (ed.) (2000) *Neurotransmitter Receptors in Actions of Antipsychotic Medications*. Boca Raton, FL: CRC Press.

Moody, E. and Skolnich, P. (eds) (2001) *Molecular Basis of Anesthesia*. Boca Raton, Fl: CRC Press.

Smith, C. M. and Reynard, A. M. (eds) (1995) *Essentials of Pharmacology*. Philadelphia: W.B. Saunders.

Snyder, S. H. (1996) *Drugs and the Brain*. New York: Scientific American Library.

QUESTIONS

1 Which of the following produced symptoms of Parkinson's disease in the early 1980s?
   a MOA
   b DMA
   c PNS

    d   NMDA

    e   MPTP.

2 Which of the following was/were responsible for demonstrating the chemical nature of neurotransmission?

    a   Rene Descarte

    b   Henry Dale

    c   Claude Bernard

    d   Otto Loewi

    e   b and d.

3 Which of the following is the primary excitatory neurotransmitter in the brain?

    a   epinephrine

    b   chloride ion

    c   acetylcholine

    d   dopamine

    e   glutamate.

4 Which of the following is responsible for inhibitory modulation of neurotransmission in the brain?

    a   norepinephrine

    b   acetylcholine

    c   gamma-aminobutyric acid (GABA)

    d   dopamine

    e   none of the above.

5 The $GABA_A$ receptor complex has recognition sites for which of the following?

    a   barbiturates

    b   steroids

    c   alcohol

    d   benzodiazepines

    e   all of the above.

6 Cocaine's principal mechanism of action in the CNS involves which of the following?

    a   increased release of epinephrine

    b   inhibition of monoamine oxidase

    c   increased release of serotonin

    d   blockade of dopamine reuptake

    e   none of the above.

7 Which of the following is credited with the discovery of the anesthetic action of nitrous oxide in 1845?

    a   Joseph Priestley

    b   William Morton

    c   Horace Wells

d   Otto Loewi
e   Henry Dale.

8 Which of the following receptors is presently the leading candidate to interact with gaseous anesthetics?
   a   epinephrine (beta$_1$)
   b   acetylcholine (muscarinic)
   c   glycine
   d   GABA$_A$
   e   serotonin.

9 Botulinum toxin acts in the CNS by which of the following?
   a   preventing the reuptake of acetylcholine
   b   preventing the reuptake of serotonin
   c   preventing the release of epinephrine
   d   preventing the release of acetylcholine
   e   none of the above.

10 Neuroleptic efficacy in schizophrenia correlates with which of the following?
   a   blockade of histamine receptors
   b   blockade of serotonin receptors
   c   blockade of adrenergic receptors
   d   blockade of dopamine receptors
   e   a and d.

Chapter 12

Cardiovascular drugs

CORONARY HEART DISEASE

Some 7 million Americans suffer from coronary heart disease (CHD). CHD is the number one killer of both men and women in the United States. Each year, more than 500,000 Americans die of heart attacks caused by CHD. Risk factors include the following:

- High blood pressure
- High blood cholesterol
- Smoking
- Obesity
- Physical inactivity
- Diabetes
- Gender
- Heredity
- Age
- Stress

Like any muscle, the heart requires a constant supply of oxygen and nutrients, which are carried to it by the blood in the coronary arteries. In CHD, plaques or fatty substances build up inside the walls of the arteries. The plaques also attract blood components (e.g., platelets) that stick to the artery wall lining. This process, called atherosclerosis, develops gradually, over many years. It often begins early in life, even in childhood. The fatty accumulation can break open and lead to the formation of a blood clot that seals the break. The presence of the blood clot occludes the vessel and reduces blood flow.

If not enough oxygen-carrying blood reaches the heart, the heart may respond adversely, producing chest pain (*angina pectoris*, or simply angina, for short). The pain often radiates to the left shoulder, neck, and arm. Anginal pain can vary in occurrence and be mild and intermittent, or more pronounced and steady. It can be severe enough to make everyday activities extremely uncomfortable, particularly if they are strenuous (i.e., aerobic) in nature. Nausea and breathlessness often occur simultaneously with the angina. If a blood clot suddenly occludes most or all blood supply to a region of the heart, a heart attack occurs. The location of the occlusion within the coronary arterial network is a major determinant of how much heart tissue is deprived of oxygen and, therefore, the extent of heart tissue death. If a major coronary vessel is involved, the result can be death.

If the symptoms of CHD give a warning (i.e., angina) and are not life-threatening, then steps can be taken to reduce symptoms and retard progression of the disease. For many people, CHD is managed with lifestyle changes and medications. Others with severe CHD may require surgery (i.e., coronary bypass) or other procedures such as angioplasty. In any event, once CHD is diagnosed, it requires lifelong management.

Medications are prescribed according to the nature of the patient's CHD and other health problems that the patient may have. The symptoms of angina are usually addressed with three major classes of drugs: beta-adrenergic receptor blockers, calcium channel blockers, and nitrites/nitrates. The tendency to produce clots is routinely treated with daily aspirin or by other platelet inhibitory and anticoagulant drugs (e.g., warfarin or heparin) depending on the situation. For those with elevated blood cholesterol that is unresponsive to dietary and weight-loss measures, cholesterol-lowering drugs may be used (i.e., the "statins") or cholestyramine and niacin (see later).

Beta-adrenergic blockers

Beta blockers competitively attenuate the effects of catecholamines at beta-adrenergic receptors. Normally, norepinephrine, for example, produces an increase in the movement of calcium into heart cells, leading to increased heart rate and contractility. Beta antagonists block this sympathetic-mediated increase in heart rate and contractility. By doing so, they decrease myocardial oxygen demand primarily during activity (i.e., aerobic) or excitement (i.e., stress, adrenal discharge). Blockers with beta$_1$ selectivity (atenolol, metoprolol, and acebutolol) are most likely to decrease myocardial oxygen demand without producing beta$_2$ blockade and, thus, fewer side effects.

Calcium channel blockers

There are four types of calcium channels in the body (L, T, N, P). The main type of voltage-dependent calcium channel in the heart and vascular smooth muscle is the L type ("long lasting"). Depolarization of cardiac muscle and vascular smooth muscle leads to contraction that is dependent upon increased cytosolic concentrations of calcium. This occurs via two mechanisms: (1) slight depolarization of the cell activates the L-type voltage-dependent calcium channels, thereby increasing calcium influx into the cell; and (2) phosphorylation of the L-type calcium channel. Endogenous beta-receptor agonists such as norepinephrine activate membrane-bound adenyl cyclase on cardiac cells, which catalyses the production of cAMP from ATP in the presence of calcium. cAMP activates cAMP-dependent protein kinases, which in turn phosphorylate proteins near sarcolemmal stores, thereby further increasing intracellular calcium and facilitating contraction, and sinoatrial/atrioventicular (SA/AV) node conduction and contraction.

Voltage-dependent L-type calcium receptors have four distinct binding sites near the pore for calcium flux. By binding to these receptor sites calcium channel antagonists block the inward calcium current through the L-type channels and antagonize increases in heart rate, SA/AV node conduction, and heart contraction. Calcium channel blockers act on cardiac and vascular smooth muscle cells; therefore, they are used in the treatment of angina and hypertension, as well as certain types of arrhythmias. Calcium blockers affect bronchial, gastrointestinal (GI), and uterine smooth muscle to a lesser extent. Calcium blockers do not affect skeletal muscle because skeletal muscle utilizes primarily pools of intracellular calcium.

The principal calcium channel blockers are nifedipine, verapamil, and diltiazem. Of the three, nifedipine is the more potent vasodilator. Calcium channel antagonists are effective in the treatment of exertional, or exercise-induced, angina. The utility of these agents may result from an increase in blood flow due to coronary arterial dilation, from a decrease in myocardial oxygen demand (secondary to a decrease in arterial blood pressure, heart rate, or contractility), or from both. Concurrent therapy with nifedipine and a beta-adrenergic receptor blocker has proven more effective than either drug given alone in exertional angina, presumably because the beta-adrenergic blocker suppresses reflex tachycardia produced by the calcium channel blocker's reduction in peripheral resistance. There is no evidence that calcium channel blockers are of benefit in the early treatment or secondary prevention of acute myocardial infarction.

Nitrites and nitrates

Nitroglycerin (NTG) is the prototypic nitrate that relaxes vascular smooth muscle via the formation of an active intermediate nitric oxide (NO), which activates guanylate cyclase to increase cGMP. NO is thought to act either directly or indirectly via endothelium-derived relaxing factor (EDRF) to produce smooth muscle relaxation. The increased cGMP activates cGMP-dependent protein kinase, which phosphorylates various proteins in the vascular smooth muscle. Ultimately, one of these activated proteins dephosphorylates myosin light chain to cause smooth muscle relaxation. By this general cellular mechanism, NTG relaxes vascular smooth muscle, but not skeletal or cardiac muscle.

Nitrates such as NTG dilate large-capacitance, peripheral veins, thereby decreasing left ventricular and diastolic volume (less resistance to work against) as well as decreasing left ventricular and diastolic pressure (once again the heart has to do less work to move blood out of it). Therefore, nitrates and nitrites improve angina by decreasing oxygen demand of the myocardium. Nitrates and nitrites do not increase total coronary blood flow, when given orally or sublingually. In fact, by decreasing myocardial oxygen demand, NTG may actually decrease coronary blood flow. Since coronary blood flow is exquisitely sensitive to myocardial oxygen demand, if demand decreases by any mechanism, coronary blood flow will also decrease. This is part of the proof that the nitrates relieve angina primarily by reducing demand rather than supply of oxygen.

Organic nitrates are extensively metabolized by a hepatic nitrate reductase that inactivates the drug. If given orally, first-pass metabolism results in > 90 percent degradation. Therefore, NTG is primarily administered sublingually or topically as an ointment or patch. Following sublingual administration the onset of action occurs within 2 minutes, but the effect declines within 30 minutes. The rapid onset of sublingual NTG is why it is used to treat *acute* angina attacks. Ointment application results in effects within 60 minutes and they persist for up to 6 hours.

Side effects from the nitrates are usually exaggerations of their therapeutic effects, particularly vasodilatation. For example, facial flushing and particularly headaches frequently occur. The latter can make patient compliance a problem. In addition, peripheral resistance can decrease to the point where orthostatic hypotension can be produced leading to syncope (loss of consciousness). The reduction in blood pressure can also lead to baroreceptor-mediated compensatory increase in heart rate and contractility.

Aspirin

In response to vessel wall injury, platelets aggregate and release granular contents, leading to further aggregation, vasoconstriction, and thrombus formation. However, platelets exposed to aspirin have diminished aggregation in response to various thrombogenic stimuli. Aspirin is able to diminish platelet aggregation by blocking the synthesis of the arachidonic breakdown product thromboxane (a potent vasoconstrictor and promoter of platelet aggregation). It blocks thromboxane formation by irreversibly inhibiting cyclooxygenase by covalently binding to a serine residue on the enzyme. While endothelial cells can synthesize new cyclooxygenase, anucleated platelets cannot synthesize new cyclooxygenase in their ~ 10-day lifetime.

In unstable angina, disruption of atheroschlerotic plaques exposes the subendothelium to circulating blood elements. This initiates platelet aggregation and formation of thrombi, as well as local vasoconstriction, release of growth factors, chemotactic factors, and mitogenic factors. These events lead to repetitive reductions in coronary blood flow. In such patients with unstable angina, aspirin reduces the frequency and severity of these episodes. Aspirin results in a 50 percent reduction in subsequent myocardial infarctions and in mortality. One baby aspirin (81 mg) is usually sufficient to inhibit platelet aggregation. However, recent evidence indicates that the concomitant administration of ibuprofen can partially negate the beneficial effect of aspirin on platelets by antagonizing aspirin's effect on cyclooxygenase (particularly if given before aspirin).

Certain surgical procedures such as hip-joint replacement or cardiopulmonary bypass, in which whole blood comes into contact with foreign materials, result in initiation of blood coagulation and thrombus formation. Here, prophylactic administration of anticoagulants, usually heparin or coumarin, is effective in diminishing unwanted thrombus formation. Commercial heparin is obtained from hog intestinal mucosa or beef lung and is a linear polysaccharide composed of alternating residues of glucosamine and glucuronic or iduronic acid.

Heparin acts by binding to antithrombin III, which serves as a major inhibitor of serine protease clotting enzymes. Abruptly ending heparin treatment can be hazardous because of reduced levels of antithrombin III. Coumarins, typified by warfarin, are structurally similar to vitamin K, which plays an important role in blood coagulation. By interfering with the function of vitamin K, vitamin K-dependent proteins such as clotting factors VII, IX, X and prothrombin are reduced.

Lipid-lowering agents

The premise for treatment of hyperlipidemia is based on the hypothesis that abnormalities in lipid and lipoprotein levels are risk factors for CAD and that reductions in blood lipids can result in decreased risk of disease and complications. Low-density lipoprotein (LDL) cholesterol directly correlates with the risk of CAD. Drug therapy is often initiated when LDL levels meet or exceed 190 mg percent. Results from clinical trials support the hypothesis that cholesterol-lowering strategies aimed at reducing cholesterol by 20–25 percent produce clinically significant reductions in cardiovascular events in patients having preexisting vascular disease. The absolute magnitude of the benefits of cholesterol lowering is greatest in those with other risk factors (i.e., family history of CAD, cigarette smoking, hypertension, and diabetes). These risk factors are the basis for recommending lower cholesterol cutoff points and goals for those who are at high risk for developing clinical CAD. The National Cholesterol Education Program and recently published studies have identified two principal groups for aggressive drug treatment: (1) those without CAD who are at high risk for developing CAD (primary prevention) and (2) those with preexisting CAD.

The relationship between elevated triglycerides (TGRs) as a risk factor for CAD is less clear. However, serum TGRs are often inversely related to high-density lipoprotein (HDL—the "good" cholesterol). Therefore, reduction in TGR levels are associated with a rise in HDL, which has a negative correlation (protective effect) with CAD.

There are four principal classes of lipid-lowering drugs used in the treatment of CAD: (1) 3-hydroxy-3-methylglutaryl-coenzyme A (HMG-CoA) reductase inhibitors, (2) bile acid-binding resins, (3) nicotinic acid, and (4) fibric acid derivatives.

Examples of HMG-CoA reductase inhibitors include lovastatin, simvastatin, and pravastatin; the so-called "statins." These drugs inhibit the rate-limiting enzyme in the synthesis of cholesterol in the liver. In addition, the reduction in the formation of hepatic cholesterol leads to a compensatory increase in the hepatic synthesis of LDL receptors on the surface of hepatocytes. These receptors bind plasma LDL leading to a reduction in plasma LDL—the "bad" cholesterol.

In 1994 the Scandinavian Simvastatin Survival Study demonstrated a survival benefit from lowering cholesterol in individuals with CAD. Interestingly, in the following year, the West of Scotland Coronary Prevention study examined 6595 men without CAD who had LDLs of 155–232 mg percent and who received Pravastatin. They found a 33 percent reduction in deaths from CAD compared to the placebo group. These data indicate that aggressive, prophylactic treatment with HMG-CoA reductase inhibitors may be beneficial in men without CAD as well as in those with preexistent CAD. HMG-CoA reductase inhibitors are the most effective drugs for reducing both total and LDL cholesterol and can be used in conjunction with other lipid-lowering strategies.

Approximately 2 percent of patients have to discontinue taking these drugs due to side effects. The most common include the gastrointestinal tract (abdominal pain, diarrhea, constipation, and flatulence). Occasionally, patients may also develop muscle pain. Nevertheless, in summary, HMG-CoA inhibitors are the lipid-lowering drugs of first choice for treatment of most patients at risk for CAD. A long-term decrease in the rate of mortality or major coronary events has been documented with pravastatin, simvastatin, and lovastatin.

The prototype of a bile acid-binding resin is cholestyramine. Cholestyramine is the chloride salt of a basic anion-exchange resin. Its mechanism of action involves exchanging its chloride ion for bile acids in the intestinal lumen. By binding these bile acids, cholestyramine prevents them from being reabsorbed and, hence, they are excreted; up to a 10-fold increase. Normally, bile acids exert a negative feedback effect on the conversion of cholesterol to bile acids in the liver by inhibiting a microsomal hydroxylase. As bile-acid levels fall, therefore, more cholesterol is catabolized to bile acids. Furthermore, as the amount of cholesterol falls in the hepatocytes, these cells attempt to compensate by increasing their LDL receptors to remove cholesterol from the plasma. Like the statins, bile-acid sequestrants show a linear relationship between the degree of cholesterol lowering and the reduction in clinical coronary events. Because these drugs are not absorbed from the GI tract, they are relatively nontoxic. Bloating and constipation do make patient compliance a problem, however.

Nicotinic acid (niacin) is a water-soluble B-complex vitamin that is converted in the body into nicotinamide before being subsequently modified to NAD (nicotinamide adenine dinucleotide) or the phosphate NADP. Nicotinic acid's mechanism of action is not clear. It is believed to reduce the secretion of very low-density lipoproteins (VLDLs) from the liver. VLDL is the major carrier for TGRs. Reduction in LDL, on the other hand, may be a product of lowered VLDL since VLDL is a precursor of LDL. Many people who take nicotinic acid experience cutaneous vasodilatation resulting in skin flushing. Tachyphylaxis can also occur within a few days, creating problems with patient compliance. Other commonly occurring side effects include GI disturbances and elevated blood uric acid and glucose. These side effects are so prevalent that the drug is not recommended in persons with peptic ulcer disease, gout, or diabetes.

Fibric acid derivatives (aryloxyisobutyric acids) include the prototypic drug gemfibrozil. These types of drugs are used mainly to lower triglycerides and to increase HDL. A large placebo-controlled primary prevention trial in hypercholesterolemic men showed that patients treated with gemfibrozil had a statistically lower number of myocardial infarctions, but not of deaths from all causes.

ANTIHYPERTENSIVES

The therapeutic goal of treating hypertension with drugs is to maintain systolic blood pressure < 140 mmHg and diastolic blood pressure < 90 mmHg. Blood pressure in the body is regulated on a moment-to-moment basis by the baroreflex system that controls sympathetic and parasympathetic innervation of the vascular smooth muscle and heart. Sympathetic fibers innervate alpha-adrenergic smooth muscle receptors in the resistance vessels (arterioles) and regulate the contractile state of the vessels. Activating the sympathetic nervous system, therefore, increases arterial vascular resistance. Under some conditions, however, sympathetic activation and consequent increased metabolic activity of the end organ (i.e., the heart) compensate for the direct vasoconstrictor effect (i.e., on the coronary arteries) to produce a metabolically induced vasodilatation.

A low level of tonic activity of the sympathetic nerves to vascular smooth muscle adrenergic receptors exists so that withdrawal of sympathetic vasomotor tone results in vasodilatation and reduced pressure. Conversely, enhancement of sympathetic vasomotor tone augments the level of vasoconstriction leading to elevated pressure. While the parasympathetic branch of the autonomic nervous system innervates some blood vessels, it does not generally play a role in regulating peripheral resistance.

Table 12.1 Possible mechanisms leading to hypertension

Local blood vessel effects (vascular smooth muscle hypertrophy)
Exaggerated activity of the sympathetic nervous system
Defect in renal excretion of sodium
Defect in sodium or calcium transport across cell membranes
Multiple interactive effects

The sinoatrial (SA) node is innervated by both the sympathetic (beta$_1$) and parasympathetic (vagus) nervous systems. Sympathetic activation increases the discharge rate of the SA pacemaker cells, and thereby increases heart rate (a positive chronotropic effect). Sympathetic nerves also innervate adrenergic receptors (beta$_1$) on cardiac ventricular cells leading to an increase in stroke volume (a positive inotropic effect). Vagal activation, on the other hand, has the opposite effect and decreases heart rate and conduction velocity. In normal adults, cardiac vagal innervation is functionally predominant, so abolition of vagal activity results in a pronounced tachycardia (increased heart rate).

The baroreflex system consists of mechanosensitive receptors in the aorta and carotid sinus that detect changes in blood pressure. The receptors give rise to afferent nerve fibers that relay impulses to the CNS. Within the CNS, the afferent signals are processed and ultimately transmitted to efferent sympathetic and parasympathetic fibers to the vasculature and heart. Increases in blood pressure will increase baroreceptors activity leading to an inhibition of sympathetic impulses to the blood vessels (thereby relaxing them) and to the heart (decreasing heart rate and contractility). In addition, parasympathetic activity to the heart is increased leading to a reduction in heart rate and possibly contractility.

In most individuals the etiology of hypertension is unknown and is simply referred to as essential hypertension. Essential hypertension is probably due to a combination of several abnormalities, including genetic predisposition, stress, environmental and dietary factors. Specific potential mechanisms are listed in Table 12.1.

Regardless of the initiating factor(s), the primary characteristic of essential hypertension is increased peripheral vascular resistance. This can be monitored with the use of a sphygmomanometer (you have probably had your blood pressure taken with such an instrument). As the blood pressure of the cuff is inflated, it begins to occlude the flow of arterial blood, which then becomes turbulent and noisy (Korotkoff sounds) as it spurts through the artery. The blood can flow past the cuff only as long as its arterial pressure exceeds that of the cuff. Therefore, in order to measure blood pressure, the cuff is inflated (and the mercury column or needle rises) until it eliminates arterial blood flow, usually in the range of 180–200 mmHg. As the cuff pressure is slowly released, the user notes the pressure at which the Korotkoff sounds first reappear (the systolic pressure). As the pressure continues to be released, arterial blood flow becomes easier and less noisy. The pressure at which the noise ceases is the diastolic pressure.

The goal of drug therapy is to return peripheral resistance to normal. Left untreated, there is increased likelihood of incapacitating stroke or death. Table 12.2 shows the principal drug categories used in the management of essential hypertension.

Table 12.2 Drug categories used in the treatment of essential hypertension

Diuretics
Beta-adrenergic receptor antagonists
Alpha$_1$-adrenergic receptor antagonists
Centrally acting alpha$_2$-adrenergic receptor agonists
Direct vasodilators
Calcium channel blockers
Agents that interact with the renin–angiotensin system

Diuretics

One of the earliest strategies for the management of hypertension was to alter sodium balance by restriction of salt in the diet. Pharmacological alteration of salt balance became practical in the 1950s with the development of the orally active thiazide diuretics. Hydrochlorothiazide is a prototypic drug. Thiazides and related diuretics make up the most frequently used class of antihypertensive agents in the United States.

Thiazide diuretics promote excretion of sodium and water by inhibiting sodium and hence water reabsorption from the luminal side of epithelial cells in the distal convoluted tubule. However, their antihypertensive mechanism of action is controversial. They initially decrease cardiac output by decreasing plasma volume. However, cardiac output returns to essentially normal within 6–8 weeks, while arterial pressure and vascular resistance remain lowered. Recent evidence indicates that thiazide diuretics may act as antihypertensives by decreasing intracellular sodium in resistance vessels. Increased intracellular sodium may contribute to vascular resistance by increasing vessel stiffness and/or by inhibiting sodium–calcium exchange mechanisms leading to increased intracellular calcium and increased resistance (see Figure 12.6 in section on digitalis glycosides).

The thiazide diuretics are primarily used for most patients with mild or moderate hypertension. Used alone they can lower blood pressure by 10–15 mmHg. In more severe hypertension diuretics are used in combination with other agents. Adverse effects include hypokalemia (lowered serum potassium), impotence, impaired glucose tolerance, hyperlipidemia, and hyperuricemia (elevated uric acid in the blood).

Beta-adrenergic receptor blockers

The common characteristic of beta blockers is their ability to antagonize competitively the effects of the sympathetic effectors norepinephrine and epinephrine on cardiac beta-adrenergic receptors. Although many beta-adrenergic antagonists have other pharmacological effects, it is clear that the blockade of cardiac beta-adrenergic receptors is largely responsible for their ability to lower blood pressure. Compounds that exhibit selectivity for the beta$_1$ subtype of adrenergic receptors (e.g., atenolol; structure shown in Figure 12.1) are effective antihypertensives; thus, one hypothesis is that all drugs in this class exert their effects on blood pressure through beta$_1$-adrenergic blockade. By decreasing force and rate of contraction cardiac output is decreased with a corresponding decline in peripheral blood pressure.

Figure 12.1 Structure of the beta$_1$-antagonist atenolol.

Figure 12.2 Structure of prazosin.

Figure 12.3 Structure of clonidine.

Alpha$_1$-adrenergic receptor antagonists

Prazosin (see structure in Figure 12.2), the prototypic drug in this class, decreases peripheral vascular resistance in arterioles and veins by blocking alpha$_1$ receptors on vascular smooth muscle. It does not decrease cardiac output. Because of this effect, patients taking prazosin are more prone (~ 50 percent) to postural hypotension, particularly following the first dose. In some cases, the hypotension is so severe that the patient may lose consciousness. In an attempt to compensate, the baroreceptors may produce an accompanying tachycardia.

Alpha$_2$-adrenergic receptor agonists (centrally acting drugs)

Clonidine is the prototypic drug in this class (see structure in Figure 12.3). The drug was synthesized in the early 1960s and found to produce vasoconstriction. However, during clinical testing of the drug as a topical decongestant, clonidine was found to cause hypotension, sedation, and bradycardia. The hypertensive response that follows parenteral administration of clonidine generally is not seen when the drug is given orally. The hypotensive response produced by clonidine is believed to result from decreased central outflow of impulses in the sympathetic nervous system. This central action has been demonstrated by infusing small amounts of clonidine into the vertebral arteries or by injecting it directly into the cisterna magna. However, the exact mechanism of action of clonidine is not completely understood. Because clonidine

Figure 12.4 Structure of hydralazine.

acts in the CNS to decrease sympathetic outflow, it decreases not only peripheral vascular resistance but also heart rate and cardiac output.

Sedation and dry mouth are most common side effects. However, sudden withdrawal can result in a hypertensive crisis ("sudden withdrawal syndrome").

Direct vasodilators

Hydralazine was one of the first orally active antihypertensive drugs marketed in the United States. Its structure is shown in Figure 12.4. Initially, the drug was used infrequently because of its propensity to produce reflex tachycardia and tachyphylaxis. However, with a better understanding of the compensatory cardiovascular responses that accompany use of arteriolar vasodilators (the drug has little or no effect on venous smooth muscle), hydralazine was combined with sympatholytic agents and diuretics with greater therapeutic success.

Hydralazine causes direct relaxation of arteriolar smooth muscle. The arteriolar vasodilatation produced by hydralazine requires an intact endothelium. Therefore, one proposed mechanism of action is that hydralazine liberates nitric oxide from the endothelium (similar to the nitrates), which in turn increases cGMP to ultimately prevent the phosphorylation of myosin light chain (which is required for smooth muscle contraction) resulting in arteriolar vasorelaxation.

Direct vasodilators frequently produce baroreflex-induced tachycardia, but rarely orthostatic hypotension. They are usually prescribed with a beta blocker or a centrally acting antihypertensive to minimize the reflex increase in heart rate and cardiac output. It should be noted that another member of the directly acting class of antihypertensives is minoxidil. This potent, long-acting drug has gained considerable notoriety for its use as a topical hair-restorer. Oral use can result in hirsutism (unwanted hair growth over the face as well as other parts of the body).

Calcium channel blockers

Depolarization of vascular smooth muscle activates the L-type calcium channels, which results in increased cytosolic concentrations of calcium and hence increased tone. Calcium channel blockers (e.g., verapamil and diltiazem) block the influx of calcium through the L-type voltage-dependent channels located on vascular smooth muscle and cardiac muscle cells as well as cardiac nodal cells. Therefore, they are used in the treatment of angina, hypertension, and certain arrhythmias.

The major toxicities are extensions of their therapeutic effects. Frequent or severe adverse effects include dizziness, headache, edema, constipation (especially verapamil), atrioventricular (AV) block, bradycardia, heart failure, and lupus-like rash with

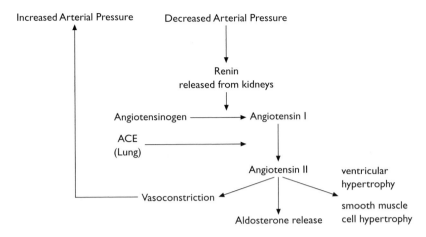

Figure 12.5 Renin–angiotensin system (courtesy of Dr Ann Bonham, UCDavis).

diltiazem. Two separate meta-analyses of 31 and 16 trials concluded that the short-acting nifedipine was associated with increased risk of reinfarction or death, in a dose-dependent manner. Therefore, nifedipine should not be used for the treatment of hypertension.

The renin–angiotensin system

In addition to baroreceptors, the body possesses an additional mechanism for affecting blood pressure. A decrease in arterial pressure, for example, causes release of the enzyme renin from the kidney into the blood. Renin then acts upon a circulating substrate, angiotensinogen, to generate angiotensin I. Angiotensin I is then converted to angiotensin II in the lung by angiotensin-converting enzyme (ACE) located in endothelial cells. Angiotensin II is a vasoconstrictor that constricts blood vessels, enhances sympathetic nervous system activity, and causes renal salt and water retention by direct intrarenal actions. In addition, the adrenal gland is stimulated to release the potent mineralocorticoid aldosterone that leads to sodium and water retention and, hence, increased plasma volume. A summary of the interrelationship between the components of the renin–angiotensin system is shown in Figure 12.5.

The main drug class derived from this scenario is that of the ACE inhibitors (see Chapter 1). Captopril was the first ACE inhibitor developed. The hypotensive response to ACE inhibitors is the result of inhibition of angiotensin II formation, especially in hypertensive patients in whom circulating blood concentrations of this peptide are increased. ACE also metabolizes the peptide bradykinin. Bradykinin is a vasodilator; therefore, inhibition of its metabolism by ACE inhibitors may contribute to the hypotensive effect of these agents. Inhibition of bradykinin by ACE inhibitors may also be related to the principal side effect of these drugs, namely, coughing. This effect is probably due to increased levels of bradykinin, which can excite pulmonary C fiber endings and irritant receptors in the lung to reflexively cause coughing.

Angiotensin II-receptor antagonists

The importance of angiotensin II in regulating cardiovascular function has led to the development of nonpeptide antagonists of the angiotensin receptor (e.g., losartan). By preventing effects of angiotensin II, these agents relax smooth muscle and thereby promote vasodilatation, increase renal salt and water elimination, reduce plasma volume, and decrease cellular hypertrophy. Angiotensin II-receptor antagonists also theoretically overcome some of the disadvantages of ACE inhibitors, which not only prevent conversion of angiotensin I to angiotensin II but also prevent ACE-mediated degradation of bradykinin and substance P. Cough, an adverse effect of ACE inhibitors, has *not* been associated with angiotensin II-receptor antagonists.

CONGESTIVE HEART FAILURE

Congestive heart failure (also known as congestive heart disease) is the inefficacy of the heart to pump or receive sufficient blood to maintain an adequate ejection fraction (i.e., diminished cardiac output). Chronic heart failure occurs most commonly in the presence of long-standing hypertension or a loss of myocardial tissue, whether segmental (e.g., myocardial infarct) or diffuse (e.g., cardiomyopathy or myocarditis). The primary symptoms of congestive heart disease are the following:

- Decreased exercise tolerance
- Fatigue
- Shortness of breath
- Edema
- Tachycardia
- Sweating

The symptoms result from compensatory mechanisms in the body set in motion to try to restore cardiac output. The decrease in cardiac output from the diseased heart causes a corresponding decrease in blood pressure that leads to (1) activation of the sympathetic nervous system with its attendant elevations in heart rate, heart contractility, arterial resistance, venous tone, and sweating; (2) activation of the renin–angiotensin system leading to increased systemic arterial resistance, release of aldosterone (which increases sodium retention), constriction of renal vasculature, ventricular hypertrophy ("remodeling"), and vascular smooth muscle proliferation; and (3) remodeling, which leads to progressive systolic failure, wherein the myocytes become distended and "fatter" and are less viable. With progressive loss of viable myocytes, systolic function continues to fail, with a corresponding progressive ventricular dilation. With progressive ventricular dilation and increases in left ventricular filling pressures, the symptoms become manifest as pulmonary congestion or fatigue caused by limited cardiac output.

The primary goals of pharmacological management of congestive heart failure are to (1) treat the cause of heart failure (e.g., antihypertensives) and (2) relieve the symptoms and delay/prevent the progression of the left ventricular dysfunction.

Strategies include improving myocardial contractility (e.g., positive inotropic agents), lower sodium retention (diuretics, ACE inhibitors), and decreasing arteriolar and venous resistance in order to decrease work load (vasodilators and ACE inhibitors) and to increase exercise tolerance.

Examples of specific drugs used in the treatment of chronic heart failure include digitalis glycosides (e.g., digoxin, positive inotropic agent), diuretics (hydrochlortiazide and furosemide), and vasodilators (nitrates such as nitroglycerin, ACE inhibitors, such as captopril, and hydralazine).

Digitalis glycosides

As mentioned previously, digitalis was discovered by William Withering for the treatment of "dropsy" (i.e., the peripheral edema produced by congestive heart failure). Digitalis glycosides are extracted from the foxglove plant, *Digitalis purpurea*, and other species. Among the cardiac glycosides, digoxin and to a lesser extent digitoxin are clinically used. As positive inotropic agents they act to enhance cardiac contractility to compensate for diminished cardiac output in congestive heart disease. These drugs selectively bind to and inhibit a membrane-bound sodium pump (sodium/potassium-ATPase). Inhibition of the sodium pump leads to an increase in intracellular sodium concentration, which in turn affects sodium/calcium exchange, leading to an increase in intracellular calcium and the force of contraction.

The relationship of intracellular sodium to intracellular calcium is such that a very small increase in sodium in terms of percentage increase leads to a disproportionately large increase in calcium. Therefore, a direct effect on the sodium/potassium-ATPase to inhibit sodium pump activity is the primary mechanism of the positive inotropic effect of the cardiac glycosides, while secondary elevation of intracellular calcium provides the ionic "punch" to increase contractility. A diagram of the relationship between sodium/potassium-ATPase and calcium is shown in Figure 12.6.

Although treatment of congestive heart failure can be palliative, cardiac output does not return to normal. The goal of therapy is to achieve as much restoration of

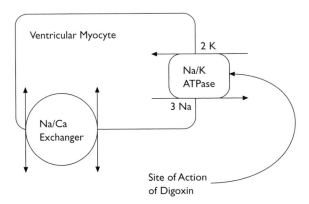

Figure 12.6 Mechanism of action of digoxin (courtesy of Dr Ann Bonham, UCDavis).

cardiac function as possible. In addition to their inhibitory effect on the sodium pump, cardiac glycosides such as digoxin can also increase the effective refractory period of the AV node by increasing parasympathetic tone to the AV node. This will prolong the effective filling time of the ventricles. Because of digoxin's effect on AV conduction, it is sometimes used in the treatment of atrial arrhythmias (to protect the ventricles, as discussed later).

A moderate inhibition of sodium/potassium-ATPase causes the positive inotropic (therapeutic) effect of cardiac glycosides, whereas an excessive inhibition produces toxicity. When cardiac muscle is exposed to toxic concentrations of a glycoside, sodium pump inhibition and cellular calcium loading become alarmingly high. This process may lead to life-threatening ventricular tachycardia followed by ventricular fibrillation. Therefore, toxicity resulting from direct actions of the cardiac glycosides on cardiac muscle is caused by calcium overload of myocardial cells. Because the therapeutic positive inotropic effect of these drugs is also caused by enhanced calcium loading of the cells and in particular the sarcoplasmic reticulum, the therapeutic and toxic effects are inseparable. Therefore, their *low therapeutic index* is an inherent property of this class of positive inotropic drugs.

With regard to adverse effects on other organs, the primary adverse effect is on the GI tract and includes anorexia, nausea, vomiting, and diarrhea. These effects result from direct inhibition of sodium/potassium-ATPase and from central stimulation of the chemoreceptor zone. The second most commonly occurring effect is in the CNS and includes visual disturbances (blurred or yellow vision), halos or flashing lights, and disorientation. While not lethal, these effects can be sufficient to decrease individual compliance in taking the drug. Because potassium competes with digoxin for binding sites on the sodium pump, elevations in serum potassium will diminish the effects of digoxin, while hypokalemia can augment the effects and result in toxicity at lower doses. The single most common cause of digoxin toxicity is the concurrent use of diuretics to the extent that potassium is depleted (except potassium-sparing diuretics, see later discussion).

Because digitoxin has a very low therapeutic index, toxicity occurs rather routinely and can be fatal; patients must be monitored closely. Moderate overdoses can be picked up by GI or CNS complaints; however, more serious toxicity on cardiac rhythm is more difficult to distinguish from the effects of heart disease. Digitalis antibody fragments are available for serious toxicity, i.e., when cardiac arrest is imminent. The fragments bind the drug and are excreted by the kidneys.

Diuretics

As mentioned earlier, thiazide diuretics promote excretion of sodium and an osmotic equivalent of water by inhibiting sodium reabsorption in the distal convoluted tubules of the kidneys. In addition, loop diuretics (e.g., furosemide) inhibit sodium reabsorption in the thick ascending limb of the loop of Henle. Because of the large absorptive capacity of this segment, these agents are the most potent diuretics. Aldosterone antagonists such as spironolactone act in the collecting tubule and are potassium sparing (see Figure 12.7). These drugs are used with other diuretics to prevent or correct hypokalemia.

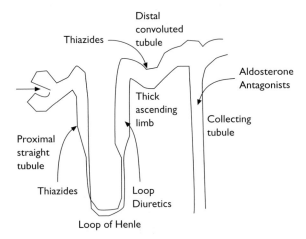

Figure 12.7 Sites of action of diuretics important in heart failure (courtesy of Dr Ann Bonham, UCDavis).

Exaggerated pharmacological effects of diuretics to decrease sodium and water retention can result in complications relating to ion changes important in congestive heart failure. Possible adverse effects include the following:

- Decreased plasma volume
- Hypokalemia
- Hyponatremia (to a lesser extent)
- Hyperlipidemia
- Glucose intolerance
- Impotence

Hypokalemia should be treated in heart failure, because either hypokalemia or heart failure can predispose individuals to experience serious arrhythmias. Therefore, potassium-sparing diuretics are sometimes used in the treatment of congestive heart failure.

Vasodilators

Vasodilators such as nitrates, ACE inhibitors, and hydralazine have been discussed previously. These agents are used to decrease arteriolar (afterload) or venous resistance (preload). A discussion of cardiodynamics is beyond the scope of this book. However, by decreasing preload and afterload these drugs decrease the work that the heart has to do to increase cardiac output; this improves perfusion pressure on the arterial side and venous return on the venous side, which contributes to reduced peripheral edema.

In summary, many patients with symptoms of heart failure take a cardiac glycoside, a diuretic, and an ACE inhibitor. Diuretics and a glycoside such as digoxin improve symptoms, but have little effect on survival. ACE inhibitors improve symptoms and prolong survival, but the disease still progresses.

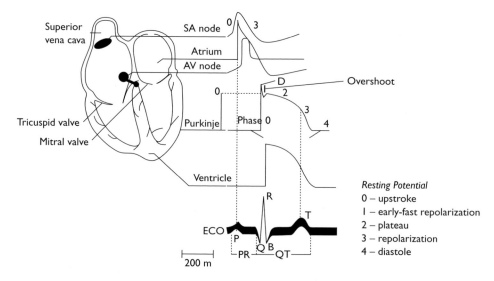

Figure 12.8 Normal impulse conduction throughout the heart (courtesy of Dr Ann Bonham, UCDavis).

ANTIARRHYTHMIC AGENTS

In the normal heart, electrical impulses that trigger normal cardiac rhythms originate in the SA node, spread rapidly through the atria to the AV node, and then propagate over the His–Purkinje system to invade all parts of the ventricles. Depolarization results in contraction and repolarization results in relaxation of myocardial cells. The relationship between normal impulse conduction throughout the heart and electrical events is shown in Figure 12.8. Arrhythmias may be caused by electrolyte disturbances, ischemia, trauma, drug overdoses, etc., but the fundamental problems are abnormal generation of action potentials (from nonpacemaker cells) or abnormal conduction (as observed with reentry arrhythmias).

Arrhythmias are characterized by abnormal formation or abnormal conductance of electrical impulses in the heart. The sodium channel is particularly important in generating action potentials and hence contraction of the ventricular myocytes. The state of the sodium channel is voltage dependent, so the resting membrane potential of the cell influences the number of sodium channels open. The state of the sodium channels can determine whether a ventricular myocyte can generate an action potential and hence contract. The sodium channels exist in three states (Figure 12.9): (1) rest (available for activation; **m** gate closed); (2) activated (both gates open); and (3) inactivated (**h** gate closed).

The number of sodium channels available for activation determines the conduction velocity of the action potential in cardiac cells. The more sodium channels available for activation, the faster the conduction velocity occurs. At resting membrane potential of ventricular, atrial, and Purkinje cells (−85 mV), the **m** gate is closed, preventing any influx of sodium; therefore, no action potential develops (Resting). With an

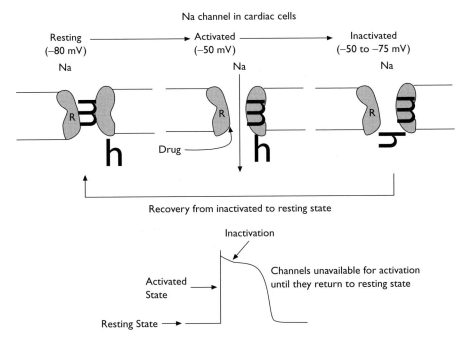

Figure 12.9 The role of the sodium channel (courtesy of Dr Ann Bonham, UCDavis).

appropriate activating stimulus (slight depolarization), the **m** gate opens, sodium rushes in, and an action potential develops (Activated). A few milliseconds later and as the membrane repolarizes to –55 to –75 mV, the **h** gate closes, inactivating the channel and halting sodium influx (Inactivated). The channel must be in the resting state to be available for promulgating an action potential. During the time in which it takes the channels to go from the "inactivated" state to the "resting" state, the cell is refractory to incoming stimuli, so no action potential develops.

The state of the sodium channel varies in healthy ventricular cells and those damaged by ischemia. This variability in the state has implications for antiarrhymic therapy with sodium channel blocking agents. In "sick" or damaged ventricular cells (i.e., from ischemia or blockade of the sodium/potassium-ATPase [sodium/potassium pump]), the resting membrane is more positive than the healthy resting membrane potential (Figure 12.10).

In healthy cardiac cells, the recovery time from inactivation of sodium channels (back to the resting state) is quite rapid, so that the maximum number of channels is available for activation. In contrast, in sick cells, the recovery time is quite slow. In these sick cells, the action potential develops from the opening of fewer sodium channels, so the action potential is a slow sluggish upstroke as opposed to the fast upstroke in a healthy cell. A slow sluggish upstroke results in poor and perhaps no propagation of the action potential. Chronically depolarized or ischemic cells may (1) fail to conduct an action potential and therefore fail to contract or to transmit the action potential to neighboring cells or (2) become an ectopic pacemaker (due to a

Figure 12.10 Comparison of healthy and diseased ventricular myocyte depolarization (courtesy of Dr Ann Bonhan, UCDavis).

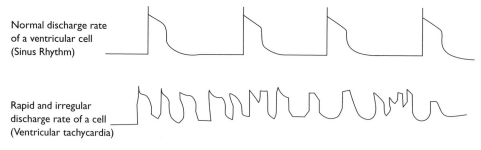

Figure 12.11 Example of a string of ectopic ventricular beats leading to ventricular tachycardia (courtesy of Dr Ann Bonham, UCDavis).

slow sodium leak in phase 4) so that it overrides the normal pacemaker activity to cause either an occasional ectopic contraction or a string of ectopic beats, which become a tachyarrhythmia (see Figure 12.11).

Electrical impulses in each cardiac cycle begin in the sinus node (SA) and continue until the entire heart has been activated. When all the cells have been discharged and are refractory, the electrical impulse dies out; it has nowhere to go. If, however, a group of cells that are not activated because of unidirectional block during the initial wave of depolarization recover their excitability before the impulse dies out, then those cells may serve as a link to reexcite areas that were just discharged but have recovered from the initial depolarization. This event is described as reentry, reentrant tachycardia, circus movement, or echo beats. Reentry depends on two pathways with different electrophysiological properties, i.e., a refractory period longer in one pathway than another, slower conduction, and/or decreased excitability in one pathway. The different electrophysiological properties are caused by local damage within an area of conduction. Figure 12.12 illustrates reentry.

In Figure 12.12, zone B contains a unidirectional block so that it is refractory to the forward-moving (anterograde) impulse. The impulse travels only through branch A (fast pathway) to depolarize the ventricle. As the impulse spreads back toward B it is propagated retrogradely (toward the AV node) through branch B to spread depolarization through the atria (i.e., to produce an echo beat in the atria) and/or provide early reexcitation (reentry) at the AV node and through A. A single reactivation of branch A will produce a single premature ventricular beat; continuous conduction will cause AV nodal tachycardia. Antiarrhythmic drugs can abolish reentry activity

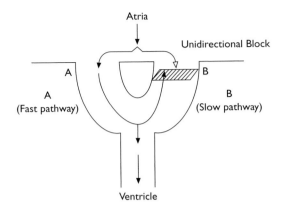

Figure 12.12 Example of reentry at the AV node (courtesy of Dr Ann Bonham, UCDavis).

Table 12.3 Comparison of various antiarrthymic drugs

Class	Action	Drugs
I	Blocks Na channels	
A	Moderately depresses phase O and lengthens APD, ERP	Quinidine[a], procainamide
B	Minimally depresses phase O and shortens APD, ERP	Lidocaine, phenytoin
C	Maximally depresses phase O and does not change APD, ERP	Encainde, lorcainide, liecainide
II	Beta-adrenergic receptor blockade	Propranolol
III	Prolong ERP, blocks K	Bratylium, sotalol[b] amiodarone[c]
IV	Calcium channel blockade	Verapamil, diltiazem

Notes
a   Quinidine and most class A agents also block the delayed K channels.
b   Sotalol also has beta-adrenergic blocking properties (II).
c   Amiodarone blocks Na channels (I) prolongs depolarization (III): noncompetitively blocks beta receptors (II), and is a weak Ca channel blocker (IV).
This table courtesy of Dr Ann Bonham, UCDavis.

by (1) decreasing conduction in branch B (slow pathway) to produce a bidirectional block and (2) increasing the refractory period in the fast pathway, so the reentrant current becomes extinct in the refractory tissue. The goal of antiarrhythmic therapy is to suppress ectopic pacemakers or reentry pathways.

Antiarrhythmic drugs have been classified by their predominant effects. However, drugs within a class do differ significantly. The presence of heart disease and arrhythmic states may modify their actions, and some drugs have more than one effect. Table 12.3 compares the drugs in the various classes.

Class I antiarrthymic drugs block sodium channels and have varying effects on action potential duration (APD) and end resting potential (ERP). Quinidine and procainamide are the prototypic drugs in this class. These drugs act to (1) slow conduction velocity (phase 0), particularly in chronically depolarized cells, and (2) decrease abnormal automaticity (phase 4) in ectopic foci, and (3) may also decrease

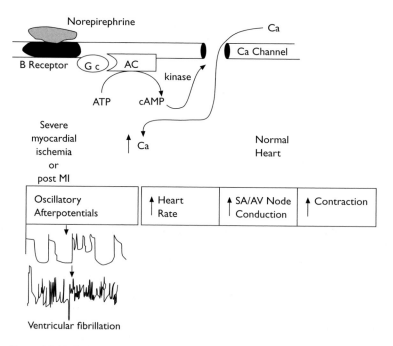

Figure 12.13 Role of beta receptor in affecting cardiac arrhythmias (courtesy of Dr Ann Bonham, UCDavis).

normal automaticity (phase 4) in Purkinje fibers. They are frequently used for chronic arrhythmias due to their oral availability and efficacy. Most common side effects are in the GI and CNS. As mentioned earlier, in some cases of AV or His–Purkinje conduction problems, quinidine can slow conduction to the extent of causing complete block. The most common problem with procainamide is lupus-like syndrome. Sixty-five percent of patients will develop antibodies within 12 months; only 12 percent will show symptoms that are reversible when the drug is stopped. Procainamide can be given intravenously more safely than quinidine.

Endogenous norepinephrine stimulates cardiac beta receptors. Receptor-linked cAMP-dependent protein kinases phosphorylate calcium channels to increase intracellular calcium. Elevated intracellular calcium increases conduction velocity (phase 0) and decreases the threshold potential in normal SA and AV node cells (see Figure 12.13). Beta blockers slow spontaneous conduction velocity in the SA node by approximately 10–20 percent. In addition, beta blockers can slow conduction velocity while increasing the refractory period of the AV node. These effects control the ventricular rate in atrial fibrillation or flutter and terminate paroxysmal supraventricular tachycardias. They are also safer, although somewhat less effective, than other drugs for suppression of premature ventricular complexes (PVCs). Drugs in this class approved by the FDA for treatment of various arrhythmias include propranolol, acebutolol, and esmolol. Problems with the beta blockers include drowsiness, fatigue, impotence, and depressed ventricular performance.

Figure 12.14 Effect of potassium blocker on cardiac action potential.

Potassium channel blockers (sotalol, amiodarone, bretylium, and dofetilide) block the outward-flowing potassium channel, decreasing potassium conductance, which prevents or delays repolarization (prolongation of APD and ERP) (see Figure 12.14). These drugs can be used in life-threatening ventricular tachyarrhythmias. Controlled clinical trials in patients with a history of sustained ventricular tachycardia or ventricular fibrillation indicate that amiodarone and sotalol are more effective than older drugs such as quinidine or procainamide. Both drugs, especially amiodarone, have become drugs of choice for these serious arrhythmias. In a clinical trial of sotalol in which it was compared to six class I drugs, it was found to be more effective in preventing death and recurrence of arrhythmias. Orally administered amiodarone can suppress PVCs and nonsustained ventricular tachycardia or fibrillation.

Amiodarone has a higher incidence of side effects than sotalol. Seventy-five percent of patients report side effects over 5 years with 15–35 percent requiring discontinuance of the drug. Severe adverse effects, including pulmonary fibrosis, can occur with usual doses of amiodarone and may be lethal or irreversible or persist for months after treatment is stopped.

Verapamil and diltiazem are prototypic calcium channel blockers. As indicated previously, these drugs influence cardiac function by blocking inward calcium movement through L channels. In so doing they block conduction velocity in SA and AV node cells. They are used therapeutically to treat reentry arrhythmias through the AV node as well as paroxysmal supraventricular tachycardias. In fact, verapamil has been reported to terminate 60–80 percent of paroxysmal supraventricular tachycardias within several minutes. However, because of their potent effect on AV conduction, these drugs are contraindicated in patients with preexisting conduction problems since they may produce complete AV block.

SELECTED BIBLIOGRAPHY

Hardman, J. G., Limbird, L. L. and Gilman, A. G. (eds) (2001) *Goodman and Gilman's The Pharmacological Basis of Therapeutics*, 10th ed. New York: McGraw-Hill.

Katzung, B. G. (ed.) (2001) *Basic and Clinical Pharmacology*, 8th ed. New York: McGraw-Hill.

Safety of calcium-channel blockers (1997) *The Medical Letter* 39: 13–14.

QUESTIONS

1 Quinidine can produce all except one of the following?
   a   depressed myocardial excitability
   b   vagal stimulation
   c   slowed myocardial conduction
   d   decreased slope of diastolic depolarization of pacemaker cells
   e   prolonged myocardial refractory period.

2 The site responsible for the pharmacological and toxic actions of digitalis glycosides is associated with which of the following?
   a   beta-adrenergic receptors
   b   sodium/potassium-ATPase
   c   protein kinase C
   d   cAMP-dependent protein kinase
   e   calcium pump.

3 The system or function *not* affected by the cardiac glycosides is which of the following?
   a   the sodium channel
   b   the calcium channel
   c   the sodium pump
   d   calcium loading of the sarcoplasmic reticulum
   e   atrioventricular conduction.

4 The following limit the clinical usefulness of digitalis *except* which of the following?
   a   narrow margin of safety
   b   low potency
   c   tendency to produce arrhymias
   d   variations in bioavailability
   e   patient-to-patient variability.

5 All of the following about calcium antagonists are true except?
   a   they decrease peripheral vascular resistance
   b   they increase coronary blood flow
   c   they decrease cardiac afterload
   d   they decrease serum calcium concentration
   e   they may cause hypotension.

6 Calcium antagonists act by inhibiting which of the following?
   a   calcium influx through L-type channels
   b   calcium influx through T-type channels
   c   calcium influx through N-type channels
   d   calcium influx through P-type channels
   e   calcium influx through M-type channels.

7 All of the following actions of nitrovasodilators are correct except?
   a   they inhibit phosphodiesterase
   b   they generate nitric oxide
   c   they increase cGMP
   d   they are similar to EDRF
   e   all are correct.

8 The loop diuretics have their principal diuretic effect on which of the following?
   a   ascending limb of loop of Henle
   b   distal convoluted tubule
   c   proximal convoluted tubule
   d   collecting duct
   e   b and c.

9 Which of the following statements for cholesterol and cholesterol metabolism is
   not true?
   a   the liver is the primary organ for cholesterol uptake and degradation
   b   most cholesterol is converted to bile acids
   c   the transport of cholesterol is primarily accomplished by binding to lipoprotein
   d   the major source of cholesterol in the body is via dietary intake
   e   none of the above.

10 Epidemiological studies on the incidence of atherosclerosis indicate which of the
    following?
    a   the greatest correlation exists for LDL cholesterol
    b   there is an inverse correlation between LDL and HDL cholesterol concentrations
    c   there is usually a consistent increase in LDL cholesterol and total cholesterol
        concentrations
    d   all of the above are correct
    e   none of the above are correct.

Part 4

Drug development

Chapter 13

Drug discovery by the pharmaceutical industry

INTRODUCTION

Throughout history, certain plants, as well as virtually every anatomical component of animals and humans, have been ascribed some curative property: earthworms rolled in honey for the treatment of gastritis; owl brain for headache; sheep brain for insomnia; deer heart for heart disease; fox lung for tuberculosis; goat liver for jaundice; powdered human skull or the fresh blood of a dying Christian gladiator for epilepsy; rabbit testicles for bladder disease and, of course, for impotence; and cow dung for eye infections, to name but a few.

These beliefs led to the creation of an extensive development of folk medicine that prevailed for many centuries. However, with the publication in 1661 of Robert Boyle's *The Skeptical Chemist*, the foundations for the application of chemistry to the development of drugs were laid down. The archaic ideas of Aristotle (regarding the four elements—earth, air, fire, and water) and Hippocrates (the body's four fluids "humors"—blood, black and yellow bile, and phlegm) were finally swept away, and a chemical element was defined as a substance that could not be broken down into simpler substances.

It was also during the seventeenth and early eighteenth centuries that the roles of chemists and druggists began to merge, and with this amalgamation several English pharmaceutical companies had their origins. For example, Allen and Hanburys (now part of the giant GlaxoWellcome Group) began as a simple apothecary shop in 1715. Early entrepreneurs such as these imported large quantities of raw materials from around the world, which were converted into such widely used preparations as tincture of Peruvian bark (for malaria) and cod liver oil (for rheumatism and rickets).

Further significant advances in chemical knowledge occurred at the end of the eighteenth and beginning of the nineteenth centuries, among which were newer extraction procedures that allowed the isolation of purer drugs from natural sources. For example, Sertürner reported the first isolation of a plant alkaloid in 1806 (morphine), which was soon followed by codeine in 1832 and papavarine in 1848. By the middle of the nineteenth century, the use of pure alkaloids rather than crude preparations began to spread throughout the medical world.

Starting in the mid-nineteenth century, important new synthetic drugs made their appearance: nitrous oxide (1844), ether (1846), and chloroform (1847) as anesthetics; amyl nitrite (1867) and nitroglycerin (1879) for anginal pain; chloral hydrate (1869) for sedation; and antipyrene (1883), acetanilid (1886), and acetophenetidin (1887) for the control of pain and fever. Introduction of the last three drugs marked the entry of the German chemical industry into the pharmaceutical field and changed it for ever. With their vast experience in organic synthesis, they set the standard for pharmaceutical chemistry until World War II.

However, the development of the giant multinational drug companies of today, with their tremendous capacity for the synthesis of organic molecules, did not occur overnight. In fact, most of the early pharmaceutical companies made their profits based upon the sale of *inorganic* preparations (e.g., Beecham's liver pills were bismuth salts while Boots' Epsom salts were basically magnesium sulfate).

The German company Bayer was the first to widely commercialize a *synthetic* drug (acetylsalicylic acid) in 1899. The company was not looking for a drug to relieve the pain of rheumatism 100 years ago, but a 29-year-old Bayer chemist and pharmacist, named Felix Hoffman, was looking for a way to relieve his father's suffering. Sodium salicylate, which was used to treat rheumatism victims at the time, not only did not taste pleasant but the acid also attacked the mucosal linings of the mouth and stomach.

In the 1830s, chemists succeeded in extracting salicin from willow and converting it to salicylic acid for use in treating fevers. In the 1870s, researchers discovered that salicin derivatives also relieved pain and inflammation. Sodium salicylate became the preferred form for treating arthritis. When Felix Hoffman began experimenting with salicylic acid in the 1890s, he started with the assumption that acidity was responsible for its gut-wrecking effects. Hoping to moderate this acidity, Hoffman uncovered the long-ignored synthesis of acetylsalicylic acid in 1853 by Charles Gerhardt, who acetylated the hydroxyl group of sodium salicylate at position 1 of the benzene ring. But Gerhardt had not pursued acetylsalicylic acid because its synthesis proved difficult. Hoffman devised a better way to synthesize acetylsalicylic acid by choosing acetic anhydride as the acetylating agent instead of Gerhardt's use of acetyl chloride.

Working in Bayer's pharmaceutical laboratory in Elberfeld, Germany, Hoffman acetylated salicylic acid in August 1897. The resultant acetylsalicylic acid powder had few of the drawbacks of sodium salicylate, and besides relieving father Hoffman's rheumatoid aches and pains, it had some additional benefits as well. Bayer scientists found aspirin helped to relieve headaches and toothaches, reduced fever, and decreased inflammation.

Bayer first sold aspirin powder to the public in 1899, and introduced a water-soluble tablet in 1900. The company estimates that 50 billion tablets are now consumed yearly on a worldwide basis. In addition to tablets, the French prefer their aspirin in suppository form, while the Italians prefer it fizzy. Aspirin is no longer just taken for headaches and aches and pains. According to Bayer market research, palliation of heart disease is now the number one use of aspirin.

The development of acetylsalicylic acid by Bayer also began a battle of trade names that lasted well into this century. Bayer christened their new drug aspirin, the name originating from the "a" of acetyl and "spir" of *Spirea ulmania*, the plant from which salicylic acid had originally been isolated. Bayer registered the trade name and argued that if aspirin was prescribed in Germany, their product should be dispensed.

With the outbreak of World War I, the international pharmaceutical situation suddenly changed. England, France, and the United States, cut off from their normal supply of German drugs and other important chemicals, were pressured to create their own drug/chemical industries. Until this time, American contributions to drug development had been modest though very important. For example, the anesthetic agents nitrous oxide and ether were both developed in the United States. At the end of World War I, Bayer lost their exclusive right to the name aspirin when the Allies assumed control over the company.

As mentioned previously in Chapter 10, the discovery of sulfanilamide during the 1930s ushered in a new era in drug therapy. As a result of worldwide publicity in medical journals, magazines, and newspapers, the demand for the new drug skyrocketed. Drug companies in England, France, and the United States, quick to see the potential sales in this new field, began to synthesize, test, and rush to market a vast array of sulfanilamide derivatives which could be patented and promoted. This approach was intensified by the relatively widespread introduction of the more effective penicillin in the mid-1940s.

It was World War II that really provided an additional "jump start" for the involvement of American pharmaceutical companies in antibiotic production. As mentioned previously, following the discovery of penicillin, there was general apathy on the part of the drug industry to devote resources to its commercialization. However, with the obvious implications of wartime injuries and their attendant infections, Britain's Howard Florey continued his drive to develop penicillin by turning his attention to the United States. With dogged determination he succeeded in obtaining help from the Bureau of Agriculture in Peoria, Illinois—which took on the task of developing a commercial-scale fermentation process in response to America's entry into the war in 1941.

Eventually, 100,000 units of penicillin were produced by a consortium of American drug companies (Merck, Squibb, and Pfizer) by the middle of 1944. A tremendous improvement in yield was made possible by the use of a new strain of mold, as well as the use of deep fermentation tanks similar to those used in the brewery industry. Interestingly, the new strain of mold discovered was serendipitously found on a decaying cantaloupe in a Peoria food market.

It was also during the 1940s that American drug companies began a very successful relationship with steroids. The first major steroid that received attention during this period was cortisone. Cortisone is normally produced by the adrenal glands. Its interest to pharmaceutical companies emanated from several factors. The first is that it was rumored to be a secret chemical used by the Germans to assist in high-altitude flying. In addition, it was also identified as the elusive "compound E" that was responsible for ameliorating arthritis in pregnant women. By 1948, a complicated 36-stage process had been developed for its synthesis. Unfortunately, 1 gram of cortisone produced in this manner cost approximately $200.

As a result of the need for more of this very effective anti-inflammatory drug, several pharmaceutical companies began major efforts to produce large quantities of the steroid, utilizing different strategies. For example, Searle attempted to extract cortisone from cattle adrenal glands, while Syntex and Upjohn focused on a more straightforward chemical conversion of progesterone into cortisone. Syntex eventually reported the successful synthesis of cortisone in 1951 using hecogenin (from the agave plant) as a starting material. Although cortisone itself did not eventually prove to be particularly successful (primarily due to side effects), structural leads were obtained that have led to the development of numerous highly effective steroid drugs over the past 50 years.

Perhaps the most significant steroid-based drug developed over the past five decades was the birth control pill. It is a relatively unique drug in that it is typically taken by healthy individuals who are not suffering from an illness. In 1950, the first oral contraceptive was designed based upon a regimen of progesterone for 3 weeks followed by withdrawal of the drug for 1 week to allow menstruation to occur. However, because of "breakthrough bleeding" a more potent progestin was needed.

By 1951, chemists at Syntex and Searle had produced analogs of progesterone called norethindrone and norethynodrel, respectively. Because they were more resistant to hepatic first-pass metabolism they were able to achieve higher potency. A large-scale clinical trial began in Puerto Rico in 1956 involving 221 women who received norethynodrel *and* a synthetic estrogen (mestranol—given to minimize "breakthrough bleeding") over a 2-year period. After the results of this trial and a subsequent larger-scale study were evaluated, Searle was given permission to market the first combination oral contraceptive in 1960.

It should be clear at this point that the basic steps in drug development involve a sequence: (a) the discovery of some pharmacological effect produced by a source material (plant or animal); (b) isolation and identification of the active ingredient; (c) determination of structure–activity relationships (SARs); and (d) the synthesis of more active congeners. Once a drug can be synthesized or isolated to complete purity, then its pharmacological profile can be quantified on a mass basis in some model system. This is referred to as drug screening.

DRUG SCREENING

Historically, the major source of chemical diversity for screening purposes has been natural products. In a 1997 survey, it was estimated that 39 per cent of all 520 approved drugs between 1983 and 1994 were natural or derived from natural products, and 60–80 percent of antibacterial and anticancer drugs were derived from natural products. However, because there has been a decrease in the number of new drugs introduced to the world market during the 1990s, efforts are being made to improve the efficiency of the drug discovery process by using high-throughput chemistry and screening.

The discovery of new drugs has traditionally depended, more or less, on the trial and error synthesis of potential lead compounds and their assay for pharmacological effect in some physiological system (e.g., intact animal, isolated organ, or receptor-binding assays). Examples include drugs such as morphine, quinine, and ephedrine, which have been in widespread use for some time. Lead compounds can also be suggested to the investigator through empirical knowledge of biochemical pathways or through success in the assay program itself. Examples include tubocurarine, propranolol, cimetidine, and the histamine H_2 antagonists. Following identification of such lead compounds, the chemical structure and physical properties of the drug have been traditionally optimized in a very painstaking and time-consuming manner by synthesis of a succession of variants with subsequent testing for pharmacological activity.

Classically, the entire process has been found to be protracted, challenging, and extremely demanding of resources because a correlation between the chemical structure of a drug and its pharmacological effect is often very difficult to discern. In addition, even if success is demonstrated in some non-whole-animal system, a drug's usefulness is often compromised by side effects and transport problems revealed when the drug is administered to the whole animal. In general, the successful development of a new drug is a relatively rare event and may require the synthesis and evaluation of thousands of candidate compounds. However, once a lead compound is discovered, then structural derivatives can be evaluated and the SAR determined.

One of the earliest examples of this SAR approach was the development of synthetic local anesthetic agents. These drugs were developed based upon the structure of cocaine, whose local anesthetic property was championed by Carl Köller, who introduced cocaine into clinical practice in 1884 for ophthamological surgery. The many local anesthetics used in clinical practice today all emanate from these early observations.

Because of cocaine's toxicity and addictive properties, a search began for synthetic substitutes for cocaine. In 1905, procaine was synthesized and became the prototypic local anesthetic for half a century. Newer derivatives include mepivacaine and tetracaine (Figure 13.1). Briefly, the SAR of local anesthetics revolves around their hydrophobicity. Association of the drug at hydrophobic sites, such as the sodium channel, is believed to prevent the generation and conductance of a nerve impulse by interfering with sodium permeability (i.e., elevating the threshold for electrical excitability).

Newer anti-inflammatory drugs have also been designed to combine the useful properties of the prototypic drug aspirin with a reduced level of gastric toxicity in derivatives. Typical of the structural modification experiments were those carried out by the Boots Company in England, which involved the synthesis and screening of numerous structural analogs of aspirin. Surprisingly, as is often the case, their "lead" or "parent" compound (Boots 7268) had originally been synthesized for use as an agricultural weed-killer. In fact, it proved to be twice as potent as aspirin when tested in an anti-inflammatory screen (companies routinely test for a wide spectrum of pharmacological activity in multiscreen assays). The chemists at Boots synthesized approximately 600 similar compounds, one of which proved to be 6–10 times more potent than aspirin. Eventually, after additional structural modifications, the highly effective drug ibuprofen was developed, which possesses 30-fold greater anti-inflammatory activity than aspirin (Figure 13.2).

More recent advances in anti-inflammatory drug research dealing with nonsteroidal anti-inflamatory drugs (NSAIDs) resulted in the development of an even newer class of compounds. Anti-inflammatory drugs such as aspirin and ibuprofen are believed to produce their effect by inhibiting an enzyme present in cell membranes (cyclo-oxygenase; COX). Aspirin inhibits COX by irreversibly (covalent) acetylating an active-site serine residue. Aspirin is distinctive among other NSAIDs in that the latter function as competitive inhibitors. COX is a necessary enzyme involved in the production of inflammatory mediators such as prostaglandins and leukotrienes when the membrane is damaged (Figure 13.3). Unfortunately, these over-the-counter (OTC) remedies do not possess sufficient potency to adequately deal with the severe joint inflammation that accompanies disorders such as arthritis. In addition, painful gastric side effects are all too common with stronger, alternative medications such as Naproxen® (the result of COX-1 inhibition).

Figure 13.1 Structural relationship between local anesthetics.

Based upon studies carried out during the early 1990s, it was discovered that there are at least two isozymes of COX. COX-1 is apparently involved primarily in protecting the stomach lining and performing other protective functions. COX-2, on the other hand, is the form that initiates the arachidonic cascade producing prostaglandins and leukotrienes. Aspirin and other similar pain relievers appear to have the capacity to inhibit both forms of the enzyme—hence their damaging as well as ameliorating effects. A major shortcoming of the 20 anti-inflammatory drugs that preceded the COX-2 inhibitors, the NSAIDs, which included ibuprofen and aspirin, was that they suppressed both enzymes causing the well-known side effect of gastrointestinal (GI)

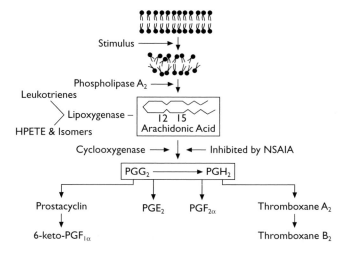

Figure 13.2 Structural relationship of the analgesic drugs ibuprofen and aspirin.

Figure 13.3 Arachidonic acid cascade and sites of nonsteroidal anti-inflammatory drug action.

Note: For more in-depth explanation of the cascade see J. G. Hardman, L. E. Limbird and A. G. Gilman, (eds) (2001), *Goodman and Gilman's The Pharmacological Basis of Therapeutics*, 10th ed., Chapter 26. New York: McGraw-Hill.

damage. In fact, 7500 to 15,000 deaths a year have been attributed to the side effects of NSAIDs. Because GI toxicity is associated with inhibition of COX-1, attempts were made to develop drugs with more selective action on COX-2.

Ongoing research led to the development of COX-2 selective inhibitors (e.g., rofecoxib and celecoxib). Celecoxib (Celebrex®) was approved by the FDA in 1998 to treat osteoarthritis and rheumatoid arthritis. Rofecoxib (Vioxx®) was approved in May 1999 to treat osteoarthritis, acute pain, and dysmenorrhea. Sales for the two drugs in 1999 were $1.5 billion and $373 million, respectively. Clinical studies have indicated a significant reduction in GI perforation, ulceration, or bleeding with the COX-2 inhibitors. The recognition of multiple COX isoforms has had one of the greatest impacts on the development of NSAIDs since the original synthesis of aspirin more than a century ago.

Despite the problems associated with classical screening programs, they have continued to yield numerous novel, important biologically active molecules. Among the most important recent examples is the discovery and development of drugs for the treatment of hypercholesteremia (see Chapter 12). In the early 1950s, scientists at Merck had begun researching the biosynthesis of cholesterol and by 1956 had demonstrated that mevalonic acid could be converted into cholesterol. In fact, the formation of mevalonic acid via 3-hydroxy-3-methylglutaryl-coenzyme A reductase was subsequently found to be the rate-limiting step in cholesterol synthesis. In the 1970s Merck scientists set up a cell culture assay in an attempt to identify substances that could inhibit the enzyme. In 1979 an inhibitor, lovastatin, was isolated from the fungus *Aspergillus terreus*. Following clinical trials, the drug was made available to selected patients with severe hypercholesteremia in 1982 under the trade name Mevacor. In 1987, the FDA approved its use for patients in the general population who had high cholesterol levels. Over the next decade a second generation of inhibitors was developed with fewer GI side effects.

In the past, most pharmaceutical companies maintained their own in-house facilities for screening drugs in whole animals. Today, with an emphasis on minimizing the use of experimental animals and their attendant cost, many companies "farm out" their drug leads to smaller companies that specialize in certain types of screening. Furthermore, with the advent of molecular pharmacology, companies can now screen drugs not initially in animals but, alternatively, on isolated receptors. Here again, there are companies that specialize in this service. It is only after a candidate drug has demonstrated desirable characteristics that it will undergo further evaluation in isolated tissues or organs as well as in whole animals. In this manner, thousands of candidate drugs can be assessed at their target endpoint without requiring the use of animals.

Increasingly, drug discovery is taking advantage of mechanistic, in vitro assays to broaden the search for therapeutic compounds. Examples include leukotriene B receptors, ionotropic excitatory amino acid receptors, epidermal growth factor receptors, histamine receptors, interleukin receptors, tyrosine kinase, and numerous others where affinity as well as inhibitory constants can be determined. An advantage of in vitro assays is that they are able to be adapted to allow high-throughput screening (HTS). For example, the National Cancer Institute (NCI), which first began screening compounds as potential anticancer drugs back in the 1960s, used to evaluate hundreds of drugs a year; now it can do thousands. HTS facilities offer the potential to readily screen hundreds of thousands of candidate drugs per year with robotics.

The database generated from HTS, when combined with other relevant information, can provide a powerful method for the identification of trends in SARs. In addition, this approach has had an impact on the very nature of the drug discovery process. Historically, pharmacology and drug discovery have been driven by the availability of a lead compound that suggested a specific receptor or binding site and a therapeutic potential if the activity was augmented or inhibited. Increasingly, this scenario is being reversed, with the discovery of the drug targets (e.g., receptors) stimulating the search for appropriate agonists and antagonists.

Opportunities in the screening process provided by access to a "pure" supply of a drug target (e.g., receptor) include the possibility of identifying a specific drug without the prior availability of a specific lead compound. For example, the metabotropic glutamate receptor family appears to be a promising therapeutic target for which specific ligands have not been identified for any of the seven cloned receptor subtypes. However, potentially restricting the application of increasing knowledge of drug targets is the intention of some groups to patent the relevant genes, their expression systems, and their use within assays for drug discovery. Within the excitatory amino acid group of receptors alone, patents have been processed for the use of ionotropic receptors in general, as well as N-methyl-D-aspartate (NMDA) and metabotropic glutamate receptors.

With the capacity for high-volume mass screening, the availability of new substances to screen is becoming the rate-limiting factor in drug discovery. Because synthetic chemists are not able to keep up with demand, drug companies have turned to other strategies such as the vast supplies of marine and plant resources. In addition, the pharmaceutical industry has committed substantial resources of its own to an alternative strategy of drug discovery, namely rational drug design.

Rational drug design has been defined as "a reasoned approach to developing medicines." This involves an understanding of both the molecular pathophysiology of the disease process and molecular and structural nature of the target molecule. Biological approaches to rational drug design exploit an understanding of disease pathogenesis, while structural approaches to rational drug design describe the application of the tools of structural biology to pharmaceutical development.

BIOLOGICAL APPROACHES TO DRUG DESIGN

Stroke

One area that illustrates drug development predicated upon an understanding of the underlying disease pathogenesis is the treatment of stroke. Stroke is the third leading cause of death in the United States, killing approximately 150,000 people annually. In addition, another 400,000 stroke victims survive, but only a fortunate third of these are left with little or no physical or mental impairment. Approximately 80 percent of all strokes occur when a blood vessel becomes blocked by a clot that interrupts blood flow to a region of the brain and induces localized ischemia. The remaining 20 percent of strokes are caused by rupture of a blood vessel. Among the cascade of deleterious events initiated by a stroke of the first type is a deadly influx of calcium ions into nerve cells.

When a thrombotic type of stroke occurs, ischemic nerve cells rapidly deplete their energy supplies and can no longer maintain a normal resting membrane potential. As a consequence, the cells burst open their stores of "excitatory" amino acids (e.g., glutamate), which activate calcium ion channels in adjacent neurons by interacting with NMDA and DL-α-amino-3-hydroxy-5-methyl-4-isoxazole propionic acid (AMPA) receptors. The subsequent elevation of intraneuronal calcium drives a number of calcium-dependent processes into excess (e.g., calcium-dependent enzymes such as protein kinases and phosphokinases). A consequence of this hypermetabolic state is the formation of free radicals, which are believed to propagate the degenerative effect.

Among the drug strategies currently being pursued to arrest this process is the development of neuroprotective drugs that, if given soon enough, might prevent the inflow of calcium or reverse cell-membrane destruction. For example, in view of the fact that glutamate (as well as glycine and polyamines) can activate calcium channels, research is currently under way to develop effective antagonists of these substances that are free of significant side effects. Unfortunately, to date, clinical trials of such antagonists have been associated with patients developing hallucinations. As it turns out, this is not particularly surprising, since the recreational drug of abuse phencyclidine, which is also known to bind to a site within the NMDA receptor, also induces psychosis. Therefore, it may prove difficult to separate these properties.

Citicholine is a drug being developed from a somewhat different perspective. It is aimed at reversing cell-membrane destruction by supplying the membrane bilayer component choline to the brain. Phosphatidylcholine, the backbone of the cell membrane, breaks down as nerve cells are damaged; thus, in theory, delivering excess choline to the brain may facilitate membrane repair. In addition, choline may also function to "mop up" free fatty acids that could be oxidized to generate free radicals. It remains to be seen whether this approach will be successful, but it does illustrate how multiple drug strategies can be developed to attack a single medical disorder.

Antisense deoxynucleotides and ribozymes

The controlled expression of genes is a cornerstone in the regulation of growth and development of cells and organisms. The transcription of DNA into RNA and its subsequent translation into a peptide is a fundamental requirement in all living beings. Interruption in the controlled progression from one step to the next can have dramatic consequences to a cell. Although numerous anticancer drugs have operated in this mode for decades, new drug candidates are being investigated that function via significantly new mechanisms. One of the more novel means of modifying gene expression is to specifically target an RNA molecule and inactivate it, thereby preventing expression of its encoded message. Two theoretical ways of accomplishing this objective involve antisense deoxynucleotides and ribozymes.

Antisense technology allows researchers to devise strategies to reduce the expression of specific proteins in cells and whole animals without having to create transgenics (discussed later). Using Watson and Crick base-pairing rules, it is possible to design oligonucleotides that will selectively hybridize with mRNAs for specific gene products, thus inhibiting the translation of mRNA and reducing protein expression. This specificity can be exploited for design of therapeutic agents and selective inhibitors of gene expression for research applications. The use of antisense technologies provides the scientist with a means of specifically inhibiting gene expression without having to manipulate the genome. Antisense molecules have shown activity against viral genes and may have potential use in the treatment of cancer. Several candidates are undergoing clinical trial.

The information necessary to produce proteins in cells is contained in genes. Specific genes contain information to produce specific proteins. The information required for the human body to produce all proteins is contained in the human genome and its collection of thousands of genes. Genes are composed of DNA, which contains information about when and how much of which protein to produce, depending upon what function is to be performed.

The DNA molecule is a "double helix," a duplex of entwined strands. In each duplex, the bases or nucleotides (adenine, thymidine, guanosine, and cytosine) are weakly bound or "paired" by hydrogen bonds to complimentary nucleotides on the other strand (A to T, G to C). Such highly specific complimentary base pairing is the

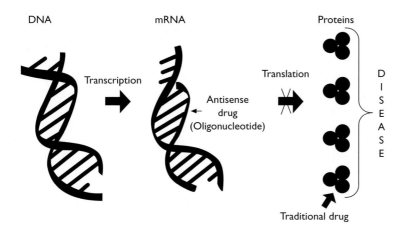

Figure 13.4 Mechanism of action of antisense drugs.

essence of information transfer from DNA to its intermediary, messenger RNA (mRNA), which carries the information, spelled out by the specific sequences of bases, necessary for the cell to produce a specific protein.

During transcription of information from DNA into mRNA, the two complimentary strands of the DNA partly uncoil. The "sense" strand separates from the "antisense" strand. The "antisense" strand of DNA is used as a template for transcribing enzymes that assemble mRNA (transcription), which, in the process produces a copy of the "sense" strand. Then, mRNA migrates into the cell, where other cellular structures called ribosomes read the encoded information, its mRNA's base sequence, and in so doing, string together amino acids to form a specific protein. This process is called "translation."

Antisense drugs are complimentary strands of small segments of mRNA. To create antisense drugs, nucleotides are linked together in short chains (called oligonucleotides). Each antisense drug is designed to inhibit production of the protein encoded by the target mRNA. By acting at this earlier stage in the disease-causing process to prevent the production of a disease-causing protein, antisense drugs have the potential to provide greater therapeutic benefit than traditional drugs, which do not act until the disease-causing protein has already been produced (Figure 13.4).

Perhaps even more esoteric than antisense nucleic acids are RNA molecules that are able to specifically cleave other RNA molecules. Until several years ago, it was generally thought that all cellular processes were dictated by DNA through the structure of polypeptides, which performed all the functions. During studies conducted on RNA, it was discovered that some RNA strands had catalytic properties. These nonprotein biocatalysts are referred to as ribozymes and combine the properties of antisense RNA with the ability to cleave target RNA.

An early hint of such a phenomenon occurred when the RNA "cofactor" of ribonuclease P was found capable of catalyzing the specific cleavage of pre-tRNAs in the absence of protein. However, the first real report of the ability of RNA to act as a catalyst was made from Thomas Cech's laboratory in 1982, for which he subsequently shared the Nobel prize (1989). Cech and colleagues examined the removal of a nucleotide sequence from the preribosomal RNA of *Tetrahymena* and found that the reaction was autocatalytic for the rRNA itself. Eventually, an L19 form of ribozyme (from the group I introns) was the first ribozyme discovered. (There are currently five classes of ribozymes: (1) the group I intron; (2) Rnase P; (3) the hammerhead ribozymes; (4) the hairpin ribozymes; and (5) the hepatitis delta virus ribozymes.) These types of studies have generated significant interest in ribozymes as potential therapeutic agents for controlling gene expression. Scientists have since discovered more than 500 ribozymes in a diverse range of organisms and have found that they share many similarities with their more widespread cousins, enzymes.

An example of the type of research that is currently being carried out deals with the in vitro evaluation of ribozymes on gene expression. Hammerhead ribozymes have been shown to have the ability to attack the coding region of mRNA of interleukin 6 (IL-6). In this manner, theoretically, downregulation of IL-6 may be a potential treatment of those diseases in which IL-6 overexpression is involved.

Although ribozymes have been shown to work *in vitro* in cellular assays, there are few reports demonstrating their efficacy *in vivo*. One such success utilized the rabbit model of IL-1-induced arthritis. In this model, IL-1 is believed to generate the formation of a proteinase mediator called stromelysin, which participates in the inflammatory condition. The intra-articular administration of ribozymes directed against stromelysin mRNA has been reported to produce a reduction in the message for this mediator in synovial fluid.

In 1998, researchers at the University of Florida demonstrated that a custom-made ribozyme could successfully cleave the faulty (bad) mRNA in a rat model of retinitus pigmentosa (RP). RP has a frequency of approximately 1 in 3000 Americans. As the disease progresses, night vision and peripheral vision decrease, and ultimately all sight is lost. Currently, there is no way to halt the destruction of sight.

In RP, a mutant gene codes for the formation of a protein that damages the eye's light-sensitive rod cells. Approximately 40 percent of people with RP have the "autosomal-dominant" form; that is, they inherited a defective gene from one parent who has the disease, but also received a normal gene copy from the other parent. The University of Florida research targets the autosomal-dominant form of the disease in their rat model. Significant protection was observed for up to 3 months.

One of the shortcomings of ribozymes is that they are short single-stranded RNA moieties with a simple secondary structure. It is possible that their use in gene therapy could be limited because they could be highly susceptible to cellular nucleases. Present research is aimed at producing ribozymes that are more resistant to degradation.

Membrane fusion

A particularly timely example of biologically based drug design involves a novel strategy directed toward treating viral infections. Instead of developing an antiviral drug to attack a virus after it has infected a cell (the more traditional approach), compounds are being developed that are aimed at blocking the virus from entering the cell in the first place. Researchers are focusing on the process by which a virus fuses with the membrane of a cell, permitting it to inject its genetic material. Viral proteins from influenza virus, HIV-1, and Ebola virus are composed of two distinct subunits, namely a receptor binding domain (gp120) and a fusion competent subunit (gp41).

The process of membrane fusion is a ubiquitous process that can occur in all eukaryotic cells but has particular significance in virally transmitted diseases such as HIV. Research in HIV-1 fusion with human lymphocytes has revealed that the virus contains an oligomeric complex of glycoproteins, gp120 and gp41, on its surface that play a central role in the fusion and transference process. In its native resting state, a heterooligomer of two gp120s and two gp41s is held together by noncovalent protein–protein interactions. A portion of gp41, known as the "fusion domain," is buried within this complex and mediates fusion with cells.

When HIV-1 encounters a human lymphocyte displaying a CD4 receptor on its cell surface, for example, the gp120 oligomer binds to the CD4 receptor. The result of that binding is a series of important events: (1) a conformational change occurs within the gp120–gp41 complex; (2) that conformational change triggers an intramolecular rearrangement of domains within the gp41 that releases a "fusion protein" from its bound configuration; and (3) the formation of a "membrane attack complex" occurs that permits insertion of the fusion peptide into the host cell membrane.

Researchers studying the viral fusion process recognized that two coiled regions in gp41 were highly conserved among all HIVs, so they synthesized a number of peptides containing this region's respective peptide structure. Assay of these peptide fragments demonstrated that one was particularly potent in selectively inhibiting the fusion event of native, intact HIV-1 to lymphocytes. Apparently, the drug candidate binds to the other coiled region of gp41 and prevents the membrane attack complex from forming when gp120 binds to the CD4 receptor. The company developing this potential drug is also utilizing a proprietary computerized antiviral searching technology to identify key sequences within fusion proteins in other medically important viruses, thus also utilizing a structural approach to drug design.

STRUCTURAL APPROACHES TO DRUG DESIGN

Background

As mentioned previously, one of the first steps in the process of drug development is the identification of lead compounds. These compounds generally have affinity for the target molecule as identified after extensive screening using receptor binding or biological assays, and are then modified to possess pharmacologically useful properties. These traditional methods of drug discovery are now being supplemented by a more direct approach made possible, in part, by increased understanding of the molecular interactions that underlie diseases.

The new approach is referred to as structure-based drug design. The starting point is not necessarily the drug, but can alternatively be its molecular target in the body. If the three-dimensional structure of a substance known to be involved in a disease can be ascertained, then conceivably a chemical could be designed that interacts with a key region producing altered function. For example, the catalytic site of a viral enzyme essential for replication might be designed. In fact, many contemporary research programs are focused on the development of inhibitors of HIV protease, a key enzyme in HIV replication. Figure 13.5 shows a representative, computer-generated interelationship between a candidate ligand and the binding domain of the protease.

Figure 13.5 Computer-generated modeling of the relationship of a protease inhibitor with a binding domain.

Protease inhibitors work by preventing cleavage of viral polyproteins into active proteins, which takes place during HIV's insidious and complicated replication process. The drug binds to the enzyme's active site, blocking cleavage of the polyprotein.

Inhibitors of purine nucleoside phosphorylase

The theoretical advantages of structure-based methodology include the creation of more lead compounds at less expense. The analogy has been made that this approach is similar to designing an effective key if the shape and arrangement of tumblers in a lock are already known. Presumably, because the final designed drug is "custom-tailored" to its target, it will be more specific and less toxic. An example of such an approach is research carried out during the 1980s dealing with the design of inhibitors of the enzyme purine nucleoside phosphorylase (PNP).

PNP normally operates in the "purine salvage pathway" of cells and is responsible for cleaving nucleosides into their respective purine and sugar components. Unfortunately, PNP can also cleave certain anticancer and antiviral drugs that are synthetic mimics of endogenous nucleosides. An example is the antiviral drug 2′,3′-dideoxyinosine (ddI) used in the treatment of AIDS. A successful candidate for inhibiting PNP was achieved in less than 3 years by a small group of chemists who prepared approximately 60 compounds aimed at blocking the purine binding site. The result was a PNP inhibitor 100 times more effective than the best inhibitor found by traditional methods of drug discovery. In traditional practice, the development of enzyme inhibitors often takes more than 10 years and can cost tens of millions of dollars for the screening of hundreds or thousands of candidates.

X-ray crystallography

X-ray crystallography is the oldest and most widely applied technology for determining macromolecular structure to atomic resolution. Three-dimensional atomic models of proteins and nucleic acids are the basis of much of our modern understanding of biology and medicine. Until relatively recently, receptors were hypothetical macromolecules whose existence was postulated on the basis of pharmacological experiments. However, during the 1970s and 1980s new methods became available for obtaining pure samples of many receptors as well as providing an insight into their structure. For example, advances in molecular biology have led to the cloning and expression of many receptors. In addition, improvements in X-ray crystallography revealed more insight into their structure. In this technique, pure receptors in their crystalline form are bombarded with X-rays. The crystal defracts the X-rays according to its molecular structure, creating a pattern of spots on photographic film or on newer types of electronic detectors. While X-ray crystallography has proven to be a major technology in determining structure, newer techniques such as nuclear magnetic resonance (NMR) spectroscopy and neutron diffraction are also being utilized.

Enzymes are often the targets of drugs, and thus protein's are of particular interest to pharmacologists. Knowing a protein's structure gives deep insight into its function. And understanding how proteins work, and what happens when they don't, is a key to uncovering the molecular basis of disease. In the application of structure-based rational drug design, analogs of natural substrates are modeled by computer graphics to the active site of the enzyme. The structure and geometry of the protein is generally well established at the atomic level through the use of X-ray diffraction techniques. The approach of rational drug design based on knowledge of target macromolecules is made all the more powerful by the ability to actually visualize the complex that is formed between the drug and enzyme. In this situation, there is the added bonus of actually seeing conformational changes that occur by virtue of the interaction.

The first successful exploitation of X-ray crystallography in drug discovery was the development of the antihypertensive drug captopril in 1975. Although the investigators at the Squibb Institute for Medical Research (now Bristol-Myers Squibb) did not know the precise architecture of their target (angiotensin-converting enzyme), they utilized the known conformation of a closely related enzyme. This type of homology modeling is still presently utilized. For example, many models of the various G-protein-coupled receptors have been built based on homology with bacterial rhodopsin, while models of human renin and HIV protease have been built from crystal structures of aspartyl proteinases.

Three-dimensional databases

Since Christian B. Anfinsen and colleagues demonstrated during the 1950s and 1960s that the amino acid sequence of a protein directs its folding, significant research has focused on understanding the molecular basis of the protein folding process and on determining the inherent information in protein primary structures to predict protein tertiary structure. The importance of structural biology is illustrated by the awarding of 10 Nobel prizes in this area since 1962. Recipients of the award include the following: the first three-dimensional structure of a biopolymer was the DNA model built by J. D. Watson and F. H. C. Crick in 1953, taking into account fiber diffraction data provided by M. H. F. Wilkins; the first three-dimensional protein structures (myoglobin and hemoglobin) were determined by M. F. Perutz and J. C. Kendrew; and the structure of the first membrane-bound protein was resolved by J. Deisenhofer, R. Haber, and H. Mechel.

Medicinal chemists have long recognized the potential of searching three-dimensional chemical databases to aid in the process of designing drugs for known, or hypothetical, receptor sites. Several databases are well known, such as the Cambridge Structural Database, which contains nearly 90,000 structures of small molecules. In addition, the Protein Data Bank (PDB) and the Nucleic Acid Data Bank (NDB) contain the crystal coordinates of proteins and other large macromolecules. The IMB Jeva Image Library of Biological Macromolecules provides access to all structures deposited at the PDB and the NDB as well as basic information on biological macromolecules.

The terms bioinformatics and cheminformatics refer to the use of computational methods in the study of biology and chemistry. Information from DNA or protein sequences, protein structure, and chemical structure is used to build models of biochemical systems or models of the interaction of a biochemical system with a small molecule (e.g., a drug). There are mathematical and statistical methods for analysis, public databases, and literature associated with each of these disciplines. However, there is substantial value in considering the interaction between these areas and in building computational models that integrate data from both sources. In the most general sense, integrating bioinformatics and cheminformatics leads to models that relate features of biological systems (sequences, protein structures, motifs) to features of the chemical structures, including small organic molecules (e.g., drugs) that interact with them. This information is useful for drug design in order to identify pharmacophores.

The three-dimensional orientation of the key regions of a drug that are crucially important for molecular recognition and binding is termed the pharmacophore. Investigators can search the three-dimensional database using a query for fragments that contain the pharmacophoric functional groups in the proper three-dimensional orientation. For example, such a process was carried out with caffeic acid phenethyl ester, an inhibitor of HIV-1 integrase. A computer search of 200,000 compounds at the National Cancer Institute yielded 19 candidates containing this pharmacophore that demonstrated in vitro activity. A statistically significant correlation was found between the presence of the pharmacophore and inhibitory potency. Using these fragments as building blocks, completely novel structures may be constructed through assembly and pruning. Pharmaceutical companies have developed substantial three-dimensional databases for their compound files to help prioritize candidates for screening.

Although observations extracted from the databases of experimentally known structures are an extremely useful empirical guide to the design of modified proteins and peptides, current biocomputational approaches to drug design are, nevertheless, limited by the relatively small subset of proteins that have been structurally characterized. Fortunately, proteins belong to a limited number of structural families whose members have very similar three-dimensional structures, thus allowing comparative modeling approaches to be used in developing databases. Various protein design software tools have been and are being developed to evaluate secondary or tertiary structures from protein sequences and to design proteins with predetermined functions and/or physical properties.

The procedure to predict protein structure has evolved from using probability profiles on the preferential localization of residues, to relying heavily on protein structure databases to define topological organization and three-dimensional relationships among proteins. The prediction of protein structure rests upon a knowledge-based approach that identifies analogies in secondary structures, motifs, domains, or ligand interactions between a protein being modeled with homologous proteins whose structures are available.

In addition to X-ray diffraction and NMR, which are direct techniques, methods based on the calculation of predicted three-dimensional structures of molecules in the range of 3 to 50 amino acids based on energy considerations are under rapid development. These approaches use what are commonly called molecular dynamics and energy minimization equations to specify the most probable conformation of polypeptides and small proteins. Often, when combined with information from other sources, such as X-ray crystallography or NMR studies, they have been demonstrated to be quite useful. However, when standing alone, their power and the accuracy of their predictive capability remains to be seen.

The multidisciplinary approach described above has been used to study protein folding phenomena and protein SARs for protein engineering endeavors, as well as protein-based and pharmacophore drug design. The validity of the predicted structure obviously depends on many factors, including the accuracy of the structures determined by the various analytical techniques, the percentage of homology in proteins used as templates, the rules used to translate amino acid alignments into geometric relationships between the template and the protein to be modeled, and the energy constraints of the resulting conformation. New discoveries regarding receptor structure, coupled with rational strategies in molecular biology and biochemical experiments, promise to speed the development of new and better drugs.

Combinatorial chemistry

One of the rate-limiting steps in the drug discovery process has always been the laborious synthesis of new entities in which a chemist makes one compound at a time. If a drug company wanted to make more compounds, it simply increased its research budget and hired more chemists. Today, because of numerous economic factors, companies are discouraged from simply increasing the payroll. However, increased competition demands that medicinal chemistry departments still increase the rate at which they produce new chemical entities. The problem of new lead development has been exacerbated by developments in molecular biology and high-throughput screening, which enable companies to screen entire libraries of archived compounds in a matter of months. One solution to this bottleneck has been the development of rapid automated procedures for the synthesis of organic molecules that can be subsequently screened.

In simple terms, combinatorial chemistry is the process whereby thousands of compounds (a library), systematic variants of a parent chemical structure, are synthesized. Although combinatorial chemistry generally refers to a single process, in reality it comprises several integrated intellectual and technological processes: computer-aided drug design and combinatorial chemistry library design; automated solid/solution-phase organic synthesis; and high-throughput screening techniques. Applied together, the synergy of these processes has been a major leap for drug development and basic medical research.

Pharmaceutical chemists can now create and test libraries of thousands, if not millions, of compounds for pharmacological properties relatively quickly. To put the results of the processes in perspective, consider that the possible number of products is defined by the number of different reagents raised to the number of synthesis steps. Therefore, for a three-step process involving 10 different reagents, the theoretical yield is 10^3 or 10,000 unique chemical combinations. For a simple pentamer peptide there are 20^5 or 3,200,000 possible combinations.

These new procedures were developed during the early 1990s and have revolutionized the rate at which new compounds can be synthesized. The first element involves the random formation of low-molecular-weight molecules (i.e. 500 daltons) via automated technology. This strategy is based on "the numbers game" or the belief that the more compounds that are screened the more likely it is that a "hit" will be found based on simple chance. The technology was pioneered by scientists at Affymax, a biotechnology company. The large number of molecules that can be prepared in this way is providing new sources of novel compounds to be screened. Instead of making one compound per week, 100 or more can be produced in a day. One important advantage of making *new* pharmaceuticals is that they are not "me-too" drugs and can be protected by patent rights—an absolute requirement of drug companies.

A second key element to evolve in combinatorial chemistry is the introduction of a rational design or bias library. Despite the huge number of potential drug-like small molecules with a molecular weight of less than 500 that can be synthesized, it appears unreasonable to assume that comprehensive representation with a "random" library will necessarily be achieved. Even relatively large compound libraries, designed with attention to molecular diversity, yield only a very small fraction of possible compounds. An example of a biased library would be a structure-based library developed around X-ray diffraction data of a ligand–protein complex, or based around an important protein motif. It is believed that a marriage of these two elements is an optimal strategy for drug discovery.

An example of using the combinatorial approach to drug discovery is the attempt to produce a "miniprotein" version of erythropoietin (EPO). As mentioned previously, EPO stimulates the body to produce red blood cells. EPO is widely used for patients with anemia, kidney disease, cancer, or AIDS and has yearly sales of approximately $1 billion. By applying combinatorial chemistry, a new 20-amino-acid molecule was discovered that successfully mimics the 165-amino-acid EPO, *in vitro*. Of particular interest is the fact that the sequence of amino acids in the small molecule is unrelated to that of the larger EPO. This research also suggests that it may be possible to make nonprotein versions of other important proteins such as insulin and avoid the need for injections.

Combinatorial libraries are generally created in the laboratory by one of two automated methods—split synthesis or parallel synthesis. In split synthesis, monomers of the starting structure are attached to small plastic bead-like particles. In a series of successive, repetitive steps, the initial monomer–bead complexes are randomly mixed and coupled with a subsequent population of monomers, creating dimers, trimers, etc., by employing the conditions necessary for appropriate organic reactions. This process can be continued until the desired combinatorial library has been assembled. Diversity is achieved by using separate reactions so the components will have an equal chance to add a new building block to a site and then mixing the compounds together again. Split synthesis greatly simplifies the isolation and identification of active agents because the beads are large enough to be observed visually and separated mechanically. Combinatorial libraries can also be made by parallel synthesis, in which different compounds are synthesized in separate vessels (without remixing), often in an automated fashion. Unlike split synthesis, which requires a solid support, parallel synthesis can be done either on a solid support or in solution.

Regardless of which method is used, the large numbers of drugs developed are usually subjected to screening in automated receptor-binding assays. According to one company, their high-throughput system allows two chemists to synthesize up to one million compounds per year. Any drug demonstrating significant affinity will proceed to the next step of evaluation. At this point in time, it is not known if the drug is an agonist or an antagonist. All that can be measured is a binding constant. It is not until the drug is assessed in some kind of "biological" system, such as isolated ion channels, that information about the nature and "effectiveness" of the drug can be determined. Success at this level may qualify the drug for evaluation in whole-animal studies. Recent developments in combinatorial chemistry have been concentrated on the use of small organic building blocks, such as benzodiazepines, in order to create libraries with more drug-like qualities.

To increase the chances of finding leads, some combinatorial chemistry companies have specialized in producing very large libraries. Often, combinatorial chemistry gives small companies chemical libraries that are on the same order of magnitude as those once the domain of only the largest drug companies. With these libraries and their proprietary technologies, small companies can leverage profitable arrangements with larger companies that can include substantial up-front and milestone payments as well as long-term royalties. These arrangements, in turn, give the small companies access to biological targets and the pharmaceutical infrastructure necessary to take drug candidates through development, clinical testing, regulatory approval, and marketing.

One new wrinkle on the combinatorial strategy involves a process referred to as combinatorial biosynthesis. In this situation, bacterial gene expression is altered in the hope of changing the structure and function of specific enzymes. For example, one class of potential bacteria-derived drugs are the polyketides, which may have antibiotic, immunosuppressant, and anticancer activity. Bacteria produce polyketides with the help of a family of enzymes known as polyketide synthases (PKSs). To date, most of the normally produced polyketides screened have shown little activity.

In order to increase the likelihood of bacteria forming new active polyketides, scientists, working like combinatorial chemists, have mixed and matched PKS genes from different organisms to create 100 different bacterial clones with unique combinations of PKS genes. Although only 25 of these clones were found to produce unique compounds, four of them proved to be as effective as the reference drug. Although such results are encouraging, it remains to be seen if this methodology will prove useful in the future.

Antibody-directed drug design

Antibodies are part of the armamentarium that physicians can use for the treatment of a range of human conditions. A few examples include injection of antibody that recognizes tumor necrosis factor to treat rheumatoid arthritis; the experimental use of monoclonal antibodies to treat metastatic cancer; injection of antibody that recognizes the antigen OKT3 to revert organ rejection after transplantation; and the use of sheep antibodies to bind the heart medication digoxin in case of an overdose. Physicians often prefer to use human antibodies, or at least animal antibodies in which parts of the antibody have been replaced with the human equivalent, to decrease the likelihood of an allergic reaction.

One of the more novel approaches to utilizing properties of macromolecules for directed drug design is that employing the recognition feature of monoclonal antibodies. In 1976 Georges Kohler, working in the laboratory of Cesar Milstein, developed a method of somatic cell hybridization in order to successfully generate a continuous "hybridoma" cell line capable of producing monoclonal antibody (mAb) of defined specificity. Briefly, hybridoma technology involves the following steps:

1   An antigen is injected into a mouse. The mouse's immune system recognizes the antigen as being foreign and directs the spleen to produce specific antibodies to attack that antigen. The spleen is then removed and the antibody-producing B lymphocytes are collected.

2 Myeloma cells are isolated from a mouse tumor. These cells have the ability to reproduce continuously in the laboratory.

3 Spleen and tumor cells are mixed together with some fusing to form "hybridomas." All the cells are transferred to a medium in which the hybridoma cells can grow while the others die. The surviving hybridomas have the spleen cell's ability to produce antibodies and the tumor cell's ability to reproduce.

4 Each hybridoma is isolated and allowed to grow into a large colony of cells that produce a single mAb.

5 Each mAb can be screened for its ability to attack the original antigen and the hybridoma colonies producing the desired antibody are kept.

The need for a successful large-scale mAb production technique is indicated by the growing commercial market for antibody-based products and the increased importance of in vivo diagnostic as well as therapeutic applications. According to market research, total sales of in vivo and in vitro mAb-based products reached approximately $8 billion in 1993 and this volume is expected to increase in subsequent years. Therefore, significant commercial production of mAbs is being emphasized. In one procedure, mAb-producing murine hybridomas are cultured in 40-liter bioreactors.

Antibody-directed drug design is based upon the concept that when a monoclonal antibody is raised against an antigen, a stereochemically *negative* image of the antigen is embedded in the structure and chemistry of the antibody's hypervariable region, a relatively small portion of the antibody composed of peptides contributed in part by both the heavy and light chains of the immunoglobin. Significantly, the antigen could be the active site of an enzyme, a viral component, or the recognition or combining site of a drug receptor, to name but a few. Obviously, the theoretical potential use of mAbs is quite substantial.

From the mAb containing the mirror image of the target macromolecule (mAb-1), a *positive* image can also be derived. This is accomplished by raising a second antibody (mAb-2) against the hypervariable region of the Ab-1. By virtue of its stereocomplementarity to the combining region of the Ab-1, a feature it shares with the original target antigen, it must, therefore, possess common structural and electrostatic characteristics. Although it may not be perfectly homologous with the target antigen, it should incorporate at least some of the essential physical disposition of key chemical groups.

Although hybridoma technology permits the production of relatively large supplies of an antibody, only the rat and mouse myeloma lines appear to be reliably stable in long-term tissue culture. Rodent monoclonals, however, have serious limitations when used as therapeutic agents in humans, especially in diseases requiring repetitive administration. For example, they are prone to induce immune responses to themselves that can neutralize their effect, and lead to rapid body clearance. In addition, murine monoclonals have a short serum half-life in humans. In view of the persistent problems in making human monoclonals by conventional fusion techniques, recombinant DNA technology has become an important mode of human antibody production.

In order to circumvent the problems associated with rodent mAbs, the concept of a chimeric monoclonal has been successfully achieved. In Greek mythology the chimera was a fire-breathing monster with a lion's head, a goat's body, and the tail of a dragon. In the lexicon of antibodies, chimeras are antibodies constructed of disparate sections. They can be constructed in various ways. For example, to reduce the immunogenicity of the rodent variable region, humanized mAbs have been created. In this case, a rat/human antibody has been produced in which only the hypervariable regions were of rat origin (i.e., only the antigen-binding site rather than the entire variable domain was from the rodent). This results in a decreased immune response in humans since 90 percent of the human immune response is directed against constant domains and 10 percent against the variable domain. Chimerization also produces up to a sixfold increase in half-life. An alternative method was published in 1999 that involves the fusion of active antibody fragments to polyethylene glycol molecules. The resulting conjugate has a much longer in vivo half-life and retains its antigen-binding activity. Successful application of genetic engineering to mAbs has produced two drugs. The FDA approved Rituxan® in 1997 for the treatment of B-cell lymphomas and Herceptin® in 1999 for certain breast cancer tumors.

Rituxan reacts with the CD2 antigen found on B-cell lymphomas. Herceptin is reactive with a growth factor receptor called HER2/neu, which is selectively overexpressed by breast cancer cells in 30 percent of women and results in abnormal cell proliferation. Neither Herceptin nor Rituxan alone can cure cancer, but combining them with other treatments, such as chemotherapy, has shown great promise for some indications.

MOLECULAR PHARMACOLOGY; RECOMBINANT DNA TECHNOLOGY—BIOTECHNOLOGY

Molecular pharmacology

The molecular approach to drug discovery is based on the availability or understanding of a molecular target for the medicinal agent. With the development of molecular biological techniques and the advances in genomics, the majority of drug discovery is currently based on the molecular approach. Modern genomics and its offspring, proteomics and gene expression profiling, offer an almost overwhelming amount of new information.

The pharmaceutical industry has rapidly integrated genomic considerations into its research and development programs. For example, target selection, a key aspect of drug development, will greatly benefit from the identification of genes that unambiguously play a role in specific diseases processes. Likewise, pharmacogenetics (i.e., genetic profiling to predict patient response to a drug) will also be of great value in clinical care. However, the most challenging step may be target validation, that is, reliably defining candidate genes with respect to disease processes. Once a target is identified, it can be rapidly addressed through combinatorial chemistry and high-throughput screening. Lead compounds emerging from the screening process must still undergo the tedious process of pharmacodynamic and toxicological profiling, however, before being considered for clinical trials.

Pharmacogenomics, the application of genotyping (determining the genetic constitution of an organism) to patient therapy, holds great promise for solving a long-standing problem: differences in individual responses to drug treatments. The ultimate goal is to maximize drug efficacy while minimizing side effects. The time when a report with each person's genetic code will guide doctors in personalized medicine is still far away, but pharmacogenomics already is allowing physicians to make treatment decisions regarding HIV-1.

Mutations in HIV accumulate and interact with each other and cause resistance to one drug and then others, one of the pivotal problems in treatment. In the past, the complexity of HIV drug-resistance testing and the limited information on its clinical utility made routine application impractical. Recent advances in automated assay technology have allowed rapid characterization of HIV in blood samples, so an increasing number of commercial laboratories now offer phenotypic and genotypic testing.

The power of new genetic screening technologies is dramatically increasing our ability to identify gene loci that might be involved in the pathogenesis of human disease. In addition, advances in transgenic technology allow the creation of animal models that reflect particular human disease states. Therefore, we can identity the role of specific genes in particular metabolic pathways and provide models for screening novel therapeutic agents. The human genome project will identify vast numbers of genes whose functions are unknown and it will not be clear whether or not they are drug targets. Thus, pharmacogenomics will allow the exploitation of genetic information to establish whether particular genes or gene loci are novel targets for drugs, and to develop cell lines or animal models as screening tools for identifying pharmacologically active molecules that will reverse the phenotypes (observable genetic expression) generated.

It has been known for approximately 50 years that individuality in response to a drug can have a genetic basis. The ability to identify individuals who might benefit or suffer as a consequence of a particular drug therapy is of considerable medical and economic importance. If drug therapy could be tailored to individuals on the basis of their genetic makeup, it would remove some of the empiricism from current drug prescribing.

The development of pharmacogenetics has evolved from understanding how the role of particular genetic polymorphisms influences the outcome of drug therapy in genes such as glucose-6-phosphate dehydrogenase and the cytochrome P450 enzymes. For example, the cytochrome P450 CYP2D6 that is responsible for the metabolism of up to 25 percent of therapeutic drugs is highly polymorphic and inactive in 6 percent of the white population. Many serious drug side effects have been ascribed to this polymorphism, particularly for cardiovascular and CNS active drugs. Future research will involve the study of polymorphisms in both candidate genes and genome-wide screens, in order to identify novel genes of pharmacological significance by screening, for example, single nucleotide polymorphisms.

Recombinant DNA

The development of recombinant DNA and hybridoma technologies has revolutionized the number and kind of pharmaceutical proteins available, and these technologies serve as two of the cornerstones of the biotechnology industry. This has been made possible, in large part, by the dramatic progress made in the methods of purification of the molecules produced. To date, there have been a number of products produced by recombinant technology (see Table 13.1).

Table 13.1 The top 10 bioengineered drugs in 1998 (sales in $ million)

1	Epogen	Red blood cell enhancement	1380.0
2	Procrit	Red blood cell enhancement	1363.0
3	Neupogen	Restoration of white blood cells	1120.0
4	Humulin	Diabetes mellitus	959.2
5	Engerix-B	Prevention of hepatitis B	886.7
6	Intron A	Bone marrow transplantation	719.0
7	Betaseron	Multiple sclerosis	409.2
8	Genotropin	Growth failure in children	395.1
9	Avonex	Relapsing multiple sclerosis	394.9
10	Recombivax HB	Prevention of hepatitis B	290.0

Although not listed among the top 10 bioengineered drugs (in 1998; Table 13.1), tissue plasminogen activator (tPA) is an important recombinant product. The clotting of blood is a normal hemodynamic function required to maintain the integrity of the vascular system. It involves a complex cascade of metabolic events involving many so-called clotting factors. The end result is the formation of proteinaceous fibrin monomers that polymerize to form the matrix of the clot, which then aggregates with platelets. This hemostatic plug normally functions to bridge ruptures within the vascular wall. In this case they are reparative. However, under certain circumstances "abnormal" clots can form transverse to a vessel, thereby forming an occlusive barrier to downstream blood flow.

Several disease states can result from abnormal blood clots. For example, strokes were mentioned previously. However, the most common and deadliest thrombotic disease is myocardial infarction (MI). Atherosclerosis has long been associated with reduced cardiac function and elevated mortality due to rupture of atherosclerotic plaques. The rupture of an atherosclerotic plaque usually results not only in blockage due to the plaque itself but also in the immediate formation of an occlusive blood clot, which results in an MI. Immediately after the initiation of an MI, a zone of necrosis begins to develop around the area as ischemia proceeds. It is during this early phase of ischemia (several hours) that therapeutic intervention not only can be life-saving but also can minimize the amount of necrotic heart tissue formed.

In addition to possessing a clot-forming system, the body has a fibrinolytic system that has the capacity to degrade the underlying fibrin in clots. One of the key activators of the fibrinolytic system is tPA. This protein functions to activate plasminogen, which subsequently activates plasmin, which is responsible for degrading fibrin. With this knowledge in mind, Genentech undertook the project of developing commercial quantities of tPA, via their recombinant technology, to be used in the acute phase immediately following an MI.

The importance of using a recombinant source is dramatized when one considers the amount of activator required for therapy. The normal concentration of tPA in the blood is approximately 2 ng/ml. Therefore, if a human dose were of the order of 100 mg, it would take 50,000 L of blood to produce a single dose of tPA, even if recovery was 100 percent. Obviously, blood is not an adequate commercial source for this material.

Genentech scientists chose to develop recombinant tPA by successfully cloning the nucleotide sequence for tPA into a Chinese hamster ovary cell line. As opposed to bacteria (see later discussion), this mammalian cell carried out the required glycosylation, disulfide bond formation, and proper folding of tPA in the same manner as human cells. The recombinant material was identical to the human-derived material in molecular weight, amino acid composition, sequence, immunoreactivity, and kinetic constants.

Additional, related work being carried out in this area by other biotechnology companies involves the creation of so-called "fusion proteins." In this case, the binding domain of an antibody, fibrin, that recognizes the major component of a clot is combined with the clot-dissolving portion of tPA. It is hoped that enhanced specificity in target interaction will translate into better therapeutic results. In fact, preliminary tests have shown these combinations to be more potent and selective than tPA alone.

In the initial recombinant work carried out in the 1980s, bacteria were used as the recipient cell-type. The underlying principle in the application of recombinant DNA is that if you insert a fragment of DNA (coded for a particular protein, e.g., insulin) into a host cell (e.g., bacteria), it will be duplicated as the cell divides and there will be a corresponding increase in the number of copies of the fragment. In order to achieve this replication the DNA fragment must be inserted into an appropriate section of the host cell's DNA, so that it will be duplicated along with the endogenous DNA during cell division.

DNA suitable for the insertion of foreign DNA is known as a vector; the most commonly used vectors in bacteria are plasmids. Plasmids are small (2–3 kb) loops of DNA found in bacteria and yeast. They were first discovered when it was observed that bacteria could pass antibiotic resistance from one colony to another. This process was demonstrated to be mediated by plasmids containing genes for enzymes that inactivated the antibiotics. In addition to the work on plasmids, other research laboratories have isolated enzymes that cut DNA at specific sequences (restriction endonucleases) and other enzymes that can rejoin these cuts again (DNA ligases).

In cloning, the plasmid vector is incubated with a restriction endonuclease that cuts open the plasmid DNA. Exposure of the open DNA to a new DNA fragment plus a ligase reconstitutes the plasmid DNA with a new nucleotide sequence. The resulting recombinant DNA is inserted into bacterial cells, which then multiply. Each cell can contain 50–100 copies of the recombinant plasmid and can duplicate every 20–30 minutes.

Transgenic animals

Transgenic animals result from genetic engineering experiments in which genetic material is moved from one organism to another, so that the latter will exhibit a desired characteristic. Scientists, farmers, and business corporations hope that transgenic techniques will allow more precise and cost-effective animal and plant breeding programs. They also hope to use these new methods to produce animals and plants with desirable characteristics that are not available using current breeding technology.

In traditional breeding programs, only closely related species can be crossbred, but transgenic techniques allow genetic material to be transferred between completely unrelated organisms, so that breeders can incorporate characteristics that are not normally available to them. Although the basic coding system is the same in all organisms, the fine details of gene control often differ. A gene from a bacterium, for example, will often not function correctly if it is introduced unmodified into a plant or animal cell. The genetic engineer must first construct a transgene, the gene to be introduced; this is a segment of DNA containing the gene of interest and some extra material that correctly controls the gene's function in its new organism. The transgene must then be inserted into the second organism.

In 1982, Brinster and Palmiter introduced by microinjection a cloned gene for rat growth hormone into the male pronucleus of fertilized mouse eggs. The gene was cloned "downstream" from an inducible promoter to increase its chances of being expressed. After insertion of the microinjected eggs into the uterus of a foster-mother mouse, a significant number of offspring expressed the gene, produced high levels of the hormone, and grew to about twice the size of normal mice. The first human drug produced by transgenics, tPA, was achieved in mice in 1987.

As mentioned earlier, genes are controlled by a special segment of DNA found on the chromosome next to the gene, which is called a promoter sequence. When making a transgene, scientists generally substitute the organism's own promoter sequence with a specially designed one that ensures that the gene will function in the correct tissues of the animal or plant and also allows them to turn the gene on or off as needed (see Figure 13.6). For example, a promoter sequence that requires a dietary "trigger" substance can be used to turn on genes for important hormones in animals; the animal would not produce the new hormone unless fed the appropriate trigger.

Copies of the transgene are usually injected directly into a fertilized egg, which is then implanted in the female's reproductive tract. However, it is difficult to control where in the chromosome the transgene will become inserted, and this sometimes causes variations in the way the gene is expressed. For this and other reasons, the process is demanding and, in general, has a low success rate. Currently, less than 5 percent of injected embryos result in offspring with the gene integrated into their DNA and able to be passed on consistently to successive generations. Researchers are therefore investigating new methods of gene transfer.

By genetic engineering, the DNA gene for a protein drug of interest can be transferred into another organism for production. Which organism to use for production is a technical and economic decision. For certain protein drugs that require complex modifications or are needed in large supply, production in transgenic animals seems most efficient. The farm animal becomes a production facility with many advantages. For example, it is reproducible, has a flexible production capacity through the number of animals bred, and maintains its own fuel supply. Perhaps most important of all, in most animal drug production, the drug is delivered from the animal in a very convenient form, the milk.

A transgenic animal for pharmaceutical production should (1) produce the desired drug at high levels without endangering its own health and (2) pass its ability to produce the drug at high levels to its offspring. The current strategy to achieve these objectives is to couple the DNA gene for the protein drug with a DNA signal directing production in the mammary gland. The new gene, while present in every cell of the animal, functions only in the mammary gland, so the protein drug is made only in

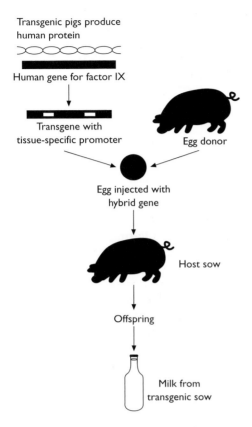

Transgenic pigs produce
human protein

Human gene for factor IX

Transgene with
tissue-specific promoter

Egg donor

Egg injected with
hybrid gene

Host sow

Offspring

Milk from
transgenic sow

Figure 13.6 Production of a transgenic pig to produce a human protein.

the milk. Since the mammary gland and milk are essentially "outside" the main life support systems of the animal, there is virtually no danger of disease or harm to the animal in making the "foreign" protein drug.

After the DNA gene for the protein drug has been coupled with the mammary-directing signal, this DNA is injected into fertilized embryos of the desired species with the aid of a very fine needle, called a micromanipulator, and a microscope. The injected embryos are then implanted into recipient surrogate mothers where, it is hoped, they survive and are born normally.

The main aim in using transgenic technology in animals, at the present time, is to improve livestock by altering their biochemistry, their hormonal balance, or their important protein products. Several companies have designed and are testing transgenic mammals that produce important pharmaceutics in the animal's milk. Products such as insulin and growth hormone that are currently produced by fermentation of transgenic bacteria (recombinant technology) or other cell types may soon be obtained by milking transgenic cows, sheep, or goats. The cost of these drugs may be much less than for those produced using conventional techniques. Drugs currently under study for transgenic production include alpha-1-antitrypsin, tPA, blood clotting factors VIII and IX, hemoglobin, and lactoferrin. An example of the potential impact of

Figure 13.7 Stereochemical relationship of the asthma medication albuterol.

transgenics on the treatment of disease is hemophilia. It has been estimated that 300 to 600 milking sows could meet the world demand for clotting factor VIII.

Chirality

While biological and structural approaches to drug design occupy most of the resources in contemporary drug development, there is an additional highly specialized area that is also receiving attention. This area deals with the fact that, as mentioned previously, some organic molecules contain an asymmetric carbon atom (i.e., a tetrahedral carbon atom that is bonded to four different atomic groupings). A molecule that contains such a chiral center can exist in two distinct mirror image-related forms called enantiomers. When both isomers are present in a 50/50 mixture, the drug is in its racemic state. The word chiral comes from the Greek word meaning hand-like.

Chemists have known about racemates since Pasteur, at 26 years of age, told the Paris Academy of Sciences how he used tweezers to separate two types of crystals of salts of tartaric acid, which rotate polarized light clockwise (D, dextro) or counter-clockwise (L, levo). Unfortunately, this correspondence does not always hold true. In fact, the magnitude and even the direction of optical rotation are complicated functions of the electronic structure surrounding the chiral center. For example, the common enantiomer of the sugar fructose is termed D because of the stereochemical orientation about the chiral atom. But this enantiomer actually rotates the plane of polarization to the left, and its mirror image, L-fructose, rotates the plane of polarization to the right.

Accordingly, an absolute convention has been developed that allows a stereochemical designation to any compound, predicated upon examination of its three-dimensional structure (essentially a rating system of groups attached to the chiral center). An example of this so-called *R–S* convention (where *R* = right and *S* = left) is illustrated by the antiasthma drug albuterol (Figure 13.7). Despite its limitations, the D–L terminology is still commonly used by biochemists and pharmacologists alike.

The *R* and *S* enantiomers of a molecule will have identical physical and chemical properties under most circumstances since they have identical energy contents and differ only at the three-dimensional level of their nonsuperimposability. However, the possibility that the two enantiomers of a chiral drug may differ in their biological effects is a phenomenon that has been recognized by pharmacologists since the beginning of the twentieth century. Table 13.2 presents some examples of chiral

Table 13.2 Examples of stereoselective differences in pharmacodynamics and pharmaocokinetics

Effect	Drug
Active absorption in GI tract	L-Dopa > D-dopa
Distribution	(S)-Propranolol selectively taken up by heart
	(S)-α-Methyldopa selectively accumulates in the brain
Plasma protein binding	(−)-Ibuprofen > (+)-ibuprofen
Potency	(−)-Hyoscyamine > (+)-hyoscyamine
	(S)-Warfarin > (R)-warfarin
Metabolism	(−)-Verapamil > (+)-verapamil
Drug interaction	Stereoselective inhibition of the metabolism of (S)-warfarin by sulfinpyrazone coupled to a stereoselective increase in the elimination of (R)-warfarin
Differential toxicity	(R)-2-Ethylhexaholic acid embryotoxicity > (S)-2-ethylhexaholic acid

factors on drug disposition and toxicity that are often overlooked. In addition, it is believed that the teratogenic effect of thalidomide resides with the *R* form. Unfortunately, even if just the *L* form is given, the body quickly converts it to the *R* form.

Because of possible pharmacological differences between drug enantiomers, the science of creating single-isomer drugs is one of the fastest growing areas in pharmaceutical research and development. In 1997 the market for chiral drugs had reached $90 billion and 50 percent of the top 100 drugs were single enantiomers. More than 80 percent of new drugs in the early stages of development are single-isomer compounds. It has been estimated that approximately 80 percent of prescription drugs now sold in the United States are single-isomer formulations. There are several reasons for this. First, regulatory pressure for chirally pure drugs has increased. Since 1992, U.S., Canadian, and European regulatory authorities have asked companies to provide information on each isomer of new racemic drugs and justify why the drug was not in its chirally pure, active form. Second, producing chirally pure drugs can often increase efficacy while decreasing toxicity.

Separating toxic effects from therapeutic effects is a constant challenge in drug development. In the case of our example of a chiral drug, albuterol, attempts are currently under way to achieve that goal. Apparently, the *S*-isomer of albuterol is responsible for increasing asthma patients' reactivity to stimuli, thereby leading to a paradoxical increased severity of asthma attacks. The "good-twin" *R*-isomer appears to be the form responsible for relaxation of bronchial smooth muscles, widening the airway, and allowing freer breathing. Clinical studies have, in fact, demonstrated that *R*-albuterol is four times more potent than the *S* form with fewer side effects. Another example is the local anesthetic bupivicaine. The racemic form of bupivicaine has been restricted to epidural use during childbirth because it is cardiotoxic if it gains entry into the bloodstream (apparently due to the *R* form). It is hoped that the left-handed isomer may reduce its cardiotoxicity and allow it to be used in a broader range of applications.

Research is also currently under way to investigate the possible advantages of D-proteins as drugs. One possible advantage is that they may be more resistant to proteolytic enzymes, suggesting that D-protein drugs may remain in the bloodstream for a longer time than conventional proteins. They also do not appear to be as immunogenic as conventional proteins, perhaps because they are not cleaved and presented to the major histocompatibility complex (part of the immune system's antigen-recognition system), a process that requires proteolysis. In addition, there are some data suggesting that D-polypeptides may be able to be administered orally without being degraded enzymatically in the GI tract.

Pharmafoods

Over the past few years, so-called "pharmafoods" have begun to appear in both the scientific literature and the marketplace. This category of agents differs from regular drugs in that they are not found in drug stores nor are they prescribed by a physician. However, the manufacturers do claim pharmaceutical effects beyond standard nutrition. The major examples being developed in this area include Benecol and Olestra.

Benecol is a brand of margarine invented by a small Finnish food company (The Raisio Group). Research published in the *New England Journal of Medicine* by Finnish researchers indicates that regular use of Benecol can lower blood cholesterol levels by an average of 10 percent "in a randomly selected, mildly hypercholesterolemic population sample." Its active ingredient is a plant sterol from Nordic pine trees known as beta-sitostanol, which apparently can block some of the body's absorption of dietary cholesterol. At present, 5 tons of wood waste are processed to produce 1 pound of the oil that is the source of the sterol.

After 20 years and more than $200 million in research and development, Proctor & Gamble received permission from the FDA in 1996 to market its fat substitute Olestra in certain snack foods (e.g., potato chips, crackers, and cheese puffs). Olestra, technically a sucrose polyester, is not digestible, so it adds neither fat nor calories to food. However, Olestra can inhibit the absorption of certain fat-soluble vitamins and other nutrients. Therefore, all products containing Olestra must be labeled with the following information: "This product contains Olestra. Olestra inhibits the absorption of some vitamins and other nutrients. Vitamins A, D, E, and K have been added." Also, as a condition of approval, Proctor & Gamble must monitor consumption and conduct studies on Olestra's long-term effects.

Other products under current development in the pharmafood sector include a salt substitute for hypertension; a yogurt-like product that adds bacteria to stimulate the body's immune system; and a drink containing docosahexaenoic acid (DHA, the baby formula additive) that Japanese consumers believe boosts brain power before exams.

SELECTED BIBLIOGRAPHY

Bugg, C. E., Carson, W. M. and Montgomery, J. A. (1993) Drugs by design. *Sci. Am.* 269: 92–98.

Christopoulos, A. (ed.) (2001) *Biomedical Applications of Computer Modeling*. Boca Raton, FL: CRC Press.

Marshall, G. R. (1995) Molecular modeling in drug design. In *Burger's Medicinal Chemistry and Drug Discovery*, 5th ed. (ed. M. Wolff) pp. 573–659. New York: Wiley.

Merchant, K. M. (ed.) (1996) *Pharmacological Regulation of Gene Expression in the CNS.* Boca Raton, FL: CRC Press.

Navia, M. A. and Murcko, M. A. (1992) Use of structural information in drug design. *Curr. Opin. Struct. Biol.* 2: 202–210.

Weiner, D. B. and Williams, W. V. (eds) (1995) *Biological Approaches to Rational Drug Design.* Boca Raton, FL: CRC Press.

Weiner, D. B. and Williams, W. V. (eds) (1995) *Chemical and Structural Approaches to Rational Drug Design.* Boca Raton, FL: CRC Press.

QUESTIONS

1 Which of the following was the first plant alkaloid isolated?
   a   codeine
   b   nitrous oxide
   c   nitroglycerin
   d   morphine
   e   heroin.

2 Which of the following was the first synthetic drug widely marketed to the public?
   a   chloroform
   b   ether
   c   amyl nitrite
   d   nitrous oxide
   e   aspirin.

3 Which of the following can be found in a birth control pill?
   a   mestranol
   b   cortisone
   c   norethynodrel
   d   testosterone
   e   a and c.

4 Which of the following techniques is/are significantly increasing the number of potential lead compounds?
   a   combinatorial chemistry
   b   computer databases
   c   high-throughput screening
   d   identification of pharmacophores
   e   all of the above.

5 Ribozymes involve which of the following?
   a   antisense deoxynucleotides
   b   protein–RNA combination
   c   catalytic RNA
   d   catalytic DNA
   e   mitochondrial DNA.

6 Which of the following is the oldest technique for determining molecular structure to atomic resolution?
   a   nuclear magnetic resonance
   b   atomic fusion
   c   differential fractionation
   d   nuclear magnetic crystallography
   e   X-ray crystallography.

7 The key region of a drug that is critical for molecular recognition and binding is which of the following?
   a   allosteric site
   b   affinity lattice
   c   two-dimensional structure
   d   amino acid sequence
   e   pharmacophore.

8 A combination rat/human antibody is known as which of the following?
   a   chiral
   b   chimera
   c   enantiomers
   d   racemate
   e   none of the above.

9 Transgenic animals involve which of the following?
   a   a gene coding for a specific protein
   b   a promoter sequence of DNA
   c   injection of the genetic material into a fertilized egg
   d   implantation of the fertilized egg into a female's reproductive tract
   e   all of the above.

10 Which of the following is/are true regarding chirality?
   a   all drugs have chiral enantiomers
   b   a symmetrical carbon atom is required
   c   the presence of a "humanized" section is required
   d   very few drugs are sold as single chiral enantiomers
   e   none of the above.

Chapter 14

Pharmaceutical development of drugs and the FDA

After a drug company has discovered what appears to be an active drug in their drug discovery program, regardless of which type is utilized, the candidate drug can then pass to the next stage of the drug evaluation process. This step will involve interaction of the drug company with the governmental agency that has responsibility for this area, the Food and Drug Administration (FDA). Over the years, the role of the FDA in drug evaluation has evolved into three main areas: (1) truth in labeling, (2) toxicity, and (3) determination of efficacy.

The roots of the FDA reach back to before the Civil War. The first national law came in 1848 during the Mexican War. It banned the importation of adulterated drugs, a chronic health problem that finally gained Congressional attention. When Congress created the Department of Agriculture in 1862, the Patent Office's chemistry laboratory was transferred to the new agency and renamed the chemical division. The first prolonged and impassioned controversy in Congress involving a pure food issue took place in 1886, pitting butter against oleomargerine. Butter won, and oleomargerine was taxed and placed under other restraints that persisted on the federal level until 1950.

In 1890 the division under went another rather insignificant name change to the Division of Chemistry and, in 1901 was renamed the Bureau of Chemistry. The Bureau of Chemistry subsequently became the Food, Drug and Insecticide Administration in 1927 and, finally, officially, the Food and Drug Administration in 1930.

While the FDA is required to review applications from drug companies for drug approval, and establish standards, the agency does not fund or conduct research to bring a drug to market. However, it does carry out highly specific applied research. In addition, the agency inspects manufacturing facilities and reviews production records. Although the agency does have responsibilities in the areas of food, cosmetics, and medical devices, its role in drug approval is the subject of this chapter. The success of the U.S. drug industry is demonstrated by sales figures for the 12 top-selling drugs in 1999 (Table 14.1).

DRUG LABELING

One of the first significant empowerments of the fledgling FDA was when Congress enacted the Food and Drug Act (also known as the Wiley Act) in 1906 directed to address unhygienic conditions in Chicago's meat-packing plants (see Upton Sinclair's

Table 14.1 Top-selling U.S. drugs in 1999

Product	Company	Indication	$ billion
Prilosec	Astra Pharm LP.	Gastroesophageal reflux disease	4.2
Lipitor	Parke-Davis	High cholesterol	3.0
Prozac	Dista	Depression	2.6
Prevacid	TAP Pharm.	Gastroesophageal reflux disease	2.4
Zocor	Merck & Co.	High cholesterol	2.3
Epogen	Amgen, Inc.	Anemia	1.8
Zoloft	Pfizer	Depression	1.1
Claritin	Schering	Allergies	1.5
Paxil	SB Pharm	Depression	1.5
Zyprexa	Lilly	Schizophrenia	1.5
Premarin	Wyeth-Ayerst	Menopause	1.1
Viagra	Pfizer	Erectile dysfunction	0.67

Source: *Pharmacy Times*: www.pharmacytimes.com/top200.html.

The Jungle) and the sale of "snake-oil" medicines of unknown composition. The act applied to drugs to the extent that preparations could be removed from the market if the concoctions could be shown to be adulterated or misbranded. As such, it dealt primarily with truth in labeling. Unfortunately, the law did little to control the sale of dangerous drugs and devices since there were no obligations to establish drug safety or efficacy. As is often the case, it took a catastrophic incident during the 1930s to induce further legislative action.

DRUG SAFETY

As mentioned previously, by the late 1930s the fame of the antibiotic sulfanilamide had spread around the world and millions of tablets of the new wonder-drug were being used each year. Always on the look-out for a new marketing ploy, one company in Tennessee, Massengill & Co., tried a different marketing strategy to set themselves apart. On the somewhat unusual theory that most people in the South prefer to take their medicine in liquid form, the company began to experiment on how to get sulfanilamide into solution. Unfortunately, sulfanilamide does not readily dissolve in water, alcohol, or any of the other common pharmaceutical solvents. However, a chemist at the company did discover that the drug was soluble in diethylene glycol (a component of antifreeze). To the sulfanilamide/diethylene glycol solution was added some coloring matter and some raspberry flavor and the mixture marketed under the name of *Elixir Sulfanilamide*. Apparently, no one at Massengill tested the elixir for safety, in any manner whatsoever, since toxicity testing was not a requirement.

Soon after marketing of the elixir began, a physician in Oklahoma reported to the American Medical Association (AMA), not the FDA, that he had recently seen six people who had died of kidney damage and who, coincidentally, had all taken Elixir Sulfanilamide. He was curious as to what the contents of the preparation were. After initial attempts to discover the ingredients in the elixir were rebuffed by the company, the presence of diethylene glycol was finally acknowledged. The situation then became clear since diethylene glycol is converted in the body to oxalic acid, a highly nephrotoxic chemical that causes a slow agonizing death from kidney failure.

Unfortunately, there were no requirements in 1937 for testing the toxicity or safety of drug products, and over 100 people died from diethylene glycol-induced renal failure, most of them children. All that could be done to the manufacturer under the law at the time was to penalize the company for mislabeling its product. Although the manufacturer steadfastly refused to accept responsibility for the debacle, its chief chemist committed suicide. This scandal followed closely on the heels of another drug-related tragedy during the 1930s. Dinitrophenol is a highly toxic poison with the ability to uncouple oxidative phosphorylation. In the process, the metabolic rate of the poisoned individual can increase markedly. It is this latter effect that led to its promotion for weight reduction. Unfortunately, there were numerous serious injuries and deaths.

The culmination of these episodes led Congress to enact the Food, Drug, and Cosmetic Act of 1938. This statute expanded consumer protection by requiring the testing of new drugs for safety prior to marketing. Toxicity studies were required, as well as approval of a new drug application (NDA), before a drug could be promoted and distributed. It was the requirement of toxicity testing that spared the United States from the tragedy of thalidomide that swept Europe during the 1960s. It should be noted, however, that no proof of efficacy was required in the 1938 legislation, and extravagant claims for therapeutic indications were commonly made.

Since its adoption, the 1938 law has been amended repeatedly, eventually extending the FDA's regulatory powers to pesticides and food additives. In 1958, the Delaney clause was incorporated into the law. This now controversial provision prohibits the approval of any food additive found to induce cancer in humans or animals.

In the relatively relaxed atmosphere before World War II, pharmacological research expanded rapidly in both industrial and academic settings. Many new drugs were introduced for a variety of illnesses. Because efficacy was not rigorously defined, a number of therapeutic claims were made that could not be supported by the appropriate scientific data. The risk-to-benefit ratio was seldom mentioned. One advancement that was made was the Durham–Humphrey Amendment of 1951. Until this law, there was no requirement that any drug be labeled safe by prescription only. This amendment defined prescription drugs as those unsafe for self-medication and that should therefore be used only under a physician's supervision. Drugs initially classified as by prescription only can have their classification changed, as illustrated by antiulcer medications such as Tagamet.

DRUG EFFICACY

In 1962, the deficiency in U.S. drug laws relating to efficacy was finally remedied when Congress put in place the third cornerstone of our current public health and consumer protection legislation. Congress stated in its new enactment that before a drug product could go on the market, it had to be both safe and efficacious. As is traditionally the case, the official act was named after the members of Congress who introduced it in the House and Senate, respectively, and is known as the Harris–Kefauver Amendments to the Food, Drug, and Cosmetic Act.

Interestingly, the question of drug efficacy evolved in its importance at the time since Estes Kefauver had originally begun investigating the drug industry in 1959 because of concerns over excessive pricing of prescription drugs. However, by the end of the Senate's investigative phase, Kefauver was convinced that not only were some drugs incredibly overpriced, but also that drugs should not be allowed on the market unless they were both safe and effective. After several years of acrimonious debate in the Senate it appeared as though a weakened version of S. 1552 (known as the "double-cross bill") was the only legislation that could be hoped for. As fate would have it, it was at that time that the story of the thalidomide tragedy swept across the country, and Congress was deluged with demands for strong legislation related to drug development that included the question of efficacy.

The new regulations were long overdue. Many useless or irrational products had already been brought to market, either by outright charlatans or by overly enthusiastic individuals or companies sincerely convinced that their product was a boon to suffering mankind. For many years, the FDA had struggled hard but often unsuccessfully to keep worthless remedies off the market and to remove those already in use. The difficulty was that the companies usually had to be proven guilty of false advertising (under the 1906 law), which often required years of effort at considerable expense. The problem had been particularly notorious for the FDA in the case of proposed cancer treatments such as Laetrile, Krebiozen, and arginases.

The 1962 amendments have proven to be significant legislation in that they require appropriate pharmacological and toxicological research in animals before a drug can be tested in humans. The data from these preclinical studies must be submitted in the form of an application for an investigational new drug (IND) before clinical studies can be initiated. Once begun, the clinical studies involve three graduated phases (discussed later) of variable drug exposure to humans. The 1962 amendments also required manufacturers to support the claims of efficacy for all drugs marketed between 1938 and 1962 (pre-1938 products were "grandfathered" in and allowed to be sold for the curious reason that they were generally recognized as safe and effective, provided no evidence to the contrary developed).

EVALUATION OF 1938–1962 DRUGS

The new law required the FDA to wait until 1964 before demanding proof of efficacy of drugs introduced between 1938 and 1962. Because of manpower constraints within the FDA, the process of independent evaluation is carried out under a contract between the FDA and the National Academy of Sciences (NAS) under its research arm, the National Research Council (NRC). Originally, some 200 experts were assembled into 30 panels to consider approximately 16,000 therapeutic claims involving more than 4000 products marketed by nearly 300 different companies. It was eventually agreed that each product would be put in one of six different categories: (1) safe and effective; (2) probably effective; (3) possibly effective—more data required; (4) effective for limited uses; (5) ineffective as a fixed combination; and (6) ineffective. Evaluation of these drugs has been ongoing for nearly 40 years.

Occasionally, new data become available that can cause reclassification of a group of drugs. For example, in May 1996 the FDA informed manufacturers that it planned to reclassify five widely used ingredients in over-the-counter (OTC) laxatives from category 1 to category 3. The five ingredients (phenolphthalein, bisacodyl, aloe, cascara sagrada, and senna) were initially marketed prior to 1962. In 1975, the NAS/NRC advisory review panel had recommended that these five ingredients be considered as safe and effective OTC stimulant laxatives and, in 1985, the FDA did, in fact, place them in category 1.

Recent studies by the National Toxicology Program (NTP) on phenolphthalein, however, have provided new data associating the laxative with carcinogenic potential in rodents. Concern for bisacodyl arises from the fact that it is structurally related to phenolphthalein (both are members of the diphenylmethane family of laxatives). FDA concerns regarding the members of the anthraquinone family (senna, aloe, and cascara sagrada) emanate from laboratory data indicating that some of the components of senna may have mutagenic properties.

Following the release of the NTP study in December 1995, the FDA's Carcinogenicity Assessment Committee met with drug manufacturers and NTP representatives to further ascertain whether this new information translated into a risk for humans. Although the FDA had never received any adverse reports linking these laxatives with cancer, the new information suggested that additional studies might be warranted. Therefore, the FDA requested that the manufacturers provide the necessary additional data to establish the safety of these five ingredients. Particular emphasis was placed on phenolphthalein.

In August 1997, the maker of Ex-Lax (which contained phenolphthalein), the nation's top-selling overnight laxative (1996 sales of $41 million), pulled three versions of the product off store shelves. The laxative had been in use since 1906. Replacement products containing senna as the active ingredient were made available several months later. The premise for forcing phenolphthalein removal was based on tests in rodents that developed a variety of tumors when fed the chemical in doses 50 to 100 times those recommended for humans.

PRECLINICAL TESTING

The process by which new drug candidates are discovered and developed is both time-consuming and expensive. This is reflected in the high rate of attrition of drug candidates that enter clinical development, such that only approximately 10 percent of drug candidates that are selected for clinical development eventually become marketed drugs.

For a drug that has never been used in humans previously, the initial step that a pharmaceutical company must take is to perform preclinical toxicity studies involving appropriate in vitro systems or whole animals. The FDA usually requires that dose-related toxicity be determined in at least two mammalian species (routinely rodents). The toxicity information obtained from these studies can then be used to make risk/benefit assessments and help determine the acceptability of the drug for testing in humans, and to estimate a safe starting dose.

Pharmacokinetic studies must be provided that document the fate of the drug, including absorption, distribution, metabolism, and excretion. In addition, the company must supply information on chemistry, manufacturing, and quality control guidelines. This ensures the identity, purity, quality, and strength of both the active ingredient and the finished dosage form.

The drug company then develops a plan for testing the drug in humans, and submits it to the FDA, along with its animal testing data, information about the composition of the drug, manufacturing data, qualifications of its study investigators, and assurances for the protection of the rights and safety of the people who will participate in the trial. This corpus of information comprises the investigational new drug application (IND). According to the *FDA Center for Drug Evaluation and Research Fact Book 1997*, the average length of time for a promising drug candidate to be synthesized, purified, and subjected to animal testing before IND submission is 18 months. Under normal circumstances, the IND must be evaluated within 30 days of submission. The FDA reviews the information in order to establish that the study participants will not be exposed to unreasonable risk or harm. If the FDA finds no safety problems with the plan or the drug, it permits the drug to proceed to the clinical phases of evaluation. According to 1996 data from the FDA, drug and biotechnology firms filed 3522 INDs between 1984 and 1993 (approximately one per day).

CLINICAL TRIALS

Prior to 1962, drug trials could often be characterized as a series of uncontrolled testimonials by clinicians associated with the studies. Today, clinical trials are much more rigorous and are traditionally conducted in three distinct phases. As each new clinical trial is started, a project manager from the drug company is assigned responsibility. The project manager selects the clinical sites, guides the preparation of the protocol, and has general oversight over all aspects of the clinical study.

Clinical trials should be carried out under the highest ethical and scientific standards possible. While this is generally the case, there have been exceptions. During the period 1964–1982, for example, FDA inquiries resulted in some 45 clinical investigators being declared ineligible to receive investigational drugs, and an additional six agreed to some restrictions on their investigational work. Some of the disqualified investigators were criminally prosecuted and sentenced to fines, probation, and imprisonment for fraud, fabrication of results, felony, etc.

The first exposure of humans to the drug, the phase I study, usually takes place in a small number of healthy volunteers, although in the case of serious and life-threatening conditions, volunteers who have the disease may be enrolled. These initial studies test the safety of the drug in humans and help to determine an appropriate dose for further investigations. In addition, pharmacokinetic data relating to absorption, distribution, metabolism, and elimination are determined. Each year, some 40,000 ostensibly healthy individuals are used by U.S. drug companies in phase I drug tests. Volunteers, often homeless, are generally paid in the range of $100 to $200 per day.

As clinical studies progress, additional animal experiments continue to be carried out in order that the safety of ongoing human studies can be ensured to the greatest extent possible. These include reproductive toxicity studies to examine the effects of the drug on fertility, reproduction, teratogenicity, and mutagenicity. In 1977 the FDA specifically restricted the participation by most women with childbearing potential from entering phase I and early phase II trials. However, in 1993 the FDA reversed this position because of the concern that the exclusion of women would prevent the accumulation of gender-related data.

The FDA's new guidelines strongly encourage inclusion of women in most early phase trials, providing that they are adequately informed of the potential risks. In fact, a characterization of drug effects by gender must now be part of all NDAs and the agency may refuse an application that does not contain such information. The 1993 guideline identifies three specific pharmacokinetic issues in women that should be considered when feasible: (1) effect of the stages of the menstrual cycle; (2) effect of exogenous hormonal therapy including oral contraceptives; and (3) effect of the drug on the pharmacokinetics of oral contraceptives.

It is important to recognize, however, that the U.S. Code of Federal Regulations does not address the question of gender in clinical trials; there is no formal requirement that women make up a significant portion of a trial's patient population or even participate at all. The reality is that unless a trial specifically mandates female participation (e.g., a test for the safety and efficacy of a new birth control pill), men overwhelmingly predominate as subjects in clinical trials. For pharmaceutical companies, there is little motivation to recruit women. The first reason for this lack of motivation has to do with attempts to limit potential liabilities. Other concerns stem from this issue and focus on economic and legal realities that are stumbling blocks to expanded inclusion of women in research.

How do concerns about company liability limit the recruitment of female patients? Two issues explain this: pregnancy and infant care. No drug developer wants to be responsible if the product it is testing turns out to have an adverse effect on fetal development or harms a breast-feeding infant through milk contamination. The result, therefore, is that most trials require participating women to be either postmenopausal or nonlactating and actively using an acceptable form of birth control. Some investigators, uncertain of what constitutes an "acceptable" birth control method, and fearful of patient noncompliance, simply refuse to enroll female patients of childbearing age to their trials. This reduces the number of women eligible to enter any given study, making recruitment that much more difficult.

From a pharmaceutical company's perspective, the costs of increasing female participation in trials are significantly greater than the odds that an approved drug, tested primarily on male subjects, will be withdrawn by the FDA because of unexpected health effects in women. Therefore, although pharmaceutical companies do not actively dissuade female participation from trials, their recruitment efforts rarely focus on women, and the lack of female participation in most research is not a point of concern.

Another issue facing clinical studies is the inclusion of children. The FDA Modernization Act of 1997 addresses the desirability of pediatric research before new drug approval when a drug is likely to be prescribed for children. The reward for such research is a 6-month prolongation of market exclusivity or patent life.

The subsequent phase in clinical studies, phase II, not only continues to evaluate the safety profile of the drug, identifying the most common side effects that might result from its use, but also begins to assess its activity for the particular disease that it was developed for. Phase II studies usually involve a few dozen to a few hundred people. By the time that phase II is completed, the drug developer knows quite a lot about the safety and activity of the drug. In fact, 80 percent of all drugs tested are abandoned by their sponsors after either phase I or II because of excessive toxicity or lack of significant efficacy. However, if the results are promising the sponsor may progress to phase III.

Phase III clinical trials represent the normal culmination of the drug discovery/ development process and are designed to establish the safety and efficacy of the putative treatment. Large, controlled phase III studies can involve thousands of people with the targeted condition scattered among numerous research sites. The studies may also examine additional uses for a drug, or consider additional population subsets, but are primarily aimed at obtaining the necessary effectiveness data. The phase III studies also continue to generate valuable safety data, including long-term effects.

The scientific evaluation of drugs in humans

At this point, it may be useful to the reader to understand some of the background that has led to the contemporary design of human clinical trials. Although the concept of a comparative trial was known in the ninth century BC, it remained for James Lind in 1774 to perform his famous trial. Lind was concerned with comparing several different recommended treatments of the day for scurvy. Lind demonstrated that when all of the proposed treatments were compared in a controlled study in human volunteers, only one proved efficacious—citrus fruit. It is important to realize that each of the treatments tested was recommended by recognized authorities of the day. It took the comparative trial to prove that citrus juice cured scurvy and the other treatments were worthless. In the process of applying this scientific method, Lind did much to destroy the credibility of testimonials.

The testimonial, someone speaking from experience, is psychologically one of the more powerful forms of persuasion. Eyewitness testimony is basic to the legal profession. However, in science, the testimonial has little evidentiary value. To illustrate this point we need only be reminded of James Woodforde and his cat. In 1791 the parson of Weston Longville in Norfolk, England, developed a painful sty on his right eyelid. Parson Woodforde, however, knew how to treat it: "As is commonly said that the eyelid being rubbed by the tail of a black cat would do it much good, if not entirely cure it, and having a black cat, a little before dinner I made a *trial* [emphasis mine] of it, and very soon after dinner I found my eyelid much abated of the swelling and almost free of pain."

Parson Woodforde concluded that a cat's tail was of the greatest efficacy for such a malady. While the good parson's reasoning was logical, his premise was incorrect. Testimonials often involve the fallacy of *post hoc, ergo propter hoc*, that is, the assumption that because two events occur sequentially, the first is the cause of the second. (In tort law, causation must be proved.) The swelling of the eyelid may have abated of its own accord even in the absence of the tail of a black cat. Moreover, there is selection bias in testimonials; a lack of consequence rarely results in a testimonial and dead men tell no tales.

Placebo-controlled trials

As mentioned previously in Chapter 1, the placebo effect can create havoc with clinical trials. The first placebo-controlled drug trial was published in 1933. The investigators evaluated drugs used in the treatment of angina pectoris. Among the comments made at the conclusion of their 4 to 26-week study was: "The value of remedies in relieving anginal pain cannot be judged unless the observations are properly *controlled* [emphasis mine]. The literature on the treatment of angina gives no indication that this side of the problem has been considered, although it is recognized that the disease pursues a varying course in regard to severity quite apart from any form of treatment."

Observer bias

The importance of observer bias was addressed in 1937 when the concept of the double-blind study was introduced, also in a study of treatments of angina patients. The authors indicate in their methods that "In a further attempt to eliminate the possibility of bias, the questioner usually refrained from informing himself as to the agent that had been issued until *after* the patient's appraisal of the period had been obtained."

Use of statistical analysis

Although the concept of patient variability had been articulated by the middle of the twentieth century, the concept that a difference between two groups could be due to chance was slow to be accepted. The first clinical trial to use a formal statistical analysis reportedly occurred in 1962. The study involved a comparison of antibody production after yellow fever vaccination by two different methods. Several years later (1966) a critique of statistical methods used in medical journal manuscripts suggested a lack of proper study design and data analysis. In this critique, the authors canonized the criterion of $P < 0.05$ for a difference between two groups to be considered not due to chance.

A problem still exists, however. Although it was established that the probability of less than 1 in 20 that a difference between two groups was due to chance meant that it was due to the drug, they did not establish criteria for how to properly interpret studies that failed to find this much difference. In other words, can this lack of evidence of effect be considered to be evidence of lack of effect? Experts in the field have settled on the convention that a clinical trial must include enough patients to have at least an 80 percent chance of finding an effect if an effect really exists. Failure to find an effect in this large a trial is considered to be evidence of true lack of an effect. This is referred to as the *power* of the study.

How can studies that lack this power be handled? Traditionally, one did a review of these studies, writing a narrative about them and drawing conclusions based on the subjective evaluation of this information by the reviewer. An alternative to this approach was introduced in 1988 and designated *meta-analysis*. Meta-analysis has been defined as "a systematic review of studies that uses quantitative statistical procedures to combine, synthesize, and integrate information across these studies." What this methodology does is take a group of different studies and analyze them together as if they were a single multicenter study following a single protocol.

The appeal of meta-analysis is that by combining a series of small equivocal studies into one analysis of all the patients, a more reliable result may be obtained. However, as one might appreciate, there are several issues inherent in a meta-analysis. One is whether all of the small clinical trials of the drug were included or only the published "positive" trials, while the small negative trials that were done were never published. This would be like excluding the data from selected centers in a multicenter trial. Obviously this would skew the data. An additional issue is whether separate studies that do not use an identical protocol can really be combined. Obviously, there is art as well as science in meta-analysis. With these limitations in mind, meta-analysis does have its place in the clinical evaluation of drug candidates.

Once phase III is completed, the sponsor submits the test results to the FDA in the form of the NDA. At this point, FDA scientists (e.g., medical officers, pharmacologists, chemists, microbiologists, and statisticians) review the application to validate the data and determine if they do, in fact, demonstrate that the drug is both safe and effective. The manufacturing facility is also evaluated in order to ensure that a consistent and high-quality product can be produced.

After the drug company has completed testing the drug, it then submits proposed labeling for the drug which must, in turn, be evaluated by the FDA. Labeling is generally reflective of the conditions of the trial in terms of indication and population. However, once the drug is approved, it may be employed by a physician in any manner he/she deems therapeutically appropriate since the practice of medicine is not regulated by the FDA. Use of a drug in this manner is referred to as "off-label" use. In some cases, additional postmarketing testing may be required by the FDA, which is often referred to as "phase IV."

While approval bestows a license to market a drug for commercial use, it also limits the marketing claims and recommendations for the doses, formulations, medical indications, and patient populations that were tested and approved during the phase III trials. If the study sponsor or the FDA wants to alter any of these parameters, a postmarketing, or phase IV, study is initiated. Because most drug companies want to expand the indications for which a medication can be prescribed, almost all drugs undergo some phase IV testing.

Phase IV studies can take almost any form as long as new questions not addressed in phases I–III are answered. Postmarketing studies can be initiated by a drug company, requested by the FDA, or conducted by third parties interested in examining a drug's application for a specific population, medical condition, or use in the home or clinic. Postmarketing studies can be performed during the new drug approval process, immediately after the drug has been approved, or even years after approval, when the FDA has had the opportunity to review consumer usage data. Such studies can last for just 2 weeks for the interaction study on food or as long as several years for compound stability.

A phase IV study initiated by a drug company is often done to expand the patient population for which a drug can be marketed. For example, Pfizer's Viagra was initially approved based on clinical trials on male patients with erectile dysfunction. Soon after the drug's 1997 approval, several physicians began prescribing it to female patients suffering from sexual dysfunction. Physicians may legally prescribe any drug for any patient or indication they think might benefit from the therapy, but drug companies are not permitted to reference, market, or publicize "off-label" uses. "Off-label" drug use increases liability and provides no advice to the patient about whether and how much of a drug is safe.

Table 14.2 Prescription drugs withdrawn by the FDA between January 1997 and January 2001

Drug	Type
Posicor	Blood pressure
Pondimin	Appetite suppressant
Duract	Analgesic
Propulsid	Heartburn
Rezulin	Diabetes
Relenza	Influenza
Baycol	Cholesterol lowering
Seldane	Antihistamine
Lotrenex	Gastrointestinal
Redux	Appetite suppressant
Raxar	Antibiotic
Hismanal	Antihistamine

Occasionally, when approved drugs enter the marketplace, unexpected, adverse effects occur. Reports of adverse drug reactions to the FDA are considered by public health officials to be the most reliable early warnings of a product's danger. The reports are filed to the FDA by health professionals, consumers, and drug manufacturers. In these cases, it is not uncommon for the FDA to rescind its approval and demand the withdrawal of the products. In fact, between 1997 and 2001, this happened on 12 occasions involving drugs cited as suspects in over a 1000 deaths (see Table 14.2).

During this same period of time, defective asthma inhalers believed to be responsible for 17 deaths were also recalled. The FDA also has a system called MedWatch (www.fda.gov/medwatch), by which consumers and health professionals can report adverse drug reactions directly to the agency. There are several reasons for drug toxicity to manifest itself after exposure to the public at large. Two reasons were identified above: exposure to women and "off-label" use. In addition, the sample size of clinical trials, although statistically significant, is small when compared to the general population that will use the drug. The statistical power of phase III trials is not believed to be able to detect adverse reactions of 1 in 10,000 drug exposures or less.

More than 250,000 side effects linked to prescription drugs, including injuries and death, are reported each year. These adverse-event reports by doctors and others are only filed voluntarily. Experts believe the reports represent as few as 1 to 10 percent of all such events. According to the *Los Angeles Times*, even when deaths are reported, records and interviews show that companies consistently dispute that their product has caused a given death by pointing to other factors, including preexisting disease or use of another medicine.

The FDA is normally the federal agency that deals with drug-related deaths. However, in 2001, the Drug Enforcement Administration (DEA) reported the results of extensive autopsy data and that the painkiller OxyContin was suspected of playing a role in 282 deaths between 2000 and 2001. Based on responses to date (October 2001) the DEA concluded that OxyContin was "directly linked" in 110 overdose deaths because either tablets were found in a person's stomach or a prescription for the drug was found on a body. DEA officials also classified 172 deaths as "OxyContin possible," cases where autopsy reports showed high blood concentrations of oxycodone (the active ingredient) without the presence of other compounds such as aspirin or acetaminophen. The review found that virtually all the deaths were of people who swallowed the pill whole or crushed rather than taking the drug by injection.

An example of a drug that has been subjected to essentially nonstop scrutiny after initial marketing is the sleeping pill Halcion. The FDA has examined Halcion periodically since 1982, lowering the recommended dose and adding warnings of such side effects as anxiety, behavioral changes, and abnormal thinking. Most recently the FDA has restricted the number of pills per package so patients will not take too many. Britain banned Halcion in 1991 and said Upjohn hid safety concerns that, had the government known, might have blocked the drug from ever being sold there. Meanwhile, at least 100 U.S. lawsuits have been filed against Upjohn relating to Halcion. Because of lingering questions about some Upjohn studies on Halcion's side effects, the FDA also intends to ask for outside experts to reevaluate the drug's safety.

EFFECT OF EFFICACY REQUIREMENTS ON DRUG DEVELOPMENT

Since the imposition of the 1962 amendments, both the drug industry and the FDA have endured a joint learning experience on the impact of the new requirements on drug development. This can be illustrated by the experience of one drug company over a period of 30 years. When Parke-Davis first marketed a particular epinephrine preparation in 1938, all it had to do was submit a 27-page report concerned primarily with safety. When it subsequently introduced a new expectorant in 1948, only a 73-page report was required. However, in 1962 when the same company requested FDA approval of its contraceptive, Norlestin, it had to submit a report totaling 12,370 pages. In 1968 when it sought approval for a new anesthetic, the required documents totaled slightly more than 72,000 pages in 167 volumes. Obviously, things were getting out of hand. In theory, one would expect that a report of two or three hundred pages would suffice if the research has been properly planned and executed and all the material submitted is cogently organized. However, as recently as 1996, the drug company Serono accumulated a 40,000-page file for its growth hormone preparation intended for use in AIDS.

TIME AND COST OF DRUG DEVELOPMENT

During the past few years, the FDA has been subjected to substantial criticism because of the length of time required for the various phases of the review process as well as the attendant costs for the drug companies. According to studies carried out at Tufts University and the Center for the Study of Drug Development, it can take approximately 12 years, from synthesis to regulatory clearance, to bring a prescription drug to market at a cost of approximately $231 million. In addition, for every 10,000 chemical entities synthesized, approximately 10 will enter clinical trial and one will gain regulatory approval. The comparative length of time normally involved in the various phases of drug development is shown in Table 14.3.

Table 14.3 Drug development and approval process

Stage	Years
Preclinical	6.5
Phase I	1
Phase II	2
Phase III	3
FDA	1–2

Source: Pharmaceutical Research and Manufacturers of America (PhRMA), Washington, DC.

In order to expedite the FDA approval stage of the process, a Prescription Drug User Fee Act was authorized in 1992. This program has allowed the FDA to collect fees from pharmaceutical companies and use the proceeds to accelerate the review process at the Center for Drug Evaluation and Research as well as the Center for Biologics Evaluation and Research. Firms were initially charged $50,000 annually, $5000 for each product on the market, and $150,000 for an IND. This user fee was $309,647 in 2000 for each new NDA. The projected income of $75 million was to be used for new staff. The companies' money now covers approximately 50 percent of the FDA's costs for reviewing proposed drugs. The results appear to be promising since the median approval time for new drugs in 1994 was 19 months, 21 percent less than in 1993. Similar improvement was also achieved with backlogged and supplemental submissions.

According to the FDA, drug companies are sending fewer novel medicines to evaluate, instead creating more "me-too" drugs similar to ones already sold. In 1999, half the drugs the FDA approved were priority drugs, breakthroughs, or medicines deemed to advance public health. In 2000, just one-third were in these categories. The FDA expects to receive applications for just 28 entirely new chemical entities in 2001. One breakthrough drug in leukemia therapy (Gleevec) set a record in the spring of 2001 when it won FDA approval in less than 3 months.

NEW FDA PROGRAMS

Over the years, the FDA has also implemented a variety of programs to make promising therapies more widely available to people with serious and life-threatening illnesses. In 1987, the FDA finalized regulations that created a "treatment IND." This was primarily in response to AIDS activists. This rule formalized the procedures that allow thousands of patients to have access to investigational drugs for treatment of serious and life-threatening diseases for which there is no satisfactory treatment prior to general marketing. The regulation allows for a treatment protocol, separate and distinct from the study protocols, while clinical studies are either still under way or completed, but the sponsor must be actively pursuing marketing approval. In addition, there must be sufficient data to indicate that the substance "may be effective," and that there are no unreasonable risks. At this point in time, the FDA is taking in excess of 2 years to review NDAs.

In the years since the treatment IND was created, a number of drugs have been subsequently approved for marketing including several for AIDS or AIDS-related conditions. In 1992, the Public Health Service published a policy statement permitting even more expanded availability of investigational drugs for AIDS through a "parallel track" mechanism. This policy outlines how promising new drugs can be made available early in the development process, once there is evidence of probable efficacy based on laboratory and available clinical data, evidence that the drug is reasonably safe, and enough data to recommend an appropriate starting dose. This policy serves people without satisfactory alternatives who cannot tolerate, or derive no benefit from, the available therapies, and cannot participate in clinical trials because they do not meet the entry criteria, or are too ill to participate, or because it would cause undue hardship, such as travel, or because the trials are fully enrolled. The parallel track differs from the treatment IND in two important regards: (1) the parallel track applies only to AIDS-related therapies; and (2) it makes drugs available earlier in the discovery process (i.e., late phase I or early phase II versus late phase II or phase III).

This accelerated program has already paid handsome dividends. In 1996, the protease inhibitor ritonavir was approved in 72 days, the fastest AIDS drug approved until that point and probably the fastest drug approval of any kind, to date, in FDA history. The FDA based its approval on data showing that it increases CD4 lymphocytes as well as decreasing the amount of HIV in the bloodstream. In addition, the cumulative mortality rate among participants on the drug was approximately 40 percent of that in the control group. Also, those on ritonavir experienced a 50 percent greater reduction in disease progression. Other protease inhibitors have also been approved in rapid order.

In 1996, President Clinton announced a "major new initiative" giving cancer patients faster and easier access to promising treatments. The FDA immediately implemented a fast-track approval process for anticancer drugs like that begun for anti-AIDS drugs. If a drug shows effectiveness in early testing, patients will have access to it even while the drug continues to undergo tests for approval. Accelerated approval is predicted to affect approximately 100 drugs now being studied, cutting FDA review time for these drugs from 12 to 6 months. From 1993 to 1999 the FDA approved 232 drugs regarded as new molecular entities compared with 163 during the previous 7 years (a 42 percent increase).

For hard-to-treat cancers, effectiveness is being redefined to include partial responses such as tumor shrinkage. Previously, before a drug was approved for marketing, it had to demonstrate such clinical benefits as increased survival or improved quality of life. Utilizing objective evidence such as tumor shrinkage will permit shorter studies for initial approval. Although abbreviated testing is not without additional risks, the risks appear acceptable for diseases such as AIDS and cancer.

In addition to expediting the availability of drugs used to treat AIDS and cancer, abbreviated new drug applications (ANDAs) have been made available for the development of generic drugs that differ little from drugs already on the market. The market share of generic drugs more than doubled from 18.6 percent in 1984 to 41.6 percent in 1996. Another important piece of legislation affecting drug development was the Orphan Drug Act of 1983. "Orphans" are drugs and other products for treating rare diseases. They may offer little or no profit to the manufacturer, but may benefit people with the rare diseases. To foster orphan product development, this law allows drug companies to take a tax deduction for about three-quarters of the cost of their clinical studies. Firms also are given exclusive marketing rights for 7 years for any orphan products that are approved. An example of such a drug is interferon β-1a, approved in 1996 for the treatment of multiple sclerosis, a chronic, often disabling, CNS disease that affects 250,000 Americans.

INSTITUTIONAL REVIEW BOARDS

Growing out of a history of U.S. scandals and reactions to Nazi medical war crimes, the U.S. government ultimately developed strict guidelines and safeguards to protect participants in clinical trials. In 1966, the Surgeon General issued a statement on the protection of human subjects, stating that no grant would be given for research involving human subjects unless the application described how the subjects would have their welfare protected, how informed consent would be obtained, and that the subjects would be protected from undue risk. This led to the formation of Institutional Review Boards (IRBs). Today, every clinical trial in the United States must be approved and monitored by an IRB to ensure that the risks are as low as possible and are worth any potential benefits.

An IRB is an independent committee of physicians, statisticians, community advocates, and others, who ensure that a clinical trial is ethical and that the rights of study participants are protected. All institutions that conduct or support biomedical research involving humans must, by federal regulation, have an IRB that initially approves and periodically reviews the research. At least five people comprise an IRB, and at least one member must come from a nonscientific discipline such as the law or the clergy.

To grant IRB approval, board members must jointly agree, for a specific trial and its investigator, that (1) patient risks are minimal and reasonable with respect to anticipated treatment benefits; (2) enrollment criteria are appropriate and patient eligibility is determined without regard to race, gender, economic background, and other such factors (unless appropriate and necessary for the trial, such as recruiting only females to test birth control pills); (3) informed consent documents meet all regulatory requirements; (4) patient consent will be obtained properly; (5) patient safety will be monitored continually; (6) collected data will be reviewed for completeness and accuracy; and (7) confidentiality will be maintained for all participants.

Periodically, the FDA can inspect IRB records and operations to certify that approvals, human subject safeguards (including informed consent), and conduct of business are what they should be. Occasionally, these inspections yield evidence of problems, such as in 1993, when the FDA imposed penalties on a large California university for infractions that included a failure to report deaths.

At any time in the clinical trials process, the FDA is allowed to issue a "clinical hold" if it is deemed necessary. A clinical hold is an order to the sponsor to delay a proposed investigation or to suspend an ongoing investigation entirely. When a clinical hold is issued, no new subjects are allowed to enter the program, and patients already in the study must be taken off the drug unless discontinuing the treatment could interfere with patient safety. During the period from 1999 to 2001, the FDA temporarily halted research because of inadequate IRB review and follow-up at two locations (Duke University and the VA Medical Center of West Los Angeles). In addition, the government suspended federally funded research on human subjects at Johns Hopkins University following the death of a healthy volunteer during an asthma experiment. Medical school officials said the patient likely died from inhaling the drug hexamethonium, which constricts airways. Hexamethonium was used widely as a tablet in the 1940s and 1950s to treat hypertension, but the FDA later withdrew its approval. It had never been approved as an inhalant, which was the way it was used in the Hopkins study.

SELECTED BIBLIOGRAPHY

National Center for Policy Analysis (1999) Policy Report No. 230, Washington, DC: NCPA.

U.S. Department of Health and Human Services, Office of Inspector General (1998) *Institutional Review Boards: Time for Reform*, Report OEI–01–97–00193. Washingon, DC: U.S. Department of Health and Human Services.

Willman, D. (2000) *How a New Policy Led to Seven Deadly Drugs*. Los Angeles, CA: Los Angeles Times.

QUESTIONS

1 Which of the following is/are true regarding phase II clinical studies?
   a   involve patients with the disease
   b   involve normal patients
   c   can involve a few dozen to a few hundred people
   d   can involve 10,000 or more subjects
   e   a and c.

2 The 1906 Food and Drug Act dealt primarily with which of the following?
   a   drug safety
   b   drug toxicity
   c   truth in labeling all of the above
   d   none of the above
   e   all of the above.

3 Which of the following chemicals was primarily responsible for the 1938 Food, Drug, and Cosmetic Act?
   a   sulfanilamide
   b   dinitrophenol
   c   thalidomide
   d   diethylene glycol
   e   Salvarsan.

4 The law requiring demonstration of efficacy for a drug occurred in which year?
   a   1906
   b   1938

c   1962
d   1977
e   1981.

5   Which of the following is required before a drug can be taken to clinical trials?
    a   IND
    b   DEA
    c   NDA
    d   NAS
    e   OTC.

6   The use of healthy volunteers usually only occurs in which phase of clinical studies?
    a   phase I
    b   phase II
    c   phase III
    d   phase IV
    e   all of the above.

7   Which of the following groups present particular problems in clinical trials?
    a   children
    b   the elderly
    c   women
    d   post-pubescent males
    e   a, b, and c.

8   The majority of all drugs tested are abandoned by their sponsors after which of the following?
    a   phase I
    b   phase II
    c   phase III
    d   phase IV
    e   a and b.

9   How many prescription drugs were removed from the market between 1997 and 2001?
    a   6
    b   10
    c   12
    d   17
    e   21.

10   IRBs are concerned with which of the following?
    a   clinical trial design
    b   informed consent
    c   proper enrollment criteria
    d   confidentiality of participants
    e   all of the above.

Chapter 15

Animals in research

The proper study of mankind is man.

Alexander Pope, 1733

I have seen numerous experiments on animals, but I have never seen an animal undergoing pain which I would not have been willing to undergo myself for the same object. Why, then, it may be asked, should not all painful experiments be done on human volunteers?

J. B. S. Haldane, 1971

Progress in the understanding and management of human disease must begin, and end, with studies of man.

Paul Beeson, MD, 1979

The use of animals for research purposes has been the subject of many articles and books, both in defense of and in opposition to, over the past 100–150 years. In some cases, opposition has been quite strident, expressing itself in both legal and illegal acts. With regard to the latter, research establishments have been raided, animals removed, records destroyed, and equipment vandalized. In fact, the uninitiated can now become knowledgeable about pursuing this line of expression by obtaining a "handbook" for animal activists. What are the reasons for such strongly held views? One major reason, of course, is that animals can be our pets. As such, they occupy a special relationship in our lives. To a certain extent, they are like children and are dependent upon our husbandry for their welfare. Most people are repulsed by the abuse of children and, hence, animals, since they are usually defenseless and are easily victimized.

Today, animals are used in scientific experiments for three general purposes: (1) biomedical and behavioral research, (2) education, and (3) drug and product testing. However, all too often those concerned with animal welfare question whether basic biomedical research has substantial clinical value and propose that alternatives should be developed for teaching and testing. Scientists answer that while all research might not have immediate value, most clinical breakthroughs are based upon multiple, fundamental studies carried out on experimental animals for which there are no appropriate alternatives. It is not the purpose of this chapter to advocate either side of the argument. Rather, the goal is to present the salient features of both sides of the issue for the reader to consider.

HISTORY

300 BC to 1800

The first recorded use of live animals for research is generally attributed to the "study of body humors" by Erasistratus in Alexandria, in the third century BC. In view of the fact that this antedates the discovery of general anesthetics by approximately 2150 years, one can only imagine the pain and suffering that "experimental" animals were subjected to in the name of science during this period. It was Galen of Pergamum, in the second century AD, who has been credited with demonstrating the significance of animal research. Galen expounded the theory that four natural humors—blood, phlegm, yellow bile, and black bile—were responsible for health. Since dissection of the human body was illegal in Rome at that time, Galen based his anatomical studies on "observations" made in "apes" and pigs.

It is extremely unlikely, however, that Galen actually carried out his research on apes. In fact, apes were not widely available for examination in Europe until about the sixteenth century. In all probability, the so-called Barbary "ape" of North Africa and Gibraltar is what Galen used. This "ape" is, in fact, a macaque monkey, which was presumably the first primate experimented upon. Among Galen's discoveries was the observation, in a live animal, that cutting a particular nerve in the neck (known to come from the lower brain) abolished movement of the larynx. After the fall of Rome, learning fell into disrepute in Europe until the thirteenth century. While this may have been a dark period for civilization, it undoubtedly served as a respite for experimental animals.

One theory advanced for the historical lack of concern regarding the infliction of pain on animals during the first millennium, or so, is that life for people of this period was often little better than their pets or the beasts of the fields. Life was basically short and hard and contained much pain and suffering. How could concern for an animal in agony be mustered when members of the family were suffering equally?

Following the Dark Ages, the Renaissance brought with it a desire for discovery in many areas including the human body. Because of this, the use of experimental animals also became popular once again. Unfortunately, influential thinkers of the day were anything but sensitive to the use of experimental animals. Francis Bacon (1561–1626), for one, championed the value of animal experimentation in his *De Augmentis Scientiarum* (The Advancement of Learning) when he asserted that "by the dissection of beast *alive*, which, not withstanding the dissimilitude of their parts to human, may with the help of a little judgment, sufficiently satisfy this inquiry."

The French philosopher René Descartes (1596–1650) was probably the most influential individual in formulating our early views regarding the status of animals in our world. According to Descartes, animals were no more than machines and were, therefore, incapable of thinking or feeling. Living in an age when clocks were at the cutting edge of technology, he wrote to the Marquis of Newcastle, "I know, indeed, that brutes do many things better than we do, but I am not surprised at it; for that, also, goes to prove that they act by force of nature and by springs, like a clock, which tells better what the hour is than our judgment can inform us." Descartes imagined insects and other creatures as elegant, miniaturized bits of clockwork "which eat without pleasure, cry without pain, desire nothing, know nothing, and only simulate intelligence as a bee simulates a mathematician" (in the geometry of its hexagonal honeycombs). Ants do not have souls, Descartes argued; automatons are owed no special moral obligations. He expressed his thoughts quite succinctly when he stated: "The greatest of all the prejudices we have retained from our infancy is that of believing that the beasts think." In Descartes' world, if an animal screamed in pain it was equivalent to the mechanical squeals of an ungreased wheel.

1800–1900

While the seventeenth and eighteenth centuries saw the growth of the scientific revolution, led by such luminaries as William Harvey (1578–1657), Anthony Van Leeuwenhoek (1632–1723), and Lazzaro Spallanzani (1729–1799), it was not until the nineteenth century that organized, systematic animal research really began in earnest; and opposition to it began to develop as a consequence. By the early 1800s the view that animals were little more than machine equivalents began to be questioned. This was particularly true in Britain, where the first Society for the Prevention of Cruelty to Animals was formed in 1824. Despite the views of Britain's Francis Bacon, alluded to previously, the overriding feeling against inflicting pain on household as well as experimental animals is one of the reasons why Britain took little part in the rapid advances in physiology that took place in the early and middle decades of the nineteenth century. Notable scientists such as Boyle and Hook, as well as other Fellows of the Royal Society, were often quite outspoken in their concern for the suffering of experimental animals, in contrast to their continental colleagues.

As a result of this Anglo viewpoint, experimental physiology did not really begin to develop in Britain until approximately 1870, by which time the use of general anesthetics had become generally available. However, despite the availability of anesthetics, some researchers were, nevertheless, selective in their use. For example, in 1875 the physiologist Emmanuel Klein was quoted as saying he had "no regard at all" for the suffering of experimental animals and only used anesthetics for his own convenience. This type of insensitivity led to the appointment of a Royal Commission in the same year and finally to the passing of the Cruelty to Animal Act of 1876. However, although this bill regulated painful research, it did not abolish it and, as a result, was strongly opposed by certain groups concerned with animal welfare. It was also during this period, in 1874, that Thomas Huxley published his critique of the Cartesian view of animals as automata. His summary conclusion was that animals were, in fact, automata but, like humans, they were conscious automata.

The situation was considerably different on the European continent, chiefly in France and Germany, where there was a heavy dependency on experiments involving major surgery on unanesthetized animals (accounts of some of these experiments have been described as "horrifying to read"). The difference in viewpoint toward the use of animals in research, particularly in France, can be ascribed to the influence of Descartes and his views on animals. Regardless of the reasons behind Descartes' position, his assertions provided the rationalization for vivisection research by the famous French experimentalists Francois Magendie (1783–1855) and Claude Bernard (1813–1878). Ironically, despite Bernard's reputation as an eminent experimentalist, his wife and two daughters became passionate antivivisectionists.

OPPOSITION TO ANIMAL USE IN RESEARCH

In general, the animal cause movement can be divided into two broad groups: (1) individuals concerned with *animal welfare*, who are not necessarily opposed to biomedical research using animals, but who do want the assurance that the animals are treated as humanely as possible (pain and suffering kept to a minimum), that the number of animals used are kept to a minimum, and that animals are used only when necessary; and (2) individuals concerned with *animal rights*, who insist that animals have moral rights, unlike Descartes' view, equal to those of humans, and are totally opposed to biomedical research using animals. People for the Ethical Treatment of Animals (PETA) and the Animal Liberation Front (ALF) have been the most vocal and visible proponents of the animal rights movement. Early opponents of animal experimentation were termed antivivisectionists (derived from the Latin *vius*, meaning living, and *sectio*, meaning cutting). Antivivisectionists are essentially abolitionists.

The roots of antivivisection as an organized movement are found in Britain, the birthplace of anticruelty crusades of all kinds. Jeremy Bentham, a Utilitarian philosopher, composed a particularly moving passage in his *Introduction to the Principles of Morals and Legislation*. In 1789 he wrote, "a full grown horse or dog is beyond comparison a more rational, as well as a more conversable animal, than an infant of a day, of a week or even a month old. But suppose the cause were otherwise, what would it avail? The question is *not* can they reason? Nor, can they talk? But, can they *suffer*? Despite this highly relevant question, it would be 87 years before British sentiment was sufficiently galvanized to pass the 1876 Cruelty to Animal Act.

In addition to the concept of suffering introduced by Bentham, Methodist theological doctrine was also a contributing factor to the British mind-set of the day because it held that animals also shared the potential of experiencing immortality with humans. This was no inconsequential tenet in a country of animal lovers. Would there be a pack of Cujos with a bad attitude at the "pearly gates"? If concern for pain and suffering in Victorian Britain, supported by arguments for the immortality of animals, were not enough, the publication of Darwin's *Descent of Man* in the midnineteenth century also served to challenge, in a far more dramatic fashion, the premise that humans and animals were different. How could Cartesian logic be depended upon if we were related in some anthropological manner to the beasts of the field?

In the second half of the nineteenth century, vivisection was actually even rarer in the United States than in Britain because of the relative paucity of experimental research. However, there were animal activists busy in North America before there was even a United States of America. In 1641, the Puritans of the Massachusetts Bay Colony drew up a list of liberties. Their formal legal code included "Liberty 92," which reads: "No man shall exercise any Tirranny or Crueltie towards any brute Creature which are usalie kept for man's use." The American Anti-Vivisection Society was founded in 1883 largely as a result of events in Britain. Their attempts to ban vivisection or significantly curtail it in several states were uniformly unsuccessful. There were a number of reasons for their failures, not the least of which was the emerging public awareness of the apparent beneficial role of animal research in the successful treatment of ravaging contagious diseases such as diphtheria. By the early

1900s, the influence of experimental medicine was growing and the humane movement, which it had become known as, receded into more mundane pursuits.

Between the two World Wars, the reputation and prestige of the medical scientist and the research establishment continued to grow. In the United States, antivivisectionist groups remained largely ineffective in implementing their concerns, despite the support of powerful backers such as William Randolph Hearst. Such was not the case in Germany, however. Although Germany had a rich history in vivisection, there existed, nonetheless, considerable opposition to this practice. In one of history's ironies, Herman Goering made the following declaration during a broadcast on August 29, 1933: "Experiments on animals for the purpose of defining an illness in human beings, for the preparation of serums and other experimental use, need legal regulation in detail and the keen control of the state. It is a sorry sign of science that during the past two decades, amply protected by law, materialistic scientists have wrought unbearable torture and suffering in animal experiments. . . . I have therefore announced the immediate prohibition of vivisection and have made the practice a punishable offense in Prussia. Until such times as punishment is pronounced the culprit shall be lodged in a concentration camp."

It was not until after World War II that the humane movement in the United States became reenergized. This was due, in part, to the sudden increase in funds available for biomedical research as well as the passage of a number of state pound seizure laws, which required release of unclaimed dogs and cats to medical research institutions to satisfy increased demand. After numerous failures to repeal these laws, humane societies turned their attention toward providing alternative shelters for homeless or lost dogs and cats. It was not until the 1980s that several states, under pressure, including New York and Massachusetts, passed laws that prohibit the release of any cat or dog from any type of shelter except for its adoption or return to its owner.

ANIMAL RIGHTS MOVEMENT

The contemporary animal rights movement had its genesis coincidental with three books published in the early 1970s. The first of these books, *Animals, Men and Morals* by Godlovitch, Godlovitch, and Harris, was published in 1971 and was an anthology that revived and presented to a new generation many long-dormant thoughts and views regarding the relationship between humans and animals. One of these was the view that animals have rights (proposed as early as 1894). This book renewed interest within the intellectual community of the relationship between human beings and animals and led to the publication in 1975 of two other important books. One of these was *Victims of Science* written by Richard Ryder, who introduced the concept of "specieism" (an elitist term similar to racism). The other book was *Animal Liberation: A New Ethic for our Treatment of Animals* by Peter Singer. It is this latter book that is generally considered to be the progenitor of the contemporary animal rights movement. Singer's expertise in the area is reflected in his joining the Princeton faculty in 1999 as a professor of bioethics. Singer has made the controversial comment that in some cases animals' lives should take precedence over humans.

Singer's book revived the classic debate that had existed for centuries between Cartesian (i.e., René Descartes—animals are machines) and Utilitarian philosophers (e.g., Jeremy Bentham—prevention of suffering) and made it an issue of the 1970s and 1980s. Singer made the disquieting suggestion that raising human infants for food is morally no different from raising pigs for the same purpose. Nevertheless, one important aspect of Singer's book was that it reintroduced to the cause of antivivisectionism an intellectual basis, a philosophical orientation, and a moral focus, regardless of one's views. These foundations gave the animal rights movement a new attraction to those who had been generally indifferent to, or repelled by, the essentially emotional appeal based on love of animals that antivivisectionism had been waging for the past century. The movement now had more legitimacy and support than ever before and its goals were consistent with other contemporary societal objectives.

Besides philosophical arguments at cocktail parties for and against animal rights, there are loose-knit groups that are proactive in asserting their beliefs. During the past 25 years, organizations such as the ALF and the Earth Liberation Front (ELF) have claimed responsibility for numerous acts involving public and private facilities. The groups have no formal structure, but espouse philosophies that support sabotage in defense of animal life or the environment. An area that they have emphasized is the release of animals.

These eco-saboteurs, as they are sometimes referred to, are suspected of at least six incidents since September 2001: (1) a firebombing at a federal corral for wild horses in northeastern California; (2) a fire at a primate research center in New Mexico; (3) release of more than 1000 mink from a farm in Iowa; (4) release of pigeons raised for research in Iowa; (5) fires at an Oregon tree farm and a laboratory at the University of Washington; and (6) a fire that destroyed a McDonald's restaurant in Tucson, Arizona. In recent years, the groups have also claimed responsibility for starting fires at a Vail, Colorado ski resort, which they say impacted a lynx habitat.

The impact of antivivisectionists has been manyfold, not the least of which has been an elevation of the consciousness of many people, including those in biomedical research, about the issue of experimental animals. As a result, a number of questions have arisen that can be justifiably directed toward those utilizing research animals. Some of these questions address scientific issues, while others are more moralistic in nature. For example, questions pertaining to science include: Is the scientific query mundane in nature? Will the data duplicate already existing data? If animals are used will their numbers be kept to a minimum? These are not, in fact, new questions. Britain's Marshall Hall (1790–1857) promulgated four related principles of animal research over one hundred years ago:

- experiments should never be done if the necessary information could be gained by observation;
- no experiment should be performed without a clearly defined and attainable objective;
- one should avoid unwarranted repetition;
- any justifiable experiment should be carried out with the least possible infliction of suffering.

While some type of answer might be presented relatively easily to the types of questions raised so far, it is the moral dilemma that appears to be more of a conundrum. After all, an experimental animal is *not* a volunteer. Animals do not have the option of consent, as their human counterparts do—they are conscripted. An animal finds itself in the constraints of a laboratory by virtue of being a "subordinate" species. As such, it is basically helpless—a victim, if you will. Intervention by appropriate review boards is not on the same level as an institutional review board (IRB) for human clinical studies. It is this exploitation, or specieism, of sentient beings that continues to challenge our moral and ethical framework. In fact, it is this particular quandary, perhaps more than any other issue, that has contributed to the internecine conflict between members of the biomedical community as well as the general public. However, rational arguments to these and other related issues have been put forth (see Nicoll and Russell, cited in the bibliography).

CONTEMPORARY STATUS

Are animals still subjected to untoward, excessive levels of pain and suffering? The answer appears to be, unfortunately, yes. In 1952 a business meeting of the American Physiological Society included the allegation from one of its members that there was much inhumane use of animals in biological and medical research. In 1957, 58 rhesus monkeys were put inside tubes set near the drop point for a nuclear bomb test. Those set in tubes along the flashpoint of the explosion were fried. Researchers have shot monkeys in the head with rifles, the barrel of the gun held just an inch from their skulls, and shot them in the stomach with a cannon impactor accelerated to 70 miles an hour to study blunt abdominal trauma. Monkeys have been crippled by having weights dropped on their spines. One of the more infamous studies during the 1960s dealt with the nature of love. Briefly, the experiments involved taking infant monkeys away from their mother and measuring their response. Remarkably, this "research" found that it is not enough for monkeys to see each other through glass partitions, they need to stroke, to hold. Such experiments were not without their challenges, however. The senior investigator in this federally funded project reported that before they began utilizing anesthetics, it sometimes took two laboratory workers to hold the struggling mother down while a third pulled the baby away. Lavish praise was bestowed on the senior investigator for this "seminal" work.

In a 1957 experiment, scientists plunged unanesthetized rats into boiling water in order to measure blood changes; in 1960, scientists wanting to study muscle atrophy immobilized the hind legs of cats with steel pins for 101 days, until the tissues withered. In 1961, researchers studied the effect of microwave blasts on dogs. Their detailed records noted that unanesthetized animals began to pant rapidly as radiation increased, their tongues swelled, their skin crisped, and if their body temperature was allowed to climb above 107 degrees Fahrenheit, the dogs died. During the early 1960s, cats were injected with acid directly into their trachea to induce mucus formation for the screening of antimucolytic drugs.

Today, most scientists and nonscientists are probably prepared to agree that standards of animal care and use have improved considerably over those of the 1950s and 1960s. However, unfortunate exceptions continue to appear periodically. In 1972, a polio researcher is credited with making the comment that "any qualms at the 'inhumanity' of injecting viruses into the spinal cords of these 'cute' creatures, who look so much like little people, is soon dispelled by their many annoying attributes." Does this reflect sensitivity to suffering? Two scientific research papers published in 1976 drew considerable criticism both from within and outside the biomedical research community for their cruel design. This research involved the use of the so-called Noble–Collup drum, within which lightly anesthetized animals were "tumbled." The interior of the drum contained shelves which projected out from the surface in order to produce injury and trauma to the tumbling animal. In other words, the experiment was designed to inevitably inflict pain. One would hope that the submission of such a paper today would result in its rejection due to violation of journal policy toward abuse of experimental animals. Fortunately, such editorial policies have become quite commonplace in scientific journals.

In 1980, the United States Department of Agriculture brought a complaint against Ohio State University concerning its care of some 40 kittens used in biomedical research. The complaint enunciated that "The kittens had lesions around their necks and many had metal tags with identification tags *imbedded* [emphasis mine] in the flesh of their necks. These injuries apparently resulted from chains being placed around the kittens' neck when they were young and not being replaced or lengthened as they grew older." The fine for this deplorable act of "husbandry" was $500, which the university reluctantly paid while denying culpability.

The existence of insensitivity during the 1980s is further illustrated by a rather remarkable statement attributed to a scientist during a meeting with an NIH grant review team in 1981. This individual argued that one cannot apply "human expectations of pain to animal surgery because pain is primarily a matter of societal conditioning to which animals are not subject." If this is, in fact, the case, how does one justify, on scientific terms, the thousands of animals that have been used over the years in pain and analgesia research? The year 1981 was also the high-water mark, or low, depending upon one's point of view, in the area of animal abuse. The alleged abuse of animals launched the precedent-setting case of the *Silver Springs Monkeys*.

Primate experiments at Silver Springs involved the procedure known as deafferentation. It requires opening of the spinal cord and slicing away selected sensory nerves, rendering the monkey crippled. In this particular case the procedure was carried out in order to "force recovery" of the affected limb. In order to make a crippled monkey use its bad limb, the investigator strapped on a straightjacket to bind the good arm, leaving the animal only the damaged one. An alternative strategy was to place animals in restraining chairs and give electric shocks if they did not move their crippled arm.

This case resulted in the first and only arrest and criminal conviction of an animal researcher in the United States on charges of cruelty to animals, the first confiscation of abused laboratory animals under a court-ordered search-and-seizure warrant, and the first hearing by the U.S. Supreme Court of a case involving animals in experiments. This type of event stimulated various organizations such as the American College of Toxicology and the Society of Toxicology, for example, to establish policy statements and guiding principles during the late 1980s relating to animal experimentation.

The point here is not to list examples ad nauseum of animal abuse in the name of science or attitudinal problems of researchers but, rather, to serve as a reminder that things are probably not perfect in our nation's laboratories despite improvement. To deny such would challenge credibility and temper continuation of necessary self-evaluation, criticism, and regulation. Constant vigilance appears to be necessary, if for no other reason than the large number of experimental animals still being used and the corresponding opportunities for negligence.

Biomedical research

Of all the industries utilizing animal research, biomedical research undoubtedly uses the greatest number of animals and has therefore been a national target for animal reform. The National Association for Biomedical Research estimates that 23 million rats and mice were used in 1998 and made up 95 percent of all laboratory animals (other estimates are of the order of 30 million). In addition to rodents, dogs and cats (1–1.5 percent) and nonhuman primates (0.5 percent) make up the majority of the remainder. According to the Institute for Laboratory Animal Resources survey, there was a 40 percent decrease in the number of animals used in research between 1968 and 1978, with the largest decline occurring with nonhuman primates, dogs, cats, and birds.

The reasons for this decrease are undoubtedly multifactorial and probably include the refinement of research techniques, development of alternatives, decrease in research funding, and animal rights/welfare activism. Funds for research have failed to increase at the same rate as costs of acquiring and caring for laboratory animals. Researchers have also lowered the incidence of spontaneous disease among laboratory animals, thus increasing their longevity. Today, the same research objectives can be obtained with fewer animals because of improved methods for breeding, rearing, genetic control, and experimental design.

As mentioned earlier, the vast majority of laboratory animals are rats and mice bred specifically for this purpose by licensed suppliers. Large animals, such as swine, cattle, and sheep, are supplied primarily by agricultural sources. Today, most nonhuman primates are obtained from scientific breeding centers and not from the wild since their exportation has been prohibited by several countries. Many cats and dogs necessary for research are "purpose-bred" animals—those bred for a particular trait or whose genealogy or physiology must be known in order for the experimental results to be valid. Such animals are bred and sold by professional dealers. Other experiments can be conducted with what are known as "random source" animals whose ancestry and physiologic history are unknown. Such animals are, in fact, preferable in some experiments because their unknown and varied backgrounds more closely approximate to those found among a human population. One source of such animals has been pounds.

Estimates vary widely, but of the approximately 16.2 to 27 million cats and dogs left in pounds and shelters each year, only about 1.1 percent (approximately 138,000 dogs and 50,000 cats) are used in research annually. The majority of these pound animals, between 10.1 and 16.7 million dogs and cats, are put to death by animal care and control agencies each year, according to the American Humane Association's 1989 statistics. The remaining animals are claimed by their owners or adopted. Animal rights groups have persuaded a number of state, county, and municipal legislatures to pass laws to prohibit the release of animals (primarily dogs and cats) from public pounds to researchers. The most comprehensive pound law, adopted by Massachusetts, bans the use of pound animals regardless of source. It is estimated that the additional cost of conducting experiments in Massachusetts will be $6 million a year.

Benefits of animal research

How does one determine if animal experimentation has been productive and justified? One criterion often quoted is the relationship between animal research and the Nobel prize, which is generally considered to be an index of scientific significance. Since 1901, approximately 75 percent of Nobel prizes awarded in physiology or medicine have been for discoveries and progress made through the use of experimental animals. More specifically, many advances in medical science in the nineteenth and twentieth centuries, from vaccines and antibiotics to antidepressant drugs and organ transplants, have been achieved either directly or indirectly through the use of animals in laboratory experiments. The result of these experiments has been the elimination or control of many infectious diseases—smallpox, poliomyelitis, measles —and the development of numerous life-saving techniques—blood transfusions, burn therapy, open-heart and brain surgery. A more extensive list of examples is shown in Table 15.1.

Behavioral research with animals has also been credited with benefit to humans. For example, fundamental information on how people learn was discovered by experiments on animals in laboratories. The behavioral modification therapies discovered or developed through such experiments are being used to treat conditions such as enuresis (bed-wetting), addictive behaviors (tobacco, alcohol, and other drugs), and compulsive behaviors, such as anorexia nervosa. In addition, information gained through experiments begun 50 years ago on "imprinting" (the tendency of an animal to identify and relate to the first species it comes into contact with) has been used to train captive-born animals to relate to members of their own species.

Although improved public health and nutrition have certainly played a significant role in advancing longevity and health, for most infectious diseases this role has been minor. Despite advances in public health and nutrition, eradication of whooping cough, measles, and poliomyelitis was not achieved until the development of vaccines and drugs through research using animals. The possible development of a vaccine against AIDS is also dependent upon continued studies conducted in animals, particularly primates (see later discussion).

An example of the role(s) that primate research has played is in the development of the poliomyelitis vaccines. Although many studies on poliomyelitis in humans were conducted in the late nineteenth century, the cause of the disease remained unknown until scientists succeeded in transmitting the virus to monkeys in 1908. There followed many years of research with primates until scientists were able, in the early 1950s, to grow the virus in human cell cultures and development of a vaccine became possible. At that point in time, in order to ensure the safety and effectiveness of the vaccines, tests were conducted with monkeys. Furthermore, in order to produce the vaccines in pure form in great quantities, it was necessary to use kidney tissue taken from monkeys. Today, an alternative to the use of monkey kidneys has been developed for the production of the vaccine.

Table 15.1 Examples of medical advances made possible through the use of animals

Pre-1900	Treatment of rabies, anthrax, and smallpox Principles of infection control and pain relief Management of heart failure
Early 1900s	Treatment of histamine shock, pellagra (niacin deficiency) and rickets (vitamin D deficiency) Electrocardiography and cardiac catheterization
1920s	Discovery of thyroxine Intravenous feeding Discovery of insulin—diabetes control
1930s	Therapeutic use of sulfa drugs Prevention of tetanus Development of anticoagulants, modern anesthesia, and neuromuscular blocking agents
1940s	Treatment of rheumatoid arthritis and whooping cough Therapeutic use of antibiotics, such as penicillin, aureomycin, and streptomycin Discovery of Rh factor Treatment of leprosy Prevention of diphtheria
1950s	Prevention of poliomyelitis Development of cancer chemotherapy Open heart surgery and cardiac pacemaker
1960s	Prevention of rubella Corneal transplant and coronary bypass surgery Therapeutic use of cortisone Development of radioimmunoassay for the measurement of minute quantities of antibodies, hormones, and other substances in the body
1970s	Prevention of measles Modern treatment of coronary insufficiency Heart transplant Development of nonaddictive painkillers
1980s	Use of cyclosporin and other antirejection drugs Artificial heart transplantation Identification of psychophysiological factors in depression, anxiety, and phobias Development of monoclonal antibodies for treating disease Discovery of HIV as causative agent for AIDS
1990s	Pancreas and liver transplantation Thrombolytic therapy for acute myocardial infarction Human gene therapy

Scientific criticisms of animal research

In 1971 the National Cancer Act initiated a "War on Cancer" that many sponsors predicted would cure cancer by 1976. Instead, this multibillion dollar research program has not achieved its goal, and the age-adjusted total cancer mortality rate has been steadily climbing for decades. This despite the use of a 5-year survival as a "cure" even if the patient died of the cancer after the 5-year period. Why has progress against cancer not been more successful? One possible explanation is the unwarranted preoccupation with animal research. Some critics have emphasized that the crucial genetic, molecular, and immunologic differences between humans and other animals have prevented animal models from serving as effective means by which to seek a cancer cure.

Animal tests for cancer-causing substances, generally involving rodents, are notoriously unreliable. A former editor of the prestigious journal *Science* has asked, "Are humans to be regarded as behaving biochemically like huge, obese, inbred, cancer-prone rodents?" Of 19 known human oral carcinogens, only seven caused cancer in nonhuman animals using the standard National Cancer Institute protocol. Even different rodent species produce conflicting results. When a comparison of carcinogenicity was made in rat and mouse for 214 chemicals, a correlation of only 70 percent was found (chance alone would have yielded 50 percent).

Despite extensive use, animal models have not contributed significantly to AIDS research. While monkeys, rabbits, and mice can be infected with HIV, none develops the human AIDS syndrome. Of over 100 chimpanzees infected with HIV over a 10-year period, only two became sick. Because chimpanzees turned out to be poor models for AIDS, and were expensive to maintain, all of the animals were faced with euthanasia (a euphemism for being killed). In 1997, the National Research Council recommended a solution. For all of the chimpanzees housed in research facilities throughout the United States, a breeding moratorium was introduced and specific steps taken toward making long-term care available for the primates. Animal rights supporters applauded the decision on the basis of moral responsibility.

Government officials have estimated that the breeding program produces approximately 25 offspring a year at a cost of $60,000 to $100,000 per animal. Most researchers are only able to afford several animals for their studies. Statisticians have pointed out that for a study to have reliable numbers, showing that a vaccine fails 10 percent of the time, for example, a minimum of 29 chimpanzees would be required.

To quote Deborah Blum, author of *The Monkey Wars*, "Rhesus macaques—or any other primates—cannot just be dismissed as simple creatures. Their abilities go far beyond the basic skills of food-finding and nest building. These are animals that teach each other negotiating skills, learn to operate computers, [and] recognize their kinfolk from a photograph. They are intelligent, capable, quick learners. They are, like us, complex beings. Once we recognize that, we must also recognize that the choices we make in using them are complex, too. It might once have been easy to toss a monkey into a research project, taking no particular thought. Today, the reverse is true. We should hesitate and we should think."

Numerous standard animal toxicity tests have been widely criticized by clinicians and toxicologists. The LD_{50} test generally requires 60 to 100 animals (usually rats and mice), most of whom endure substantial suffering. Because of difficulties extrapolating the results to humans, the test can be highly unreliable. Also, since such variables as an animal's age, sex, weight, and strain can have a substantial effect on the results, laboratories often obtain disparate data with the same test substances. In 2001, The Organization for Economic Co-operation and Development announced that it was to phase out its Test Guideline 401 (dealing with the LD_{50} test), deeming it unnecessary, inhumane, and lacking in scientific merit (http://www.oecd.org).

The Draize eye irritancy test, in which unanesthetized rabbits have irritant substances applied to their eyes, yields results that are inherently unreliable in predicting human toxicity. Humans and rabbits differ in the structure of their eyelids and corneas as well as in their abilities to produce tears. When comparing rabbit to human data on the duration of inflammation after exposure to 14 household products, they differed by a factor of 18 to 250.

Critics of animal studies contend that such studies can neither confirm nor refute hypotheses about human physiology or pathology; human clinical investigation is the only way such hypotheses can be tested. The Medical Research Modernization Committee's review of 10 randomly chosen animal models of human diseases did not reveal any important contributions to human health. In addition, the animal models differed substantially from their human counterparts in both cause and clinical course. Furthermore, the study found that treatments effective in animals tended to have poor efficacy or excessive side effects in human patients.

In contrast to human clinical trials, vivisection involves manipulations of artificially induced conditions. Furthermore, the highly unnatural laboratory environment invariably stresses the animals, and stress affects the whole animal by altering pulse, blood pressure, hormone levels, immunological activity, and other functions. Unfortunately, some laboratory "discoveries" are more of an artifact than scientifically relevant. For example, during the 1980s researchers reported 25 compounds that reduce ischemic-stroke damage in nonhuman animals, but none proved effective in humans. Animal tests can also mislead in other ways. The drug Milrinone was reported to increase survival of rats with artificially induced heart failure, but humans taking the drug experienced a 30 percent increase in mortality. The drug Fialuridine appeared safe in animal tests, but it caused liver failure in seven of 15 humans taking the drug, five of whom died and two required liver transplantation.

Animal studies failed to predict dangerous heart valve abnormalities in humans induced by the diet drugs fenfluramine and dexfenfluramine. To this list can be added the 12 drugs recently removed from the market in the United States. The General Accounting Office reviewed 198 of 209 drugs marketed from 1976 to 1985 and found that 52 percent had "serious postapproval risks" not predicted by animal tests. Animal studies are reliable at only the crudest levels—such as the ability of strong acids to damage eyes. However, such effects can be assessed relatively easily with in vitro systems. For more subtle effects, animal models are often unreliable.

It would not be fair to state that everyone in the biomedicine community agrees with all of the above conclusions, however. An article in the February 1997 issue of *Scientific American* ellicited a robust debate in this area. The article was entitled "Animal Research is Wasteful and Misleading." Critics of the article contend that the authors skewed their analysis and included inaccuracies that could produce misconceptions and mislead, particularly, layreaders of the piece. Objections to the article can be summarized by one of its critics: "In no case . . . has adequate animal research led to human illness or death, as every animal study is followed by a clinical study afterwards. The statement that use of animal models has prevented illnesses and deaths by screening out toxic drugs would be truthful." More information from responsible animal-use proponents can be researched at the American Association for the Advancement of Science (http://www.aaas.org/).

ALTERNATIVE METHODOLOGIES IN ANIMAL RESEARCH

In recent times, alternative methods in biomedical research and safety evaluation of chemicals and compounds have come under increasing scrutiny. This development represents the convergence of several factors: (1) accelerating developments in basic biologic methodology and understanding, especially in vitro; (2) increasing realization of the wastefulness of such tests as the classic LD_{50} and Draize, once useful but now considered archaic; and (3) increasing insistence from the public and animal rights groups that new understandings and methodologies be pressed into service of reducing animal use and alleviating animal suffering. An alternative to animal testing website may be found at http://www.sph.jhu.edu/~altweb.

Interestingly, although never specifically required by the government, the LD_{50} test has become the standard measuring tool for FDA approval of drugs and for meeting certain toxicity requirements of the Environmental Protection Agency (EPA). The FDA has declared that it does not require that data be based on the LD_{50} test for approval and the EPA has established circumstances in which the test can be replaced by a "limit" test that uses fewer animals (4–10 vs. 30–100) to screen for toxicity.

Animal rights organizations have been successful in changing the product testing protocols in some industries. Of particular note has been their effectiveness in the cosmetic industry. For example, an international campaign to expose the cruelty of product tests on animals led to the Benetton company's permanent ban on animal tests, a first for a major cosmetics company. Other leading companies such as Revlon, Avon, and Estée Lauder quickly followed suit. At the present time, there are more than 500 cosmetic companies that do not test products on animals. This has been particularly significant in eliminating the Draize tests for eye and skin irritancy. Companies such as General Motors (GM) have also not been immune from pressure. GM, which for a decade had been conducting crash tests on pigs and ferrets, involving an estimated 20,000 animals, finally ceased this program.

Most research organizations and scientists follow a practice known as the "three R's," which stand for replacement, reduction, and refinement in alternatives. This concept had its roots in a book published in 1959 entitled *The Principles of Humane Experimental Technique* by William Russell and Rex Burch. They wrote that scientific excellence and humane use of laboratory animals are inextricably linked. The scientific basis for the three R's has been endorsed and reaffirmed in the 1980s and 1990s by numerous national and international agencies and scientific societies (e.g. the American Society of Pharmacology and Experimental Therapeutics, the Society of Toxicology, and the American College of Toxicology).

- *Replacement* alternatives are methods that use organisms with limited sentience or that do not use whole animals. They include improved information exchange to avoid unnecessary repetition of animal experiments; physiochemical techniques and structure–activity relations; mathematical and computer models; use of invertebrates, plants, and microorganisms; in vitro methods; and human studies, including the use of human volunteers, postmarketing surveys, and epidemiology. In the biomedical sciences, in vitro methods are increasingly being used, not because they provide precisely the same information as do animal studies but because they offer the best scientific approach. Such methods often use results from past animal studies as a basis for cellular and molecular investigations. Unfortunately, for most basic researchers, replacement is problematic. Alternative methods such as tissue-culture systems simply cannot approximate the complexity of whole animals, especially in areas such as neuroscience and behavior. Neuroscientists point out that you cannot study learning and memory, or the effects of emotion or stress, except in a fully functioning animal.

- *Reduction* refers to areas where the number of animals used can be reduced. For example, the number of animals used in acute toxicity testing is being reduced as scientists have discovered ways to obtain accurate toxicity data using fewer animals. In addition, as mentioned in Chapter 13, scientists can now screen for the binding of some potential drugs by using isolated receptor preparations rather than using hundreds of animals.

- *Refinement* alternatives are methods that eliminate or minimize pain and distress or enhance animal well-being. Assessments of animal pain and distress are currently based on subjective evaluation of abnormal behavior or appearance. Because proper evaluation of pain relies largely on the ability to understand the behavior and needs of each species of laboratory animal, it is best for investigators to assume that a procedure that inflicts pain and distress in humans will do the same in animals. Much pain and distress can be diminished or eliminated with the proper use of anesthetics and analgesics. Researchers can enhance animals' well-being by using environmental enrichment techniques, such as proper handling, appropriately sized cages, and group housing of social species.

Alternatives most commonly employed in biomedicine include cell, tissue, and organ cultures, computer modeling, and the use of minimally invasive procedures that produce less stress. While more toxicological research is being carried out in vitro, the potential of culture methods in toxicological methods in toxicological protocols and hazard assessment is only in its early stages of development. Much of the emphasis in these new areas is the result of public pressure from the animal protection movement. Because of improved cell culture techniques, experimental models have been developed to assess important biological characteristics such as:

- membrane permeability;
- active and passive transport of ions and other compounds through the membrane;
- cellular respiration and energy metabolism;
- integrity of the cytoskeleton;
- growth inhibition and cell viability;
- inhibition of cell-cycle controlling factors;
- measurement of macromolecular synthesis (DNA, RNA, and proteins);
- changes in cell morphology;
- release of mediators;
- release of specific proteins;
- release or uptake of dyes or radioactive markers;
- ATP levels.

Scientists have been, and still are, searching continually for alternative methods to the use of animals in biomedical and behavioral research for a variety of reasons, including an interest in the welfare of animals and a concern for the increasing costs of purchasing and caring for animals, and because in some areas alternative methods may be more efficient and effective research tools. However, although the search for alternatives to the use of animals in research testing remains a valid goal of researchers, the chance that alternatives will completely replace animals in the foreseeable future is nil. Nevertheless, some industries, such as the cosmetic industry, are making significant strides. For example, that industry is presently involved in the organization of a database of currently available results for the evaluation of safety of cosmetic ingredients obtained or being developed with alternative methodologies. In addition, significant reduction in animal use has occurred in U.S. medical schools. This is due to (1) attendant costs and (2) the availability of new technological tools such as videos, computer models, and patient simulators.

There are signs that significant changes are being made in how the search for new drugs is being carried out. A good example is the National Cancer Institute (NCI) in the United States. Over the past 35 years, 400,000 chemicals have been injected into mice deliberately bred to develop leukemia. A few drugs were found this way but not against other forms of cancer. To become more effective, the NCI has stopped using mice. They now use 60 human tumor cell lines from seven main areas: colon, lung, melanoma, kidney, ovary, brain, and blood. By using these cell cultures they are able to screen 300 chemicals a week.

Fortunately, cell culture tests are becoming increasingly common in cancer research. Some examples include:

- A human leukemia cell line has been used to test 11 anticancer drugs to determine if they are more effective when used alone or in combination.
- Four human colorectal cancer cell lines have been used to test the effectiveness of seven drugs.
- Eight different human tumor cell lines have been used to find the most effective dose of the drug paclitaxel, and for what period it should be given.
- Human breast cancer tissue removed for biopsy has been tested with four different drugs.

Cell cultures have also been used to investigate differences between people. In one such study, four drugs were tested on ovarian tumors from 100 people. Because there was wide variability in response to the drugs, the patients were able to receive individual dosing regimens.

REGULATION OF RESEARCH ANIMALS

The status of laboratory animals in universities, hospitals, drug companies, and other research facilities is monitored by the U.S. Department of Agriculture (USDA) under the provisions of the Animal Welfare Act (AWA). The AWA has been amended three times since its passage in 1966. In 1985, an amendment was added that requires federally funded investigators to consider alternatives to animal use. Under the AWA, USDA officials make periodic unannounced inspections to ensure compliance with stringent standards for housing, feeding and watering, cleanliness, ventilation, and veterinary care. In addition, the AWA calls for the use of anesthetics and analgesics for potentially painful procedures and for postoperative care. However, the AWA excludes any other comment on how animals are used and critics characterize the AWA as a "paper tiger."

The U.S. Public Health Service (PHS) also has an Animal Welfare Policy that applies to all NIH-funded projects involving animals. The NIH requires that the institutions follow the "Guide for the Care and Use of Laboratory Animals," prepared by the Institute for Laboratory Animal Resources of the National Research Council. Any institution that receives funding from the PHS is required by law to comply with the Guide, or else it will lose funding.

Both the AWA and the Guide mandate that each research institution establish an Institutional Animal Care and Use Committee that must review in detail every proposal for research involving animals and approve each proposal before the research can begin (in fact, even before the investigator can receive funding). Among the issues covered by these requirements are standards for postoperative care and the use of anesthetics and analgesics to prevent any unnecessary discomfort to the animals.

In addition, the American Association for Laboratory Animal Science (AALAS) provides guidelines for animal care and use, operates a certification program for animal technicians, and develops educational materials. The AALAS also serves as a scientific forum for laboratory medicine and care. The American Association for the Accreditation of Laboratory Animal Care (AAALAC) offers a peer review laboratory accreditation program for research facilities. In addition, the FDA and the EPA have Good Laboratory Practice (GLP) regulations.

HUMAN EXPERIMENTATION IN MEDICINE

The magnitude of human experimentation in the United States is quite substantial. Each year more than 3000 clinical trials are carried out subject to FDA regulations. Thousands more trials are carried out in other countries. Each trial involves many volunteers, and the humans who are the first to take experimental therapies often face major risks. Yet without human experiments we would not know with any degree of certainty whether potential new preventions, such as vaccines, drugs, and surgery, are safe. Even then, these therapies can prove toxic in many ways.

In a long and continuing tradition physicians have often chosen to become the first volunteers. Examples of some of these human guinea pigs and their remarkable commitment are presented here. But, to set the mood, we need only look back to 1984. Dr Barry J. Marshall, an Australian physician, had been experimenting with ulcers and, with a colleague, had identified a bacterium, now known as *Helicobacter pylori*, in patients with ulcers. Marshall believed that the pathogen was the cause of the ulcers. In the next phase of his research, Marshall swallowed a tube, which was used for tests to document that he had neither gastritis nor an ulcer and was not harboring *H. pylori*. Then Marshall swallowed a liquid containing *H. pylori*. At 0500 h Marshall woke up vomiting and began suffering from gastritis. By acting as his own experimental subject he had proven to his own satisfaction that the bacteria could bring on ulcers and gastritis. The production of gastric ulcers by this strain of bacteria is now well established.

Not too long ago there was an unwritten code that if there was a scientific question asked, then the experimenter should first perform the appropriate experiment on themselves (e.g., Golden Rule). One of history's first self-experimenters was a Viennese physician, Dr Anton Stock (1760). Stock was particularly interested in the potential curative properties of hemlock. In his desire to experience its effects in humans he first fed samples in meat to a little dog that was hungry. After several days, seeing no adverse effects in the animal, he began to experiment on himself. Each morning for 8 days he took several hundred milligrams in tea. He noted no unusual effects. Despite the failure of this crude test to do anything, Stock and other Viennese physicians prescribed hemlock for cancers, tumors, ulcers, and cataracts, although it possessed no medicinal value.

In the nineteenth century there were several dramatic demonstrations of the efficacy of the antidotal value of charcoal in poison overdoses. In 1813, the French chemist M. Bertrand, after showing that he could use charcoal to prevent arsenic poisoning in animals, gave a public demonstration of its benefits in humans. Bertrand swallowed 5 grams of arsenic trioxide mixed with charcoal without ill effect. In 1852, another French chemist named Pierre-Fleurus Touery provided another demonstration. In front of a large audience of the French Academy of Medicine, he swallowed 1 gram of strychnine (10 times the fatal dose) mixed with 15 grams of charcoal. Other examples of nineteenth-century self-experimentation have already been mentioned, including Dr Horace Wells having his own teeth extracted under nitrous oxide and Dr Carl Koller using cocaine on his own eye as a local anesthetic.

The name of Dr Walter Reed is synonymous with self-experimentation. He was at the head of an American military medical team that went to Cuba in 1900 and proved through daring human experiments that mosquitoes were the vectors that transmitted yellow fever (now known to be a virus). However, in reality, the team actually confirmed findings made almost a century earlier by another self-experimenter that yellow fever was not a contagious disease. In 1800, an American, Dr Issac Cathrall, repeatedly placed black vomit from several yellow fever patients to his lips and tasted it. (Black vomit occurs in yellow fever victims by virtue of bleeding in their stomachs, and is subsequently expelled.) He did not become infected. A physician named Ffirth went five steps further in 1802, when he: (1) inserted black vomit into his forearm; (2) dropped black vomit into his eye; (3) boiled black vomit and inhaled the gas and steam; (4) swallowed black vomit taken directly from a patient; and (5) prepared pills made from black vomit.

The yellow fever team led by Walter Reed had three other members. One of these, Dr James Carroll, maintained till his death that he was the originator of the pact that the team test their experiments on themselves. In any event, all members agreed to the pledge. Eventually, while Reed was in Washington, DC, on August 27, 1900, James Carroll was exposed to mosquitoes known to be carrying the disease. Two days later Carroll began experiencing the early symptoms of yellow fever. Four days after the bite, the symptoms had become much more severe. For three more days Carroll's life was in the balance. Fortunately, Carroll must have had a strong constitution for he began to slowly recover and attempted to return to work on September

Table 15.2 Selected examples of human/self-experimentation

Edward Jenner (1796)	Cowpox (8-year-old boy, with permission)
Issac Cathrall (1800)	"Black vomit" (yellow fever, self)
Stubbins Ffirth (1802)	"Black vomit" (yellow fever, self)
Jaime Ferran (1884)	Cholera vaccine (self)
Louis Pasteur (1885)	Rabies vaccine (9-year-old boy, with permission)
Waldemar Haffkine (1892)	Cholera vaccine (self)
Almroth E. Wright (1896)	Typhoid vaccine (self)
Arthur Loos (1898)	Hookworm (self)
James Carroll (1900)	Yellow fever (self)
Claude Barlow (1920)	Intestinal flukes (self)
Maurice Brodie and William Park (1934)	Polio vaccine (self)
John Kolmer and Anna Rule (1934)	Polio vaccine (self)
Albert Hofmann (1943)	LSD (self)
Claude Barlow (1944)	Schistosomiasis (self)
Hilary Koprowski and Martin Kaplan (1955)	Rabies vaccine (self)
CIA (1970s)	LSD (unspecified adults, no permission)

28. The conduct of the yellow fever experiments was the forerunner of the current practice of informed consent and was cited in the formulation of the Nuremberg Code and in many other discussions about the ethics of human experimentation.

Scientists are a strange breed. We mentioned Dr Marshall at the beginning of this section for his self-experimentation with bacteria. One of the most bizarre examples of self-use occurred during World War II. Dr Claude Barlow, who had previously experimented on himself with intestinal flukes (Table 15.2), now took it upon himself to determine whether servicemen who had been infected with schistosomiasis (principally in Egypt) might pass the parasite on to previously uninfected snails in the United States. (Schistosomiasis is transmitted to humans via infected snails, whose larvae have suckers that help them bore through the skin and migrate to the liver and lungs.)

Barlow became fixated on determining whether the parasite could develop in a species of snail native to the United States. In order to accomplish this, he needed to have some viable parasites to carry out the research on. Unfortunately, while the parasite was quite happy living in foul canals, it was extremely fussy about living under laboratory conditions; laboratory models were a failure. To overcome this reality, attempts had been made by Barlow, and others, to infect animals in countries where the disease was common and send them to countries where the disease did not occur. The animals invariably died in transit. But Barlow had an idea to circumvent this challenge. He would transport the parasites himself in an environment he knew the parasites would not object to—his own body. By doing so, he would also avoid the necessity of an import permit.

Barlow began his self-experiment in Egypt on May 31, 1944. Over a 3-week period of time Barlow placed specific numbers of the chosen strain of parasite to the skin over his left forearm and to his naval. On July 4, 1944, Barlow and his freeloaders flew to the United States. The first symptom occurred on October 31 when several itching spots appeared that oozed serum containing eggs of the parasite. Ten days later, Barlow had a biopsy taken to look for the worms that had produced the eggs.

Barlow refused to take a local anesthetic because he feared the injection might disturb the worms! The biopsy revealed a pair of adult worms.

By December Barlow's condition had begun to decline. His temperature exceeded 103 degrees Fahrenheit, blood and mucus appeared regularly in his urine and stools. He could only sleep with the aid of sedatives. Being the consummate scientist, Barlow frequently examined his own specimens and kept an almost daily record of his clinical and laboratory observations. For example, in tests of his urine he found he was passing up to 12,000 eggs in each 24-hour sample. Barlow was a very sick man, so sick that he was subjected to extremely painful injections of antimony. Treatment with the heavy metal did clear Barlow of the infection by December 1944. In 1948 Barlow received the Medal of Merit from President Truman. He died at the ripe old age of 93.

One of the most remarkable examples of self-experimentation involves Dr Werner Forssmann. Although not involving drugs or pathogens, his hubris is, nonetheless, remarkable. Forssmann obtained his medical degree in 1929 and began his internship in Eberswalde, Germany. During his studies, Forssmann had been deeply impressed by a sketch in his physiology textbook that showed French physiologists standing in front of a horse, holding a thin tube that had been put into the jugular vein in the animal's neck and then guided into the heart. Forssmann became obsessed with the potential of putting a tube into the heart of a living human. Forssmann eventually approached his mentor about introducing a tube into a human heart. His mentor refused permission even when Forssmann volunteered to perform the procedure on himself.

Forssmann decided to do the experiment anyway—in secret. By befriending a nurse, who was deeply interested in medicine, Forssmann found a kindred spirit who was sympathetic to his research idea. In fact, she volunteered to be his guinea pig. Then, in a drama befitting Hollywood, Forssmann tricked the nurse in order to obtain the necessary surgical equipment, plus a ureteral catheter, the thin tubing urologists use to drain urine from the kidneys. Realizing she was going to be the first human to have a tube placed in her heart, the nurse climbed onto a surgical table and had her arms strapped down. As the nurse adjusted her body, Forssmann dabbed iodine over *his* left elbow crease and injected novacaine to numb the skin. After the local anesthetic had taken effect, Forssmann picked up the scalpel and cut through the skin. When he reached a large vein, he put down the scalpel, picked up a hollow needle, and gently pushed it into the vein. He then inserted the catheter into the needle and guided the catheter up to the level of his shoulder and left it in place.

At this point, Forssmann knew he would need documentation, as well as the nurse's cooperation. Despite her exasperation at being duped, the nurse assisted Forssman down to the basement X-ray laboratory. There, Forssmann, with guidance from the nurse, using a fluoroscopic X-ray screen, successfully placed the catheter into the right auricle. The X-ray technician snapped the picture and radiographic proof was obtained. The importance of describing the procedure in the scientific literature was obvious. However, Forssmann's mentor was concerned that it was too revolutionary to be understood by doctors. To quote the mentor: "Say that you tried it on cadavers before you did it on yourself. The reader of your paper must have the impression that it is not too revolutionary and that it was not made without a lot of forethought. Otherwise the critics will tear you to pieces." Even today, textbooks describe the fictitious, aborted first effort and the nonexistent preliminary test on a corpse.

One would have thought that self-catheterization would have been enough for Forssmann. Such was not the case. Radiopaque chemicals were just beginning to be used to help X-ray the urinary system and the stomach. Forssmann decided to investigate whether this technique could be applied to the heart. Once again, he undertook to study this question on himself. After some experiments on dogs, he eventually decided to do the experiment. At this point, he was no longer threading the catheter through the veins in his elbow crease because the most readily accessible of these blood vessels had been sewn closed after his previous catheterization experiments. Instead, he injected a local anesthetic into the skin around his groin, made an incision, and inserted a catheter into the femoral vein. He then pushed it up into the abdomen, then the inferior vena cava, and on into its connection with the heart. Unfortunately, this and several other attempts were unsuccessful. It remained for others to apply his revolutionary techniques to the everyday practice of medicine. Today, hundreds of thousands of cases of cardiac angiography are carried out yearly. Forssmann shared the 1956 Nobel prize in medicine.

During World War II, doctors in Nazi Germany invoked the name of science to justify atrocities, labeled "experiments," that involved hundreds of thousands of victims. Among the 20 Nazi doctors who were tried at Nuremberg was an eminent malaria expert. This former member of the League of Nations Malaria Commission infected more than 1000 prisoners at Dachau with the parasitic disease. More than 400 died from complications arising from the use of experimental antimalarial drugs. He was hanged.

According to the U.S. chief war crimes prosecutor at Nuremberg, additional "experiments" included: locking prisoners into airtight chambers and then rapidly changing the pressures to duplicate the atmospheric conditions that an aviator might encounter in falling long distances without a parachute or oxygen; infecting individuals with cholera, diphtheria, paratyphoid A and B, smallpox, typhus, and yellow fever and then testing experimental and mostly useless vaccines on them. Some inmates "were deliberately infected with typhus with the sole purpose of keeping the typhus virus alive and generally available in the bloodstream of the inmates"; injecting phenol or gasoline into the veins of prisoners, who died within 60 seconds; testing to determine how long humans could survive without water and after eating huge amounts of salt.

One of the most frightening cases of self-experimentation occurred at the headquarters of Burroughs Wellcome in 1944. British anesthesiologists had become impressed with the potential importance of curare in medicine. However, because of its lack of purity it was not practical to experiment with it. The giant British drug company independently prepared curare in pure form. Scientists at the drug company had carried out animal studies that indicated to them that the drug was safe. It was time for clinical tests on humans. The director of clinical research "perhaps foolishly" consented to be the human guinea pig.

For the experiment with curare, the director and his colleagues drew up a protocol. According to the protocol, the director was to lie on a table while his breathing rate, blood pressure, and pulse were being continually recorded. There would be a full tank of oxygen on hand. The experiment began with an injection of 10 milligrams. Although some paralysis was experienced, recovery began in approximately 15 minutes. A week later, the dose was increased to 20 milligrams. The paralysis was more widespread this time but recovery again began within 15 minutes. They were now ready for the third stage, a 30-milligram dose that was given about 2 weeks after the first.

Within 2 minutes, the muscles of his face, neck, arms, and legs were completely paralyzed. He could not speak or open his eyes. Within 3 minutes his breathing muscles were paralyzed. At this point, the director was unable to communicate with his colleagues who were otherwise occupied. When they did glance at him everything appeared fine. However, they had forgotten one thing in the protocol—a means of communication. The director could not communicate and he had the feeling he was suffocating. The back of his mouth and voice box were becoming clogged with saliva and mucus. There was nothing he could do about it. He could not move a limb, finger, or toe. He was terrified. His blood pressure and pulse rate, which had risen dramatically, showed fear, but his colleagues failed to realize how frightened he was. Once the medical team had collected the data it sought, a dose of the antidote (neostigmine) was given. But the dose was not large enough. For seven additional minutes the director received artificial respiration. Eventually his own breathing muscles took over and he was able to talk.

One of the better examples of self-experimentation is the development of Antabuse (disulfiram), a drug that is still used today to treat alcoholics. During World War II, at a Danish company called Medicinalco, it was customary practice for pharmacologists and technicians to experiment on themselves when a new drug was being tested. The employees who did so were admitted to an unpaid group that called itself the "Death Battalion." The medical research director believed that pharmacologists should test a drug on themselves before doing so on another human. Although not compensated monetarily, members of the battalion were offered a glass of port if they provided a blood sample. Members were also fêted to a yearly banquet with the presentation of awards.

One of the members of the director's research team, while reading an article about the use of disulfiram against the parasitic skin disease scabies in animals, wondered if the drug might prove useful against intestinal parasites as well. The drug was first given orally to rabbits, who showed no ill effects. Next the drug was given to rabbits who were infected with an intestinal parasite. There seemed to be some improvement. The inevitable question was, is the drug safe in humans? Just to be safe, two of the team decided to take some of the tablets themselves. Both of the scientists began taking disulfiram pills as a daily regimen while they continued their regular tasks.

At lunchtime one day, shortly after the pill experiment had begun, one of the researchers picked up the brown paper bag that contained the sandwiches his wife had made him that morning, and removed a beer from the refrigerator. By the time lunch was over he felt groggy, his head throbbed, and he felt nauseated. By the end of the day his symptoms had disappeared. The next day he ate an open-faced shrimp sandwich and coffee. Nothing happened.

During the next several weeks these symptoms would periodically reoccur. One day, the two collaborators met in the hall and, during the course of their discussion, discovered that they had been having the same symptoms. Comparing notes, they realized that the only common denominator was alcohol. Subsequent studies confirmed that the problem was caused by a drug–alcohol interaction. Eventually, disulfiram was introduced clinically as aversion therapy in alcoholics. Its mechanism of action proved to be inhibition of acetaldehyde dehydrogenase, which causes an accumulation of the toxic intermediate acetaldehyde during alcohol metabolism.

Out of the Nuremberg trials in 1947 came the Nuremberg Code, the first code to deal specifically with human experimentation. It created ethical guidelines for the conduct of medical research throughout the world. Although many researchers had customarily obtained consent from volunteers in the past, it was the Nuremberg Code that first established the practice formally. The code deals with self-experimentation in Article 5, which states: "No experiment should be conducted where there is an a priori reason to believe that death or disabling injury will occur; except, perhaps, in those experiments where the experimental physicians also serve as subjects."

Following the Nuremberg trials it was unthinkable that any such unethical human research could take place in a democratic society, much less the United States. Shockingly, in the 1960s, disclosures of glaring breaches of ethics were uncovered. Fifty unethical studies were cited, among them: deliberately withholding penicillin from 109 servicemen who suffered streptococcal infections, thereby exposing them to the risks of rheumatic fever; administering several chemicals of no benefit to patients with advanced cirrhosis to determine their effect on the liver disease; and exposing 26 normal newborn infants to extensive X-rays so their urinary bladder function could be studied.

Most of the post-World War II criticism about breaches of scientific ethics involved civilian researchers working in private institutions. However, governmental researchers came under attack in 1972 when the public learned that U.S. Public Health Service officials had withheld antibiotic therapy from a group of syphilis patients whose medical histories they had carefully followed for more than 40 years. The patients, who had acquired syphilis naturally, had been asked to volunteer for what came to be known as the "Tuskegee Study." Its aim was to observe the natural course of the infection and to further medical knowledge about the disease. In return for their cooperation, the volunteers—mostly poor and black—were to be given free medical care and free burials. Although penicillin is really only effective in curing the infection during the early stages of the disease, and most volunteers had already progressed to later stages, no volunteers were offered treatment.

[Note: With regard to writing this chapter, the author would particularly emphasize reading *The Monkey Wars* (1994) and *Who Goes First?* (1998), listed below.]

SELECTED BIBLIOGRAPHY

Altman, L. K. (1998) *Who Goes First?* Berkeley, CA: The University of California Press.

Anon. (1992) *Use of Animals in Biomedical Research—The Challenge and Response*. Chicago, IL: American Medical Association.

Balcombe, J. (2000) *The Use of Animals in Higher Education: Problems, Alternatives and Recommendations*. Washington, DC: Humane Society Press.

Beeson, P. B. (1979) The growth of knowledge about a disease: hepatitis. *Am. J. Med.*, 67: 366–370.

Blom, D. (1994) *The Monkey Wars*. New York, NY: Oxford University Press.

Fano, A. (1997) *Lethal Laws: Animal Testing, Human Health and Environmental Policy*. London: Zed Books.

Fox, M. A. (1986) *Case for Animal Experimentation—An Evolutionary and Ethical Perspective.* Los Angeles, CA: University of California Press.

General Accounting Office (1990) *FDA Drug Review: Postapproval Risks 1976–1985.* Washington, DC: GAO.

Kaufman, S. R., Czarnecki, T., Haralabatos, I. and Richardson, M. (1991) Animal models of degenerative neurological diseases. *Perspect. Med. Res.* 3: 9–48.

Kohn, A. (1986) *False Profits.* Oxford: Basil Blackwell.

LaFollette, H. and Shanks, N. (1997) *Brute Science.* New York: Routledge.

Loprieno, N. (1995) *Alternative Methodologies for the Safety Evaluation of Chemicals in the Cosmetic Industry.* Boca Raton, FL: CRC Press.

Nicoll, C. S. and Russell, S. M. (1992) Animal rights, animal research, and human obligations. *Mol. Cell. Neurosci.* 3: 271–277.

Paton, W. (1984) *Man and Mouse.* Oxford: Oxford University Press.

Rowan, A. N. (1984) *Of Mice, Models, and Men.* Albany: State University of New York Press.

Ryder, R. (1975) *Victims of Science.* London: Davis-Poynter.

Singer, P. (1977) *Animal Liberation—A New Ethics for our Treatment of Animals.* New York: Avon Books.

QUESTIONS

1 The first use of live animals for research is believed to have occurred in which century BC?
   a first
   b second
   c third
   d fourth
   e fifth.

2 Which of the following championed the value of animal experimentation and considered animals as nothing other than automatons?
   a Francis Bacon
   b Herman Goering
   c René Descartes
   d Jeremy Bentham
   e a and c.

3 The roots of antivivisection occurred in which country?
   a Belgium
   b France
   c Germany
   d Britain
   e United States.

4 Who is most responsible for rejecting the Cartesian viewpoint regarding the suffering of animals?
   a Francois Magendie
   b Claude Bernard

   c   Jeremy Bentham
   d   Peter Singer
   e   Richard Ryder.

5 Which of the following authors introduced the term "specieism" in the animal rights movement?
   a   Peter Singer
   b   Jeremy Bentham
   c   René Descartes
   d   Francis Bacon
   e   Richard Ryder.

6 Approximately how many million rodents are used yearly in biomedical research?
   a   10
   b   25
   c   40
   d   50
   e   100.

7 The "three R's" in biomedical research stand for which of the following?
   a   relief, regimentation, and restraint
   b   recurrence, restraint, and redundancy
   c   replacement, reduction, and refinement
   d   relief, refinement, and restraint
   e   replacement, relief, and recovery.

8 Which of the following has involved human self-experimentation?
   a   rabbies vaccine
   b   cholera vaccine
   c   typhoid vaccine
   d   yellow fever
   e   all of the above.

9 Which of the following performed the first heart catheterization on himself?
   a   James Carroll
   b   Walter Reed
   c   Claude Barlow
   d   Arthur Loos
   e   Joseph Forssmann.

10 Which of the following infected himself with schistosomiasis in order to transport the parasite to the United States?
   a   James Carroll
   b   Claude Barlow
   c   John Hunter
   d   Almroth Wright
   e   Edward Jenner.

Chapter 16

Alternative medicine

First the word, then the plant, lastly the knife

Asclepius of Thessaly, *circa* 1000 BC

If we arbitrarily designate the beginning of modern drug development to coincide with the synthesis of acetylsalicylic acid, then mankind has only been exposed to modern medicine for a century. During this period, a number of wonderful drugs have been developed. Most notable, perhaps, are the antibiotics during the 1930s and 1940s, and psychotropic agents during the 1950s. Antibiotics could actually cure certain infections. And, while the psychotropic drugs did not cure mental illness, their impact on mental health is almost incalculable. They permitted an end to institutionalization for tens of thousands of patients, with the attendant reduction in hospital costs and a resumption of more normalcy of life—a legacy that remains today. Despite these successes, 80 percent of the world's population still use herbs, according to the World Health Organization.

During the second half of the twentieth century the public developed a more jaundiced view of the contemporary pharmaceutical industry and its products: high prescription costs; criminal behavior by industry officials; the cozy relationship between authors of clinical research and the sponsoring agency; inadequate testing leading to the threat of unrecognized lethal toxicity; and drug–drug and drug–food interactions, to name but a few. To many, each new "breakthrough" is accompanied by a new "warning" and has turned much of the population to the admonition of Hippocrates, "Honor the healing power of nature." According to a 1998 study published in the *Journal of the American Medical Association*, people use alternative medicine not only because they are dissatisfied with conventional medicine, but because these health care alternatives mirror their own values, beliefs, and philosophical orientations toward health and life.

Alternative medicine includes (but is not limited to) the following: herbal medicine, homeopathy, aromatherapy, chiropractic, osteopathy, acupuncture, acupressure, yoga, tai chi, meditation, music or art therapy, shamanism, and faith healing. In this chapter our focus is on herbal medicine. The increased use of herbal medicine outside of the traditional physician–patient paradigm represents a search for other sources of health as well as an expression of assuming greater responsibility for our own health maintenance. In one sense, it is a return to an earlier period. The shift from "traditional medicine" to "modern medicine" can be traced to the Flexner Report of 1910.

This evaluation of medical training in the United States was highly critical of institutions of the day and resulted in the closing of 80 percent of the nation's medical schools, including "alternative" schools of homeopathy, herbology, and naturopathy.

HISTORY

As mentioned previously, in the introductory chapter of this book, interest in the treatment of disease can be found in documents as old as the existence of records. Folklore accumulated about presumed effects after the use of certain "medicines." The Ebers papyrus, written in Egypt around 1550 BC, was a compilation of some of this folklore. In India, Ayurveda (from ayur, meaning life, and veda, meaning knowledge or science), a whole conceptual system of living, is believed to have started around the same time. The codification of this system of medicine, including the concept of a formulary in which herbal remedies and recipes for them are described, was written in Sanskrit around 100 BC to AD 100 or possibly earlier. The written record of a Chinese herbal formulary comes from the Han dynasty (206 BC to AD 220).

In North America, our country's native inhabitants relied on this continent's indigenous plants for food as well as medicines. Native Americans were using Echinacea, or purple coneflower, as a remedy for everything from snakebites and spider bites to toothaches and burns long before health food stores began to offer it in convenient capsule form. In colonial America, many settlers earned all or part of their income as "sang" hunters, searching for wild ginseng in the woods. This plant's aromatic root brought "the surprising price of seven or eight ounces of silver," according to the writings of Swedish botanist Petr Kalm, who visited North America in the mid-eighteenth century. To colonists, the value of ginseng root lay in its reputation as a treatment for ailments ranging from asthma and bladder stones to infertility and wounds.

Perhaps the single most significant event impacting the sale of herbal drugs in the United States was the passage of the Dietary Supplement Health and Education Act (DSHEA) of 1994. This was an Act of Congress (Senate Bill 784, the Hatch–Harkin bill in the Senate) to amend the Federal, Food, Drug, and Cosmetic Act to establish standards with respect to dietary supplements, and for other purposes. The main components of the DSHEA are the following:

- To establish legal status for dietary supplements
- Protection from regulation as food additives or as drugs unless the product contains therapeutic claims
- Burden of proof that herbs and other supplements are unsafe now shifts to the FDA
- New ingredients introduced after October 15, 1994, must be shown to be safe by importer or manufacturer.

In the United States, herbal medicines exist in a regulatory limbo; they are sold as foods, food additives, or dietary supplements, although they are in fact used by the public as drugs. However, as long as no medicinal claims are made on the label, the

FDA does not regulate herbal products. However, manufacturers of supplements can make "statements of nutritional support" without FDA approval, as long as the statement is true and not misleading. Such statements usually describe the supplement's effect on the "structure or function" of the human body (known as "structure/function claims") or the effect on a person's "well-being."

Not surprisingly, manufacturers have taken great pains in product marketing to use statements that qualify as structure/function claims, not as health claims. This often requires linguistic agility. A manufacturer of saw palmetto, for example, cannot claim that its product "prevents prostate cancer," but can say instead that the product "helps maintain prostate function." Manufacturers must also include a disclaimer that the claim has not been evaluated by the FDA and that the product is not intended to treat, cure, or prevent any disease.

The 1994 Act further loosened oversight because now a product cannot be removed from the market until it has been proved to cause harm, and the burden of proof is on the government. Since 1994, the FDA has taken approximately 100 actions, mostly warning letters, against manufacturers that have violated labeling requirements. Following dozens of reports of adverse health effects and one death, the agency asked for a voluntary recall of gamma-butyrolactone, a supplement often promoted for body building. The agency has similarly targeted products advertised as "herbal fen-phen" because of implications that they replaced traditional pharmaceuticals. In February 2001 the FDA released a warning about the interaction of St John's wort with indinavir and other drugs used in combating HIV.

The government is currently in the process of attempting to regulate ephedrine use in pep pills and supplements. The proposal is the FDA's first regulatory major initiative under the 1994 Act. According to the FDA, more than 800 adverse reactions, including seizures, strokes, and heart attacks, have been linked to ephedrine capsules, tablets, and teas since 1994. The FDA puts the ephedrine-related death toll at 18 since then.

The 1994 deregulation has fueled the explosion of consumer interest in the herbal and vitamin industry. In 1990, only 3 percent of the nation used herbs as medicines, according to the *New England Journal of Medicine*. In 1994 it was 17 percent according to a Gallup survey. According to the American Council on Science and Health, more than 40 percent of Americans now use some kind of "alternative therapy." Data for supermarket sales of nutritional supplements since passage of the Act are also compelling (Table 16.1).

Consumer use of herbs and medicinal plant products in the United States over the past two decades has become a mainstream phenomenon. No longer relegated to health food stores, mail order houses, and multilevel marketing organizations, herbs and phytomedicines (advanced medicinal preparations made of herbs) have become one of the fastest growing segments in retail pharmacies, supermarkets, and other mass market outlets. In addition, major health insurance companies are beginning to include herbs as covered modalities of "alternative therapies" and herb products are being considered for use by some managed care organizations.

In general, consumers use herbal products as therapeutic agents for treatment and cure of diseases and pathological conditions, as prophylactic agents to prevent disease over the long term, and as protective agents to maintain health and well-being. Additionally, herbs and phytomedicinals can be used as adjunct therapy, to support

Table 16.1 Supermarket sales of nutritional supplements

Year	$ (millions)
1994	88.4
1995	106.5
1996	141.5
1997	191.0
1998	279.7

Source: ACNielsen.

conventional pharmaceutical therapies. This last use is usually found in societies where phytotherapy (the use of herbal medicines in clinical practice) is considerably more integrated with conventional medicine, as in Germany.

EUROPE AND HERBAL MEDICINE

Europeans have a longer history of herbal drug use than the United States. In contrast to other countries in Europe, herbal medicines have a special status in Germany, beginning with the Imperial Decree of 1901, which permitted the trade of many botanical drugs outside pharmacies. Therefore, most of the research has taken place in Germany. Because herbal medicines are usually not patentable, the profit margin on them is often much lower than for synthetic drugs. As a result, companies generally have not been willing to make the investment needed to meet the United States' stringent efficacy requirements for new drugs. However, thanks to the 1994 law many herbal products can be sold in the United States as dietary supplements, for which efficacy is essentially nonexistent. In an attempt to partially fill this void, the U.S. Pharmacopoeia (USP) is stepping in to award their "seal of approval" to products that contain what their label claims.

This seal does not claim that the product is safe or that it works. However, quality control of ingredients is an important issue. For example, researchers at the University of California, Los Angles (UCLA) studied 12 brands of body-building supplements and found only one contained the amount of androstenedione or related ingredients the bottle promised. One brand contained nearly double the amount listed, a potential danger, while another was pure fraud, it contained none. Far worse, one brand contained 10 milligrams of testosterone, a controlled substance that is supposed to be available by prescription only. Enter the certification program by the nonprofit USP that sets standards for many pharmaceuticals. It promises that supplements that win its seal will deliver the ingredients promised.

Herbal remedies consistently rank among the top 10 in drug sales in Germany and 80 percent of all German physicians regularly prescribe herbal medications. Herbal drug sales represent in excess of $10 billion in sales per year. Of the 10 top-selling herbs in health care stores in the United States in 1995, six were popularized largely on the basis of European research (Table 16.2).

Partial listings of alleged natural alternatives to the top five over-the-counter (OTC) and prescription drug categories are shown in Tables 16.3 and 16.4, respectively. It

Table 16.2 Best-selling herbal products in the United States

Rank	Product
1	Echinacea (9.9)
2	Garlic (9.8)
3	Goldenseal (7.0)
4	Ginseng (5.9)
5	Gingko (4.5)
6	Saw palmetto (4.4)
7	Aloe gel (4.3)
8	Ephedra (3.5)
9	Eleuthero (3.1)
10	Cranberry (3.0)

Note
Values in parentheses are percent of market share.

Table 16.3 Natural alternatives to the top five OTC drug categories

OTC drug	Natural alternative
Analgesics	Capsaicin, omega-3 fatty acids, vitamin E, pycnogenol
Antacids/antigas	Licorice root, probiotics
Cold remedies	Zinc lozenges, high-dose vitamin C
Allergy relief	Quercetin, pycnogenol, bee pollen
Laxatives	Fruits, vegetables, whole grain

Table 16.4 Natural alternatives to the top five prescription drug categories

Prescription drug	Natural alternative
Estrogen replacement	Isoflavones (soy foods), black cohosh
Antibiotics	Probiotics, garlic, Echinacea
Antidepressants	St John's wort, vitamin B1
Hypertension	Calcium, magnesium, potassium, garlic
Antiulcer (not caused by H. pylori)	Licorice root, bilberry

should be emphasized that the efficacy of these products is subject to question, and consumers are advised to carry out their own research.

Germany holds the lead in the amount of high-quality research carried out on herbal medicines. In 1978 the German Ministry of Health established Commission E, a panel of experts charged with evaluating the safety and efficacy of the herbs available in pharmacies for general use. The Commission reviewed over 300 herbal drugs. Results were published by the German Federal Health Agency (now the Federal Institute for Drugs and Medical Devices) in the form of monographs. A total of 380 monographs were published (254 approved; 126 unapproved), plus 81 revisions. These monographs provide guidelines for the general public, health practitioners, and companies applying for registration of herbal drugs. The process followed by

Commission E resulted in what has been called the most accurate information available in the entire world on the safety and efficacy of herbs and phytomedicines (see Bibliography).

Herbal remedies hold a different place in medical practice in many European countries than in the United States. One of the most dramatic examples of the difference is in the treatment of benign prostate disease. This very common condition affects about 25 percent of men in their forties and nearly 80 percent of men who are over 70. In Germany, several hundred million dollars are spent annually on prostate remedies, with 80 percent of that spent on herbal medications. Herbal medications dominate the market for treating nonmalignant prostate disease. They have very few side effects and cost per dose approximately 20 to 35 percent of what synthetic drugs do. Treatment with herbal preparations typically costs under a dollar a day. Four of the most popular in Germany are extracts from the fruit of the saw palmetto, pumpkin seeds, rye pollen extract, and nettle root.

NATIONAL CENTER FOR COMPLIMENTARY AND ALTERNATIVE MEDICINE (NCCAM)

In 1998, Congress established the NCCAM at the NIH to stimulate, develop, and support research on CAM for the benefit of the public. Prior to 1998, the NCCAM was the Office of Alternative Medicine. The NCCAM is an advocate for quality science, rigorous and relevant research, and open and objective inquiry into which CAM practices work, which do not, and why. Its overriding mission is to give the American public reliable information about the safety and effectiveness of CAM practices. The NCCAM focuses on the following efforts:

- evaluating the safety and efficacy of widely used natural products, such as herbal remedies and nutritional and food supplements (e.g., megadoses of vitamins);
- supporting pharmacological studies to determine the potential interactive effects of CAM products with standard treatment medications;
- evaluating CAM practices, such as acupuncture and chiropractic.

How has deregulation worked? A meta-analysis of the herb St John's wort (*Hypericum perforatum*) for mild and moderately severe depression, published in 1996 by German and American physicians, concluded that it was more effective than a placebo and was as effective as standard antidepressants but with fewer side effects. However, the authors of the analysis raised questions about the methods employed and cautioned about its efficacy in seriously depressed patients. The active chemical in the herb, they claimed, was not appropriately standardized. Furthermore, the study only compared St John's wort with antidepressant drugs that were given at or below their lowest level of efficacy. And, finally, patients were treated for only 6 weeks. An accompanying editorial concluded that "longer term studies are needed before it can be recommended in major depression."

The above report eventually led to the NIH's Office of Alternative Medicine (now NCCAM) to call for a trial comparing St John's wort with the popular antidepressant Prozac. NCCAM, the National Institute of Mental Health, and the Office of

Dietary Supplements are collaborating on a study to evaluate the efficacy and safety of standardized extract of *Hypericum* in major depression.

The NCCAM is also supporting research studies on kava. However, these have been put on hold because the FDA is investigating whether the use of dietary supplements containing kava (also known as kava kava or *Piper methylsticum*) pose a health risk. The FDA's $9 million supplement division investigates problems and tries to curb use of products it can prove dangerous. Kava is a member of the pepper family. Products containing kava are sold in the United States for a variety of uses including insomnia and short-term reduction of stress and anxiety.

Recent reports from European health authorities have linked kava to at least 25 cases of liver toxicity, including hepatitis, cirrhosis, and liver failure. The FDA is currently (2002) investigating the health risks of the herbal supplement. Under review are 38 Americans, including a liver transplant recipient, with medical problems associated with kava use. As of February 2002, sales have been halted in Switzerland and are suspended in Britain, Germany is acting to make kava a prescription product and the FDA recommends avoiding kava until safety questions are answered.

It may also be of interest to the reader to know that the "War on Drugs" has come to health food stores. As of February 6, 2002, U.S. grocery stores are no longer permitted to carry any food product containing hemp. They are subject to confiscation by the Drug Enforcement Administration (DEA). The problem with hemp is that it can contain less than 1 percent of tetrahydrocannabinol (THC). According to the DEA there is no allowable limit of THC in the United States. Unless the manufacturer can provide scientific evidence that their product contains absolutely no trace of THC, it has to go. As a result, frozen waffles, cookies, cereals, salad dressings, tortilla chips, and even ice cream have been removed from the shelves. Once again, we are protected from ourselves.

VITAMINS

Vitamins were first called *accessory factors* in 1906 when it was demonstrated that normal foods contain, in addition to the nutrients then recognized—carbohydrates, proteins, fats, minerals, and water—minute traces of other substances essential to health. The curative effects of diet on scurvy, rickets, beriberi, night blindness, etc., had been observed and speculated upon for centuries. In 1911 the antiberiberi factor that was isolated from rice polishings was believed to contain an amine and, hence, the term accessory factors was changed to vitamines to emphasize the fact that the factors are essential to life and not merely accessory to other nutrients. Eventually, the term vitamine was replaced by vitamin when it was found that vitamin A lacks an amine group. Originally, successive letters of the alphabet were assigned to new vitamins as they were characterized and isolated, although some letters were assigned out of order; vitamin K, for example, refers to the Scandinavian word *Koagulation*. The recent trend has been towards chemical names; vitamin B_1 has become thiamine; B_2, riboflavin, and so on.

Perhaps the most controversial aspects of vitamins is whether we need to take them and, if so, at what dose? Tables 16.5 and 16.6 show the recommended daily allowances (RDAs) for fat- and water-soluble vitamins, respectively.

Table 16.5 Comparison of RDAs for fat-soluble vitamins

Category	Vitamin A (µg RE)	Vitamin D (µg)	Vitamin E (mg TE)	Vitamin K (µg)
Infants	375	10	4	10
Children	400–700	10	6–7	15–30
Males	1000	10	10	45–80
Females	800	10	8	45–65
Pregnant	800	10	10	65

Source: The Food and Nutrition Board, National Academy of Sciences, National Research Council, Recommended Dietary Allowances (Revised 1989).

Table 16.6 Comparison of RDAs for water-soluble vitamins

Category	Vitamin C (mg)	Thiamin (mg)	Riboflavin (mg)	Niacin (mg NE)	B6 (mg)	B12 (µg)
Infants	30–35	0.3–0.4	0.4–0.5	5–6	0.3–0.6	0.3–0.5
Children	40–45	0.7–1.0	0.8–1.2	9–13	1.0–1.4	0.7–1.4
Males	50–60	1.2–1.5	1.4–1.8	15–20	1.7–2.0	2.0
Females	50–60	1.0–1.1	1.2–1.3	13–15	1.4–1.6	2.0
Pregnant	70	1.5	1.6	17	2.2	2.0

Source: The Food and Nutrition Board, National Academy of Sciences, National Research Council, Recommended Dietary Allowances (Revised 1989).

Opponents of emphasizing RDAs point out that these numbers are for an average person, whatever that is. And, furthermore, these numbers may be outdated and are really relevant only to avoiding deficiency states. They do not allow for the possibility of enhanced or optimal nutritional states from doses above those necessary merely to protect against scurvy, beriberi, or rickets. Vitamin C is the classic example, having gained notoriety from Linus Pauling. Dr Pauling advocated megadoses (many grams per day) for the amelioration of the common cold.

Some nutritionists believe that the processing of modern foods has left us with a less wholesome diet deficient in many vitamins and minerals (refined sugar, refined flour, and fried foods). Therefore, in order to regain the nutrients removed in these processes, it makes sense to supplement our diets with relatively high doses of vitamins and minerals. Fortunately, these are among the most nontoxic OTC products available.

SELECTED BIBLIOGRAPHY

Bisset, N. G. (ed.) (1994) *Herbal Drugs and Phytopharmaceuticals*. Boca Raton, FL: CRC Press.
Blumenthal, M., Busse, W. R., Goldberg, A., Gruenwald, J., Hall, T., Riggins, C. W. and Rister, R. S. (eds) (1998) *The Complete German Commission E Monographs: Therapeutic Guide to Herbal Medicines*. Austin, TX: American Botanical Council.
Duke, J. A. (1997) *The Green Pharmacy*. Emmaus, PA: Rodale Press.
Foster, S. (1996) *Herbs for Your Health*. Loveland, CO: Interweave Press.

Mowrey, D. B. (1986) *The Scientific Validation of Herbal Medicine*. New Canaan, CN: Keats Publishing, Inc.

Spreen, A. N. (1999) *Nutritionally Incorrect: Why the American Diet is Dangerous and How to Defend Yourself*. Pleasant Grove, UT: Woodland Publishing.

Stary, F. (1996) *The Natural Guide to Medicinal Herbs and Plants*. New York, NY: Barnes and Noble.

QUESTIONS

1 Alternative medicine includes which of the following?
  a   aromatherapy
  b   yoga
  c   chiropractic
  d   herbal medicine
  e   all of the above.

2 The transition from traditional medical training to modern medicine is believed to have occurred in which year?
  a   1906
  b   1910
  c   1919
  d   1921
  e   1933.

3 Perhaps the single most significant event impacting on the sale of herbal drugs in the United States was which of the following?
  a   encouragement from Timothy Leary
  b   the "pop" culture of the 1960s
  c   the thalidomide tragedy
  d   passage of the 1962 law requiring prescription drugs to prove efficacy
  e   passage of the Dietary Supplement Act of 1994.

4 Supermarket sales of nutritional supplements now exceed how many millions of dollars yearly?
  a   275
  b   500
  c   750
  d   800
  e   900.

5 Which of the following countries has had the greatest impact on herbal medicine?
  a   Spain
  b   United States
  c   Germany
  d   France
  e   Slovakia.

6 Commision E is/are which of the following?
   a   a German panel of herbal experts
   b   a British panel of herbal experts
   c   a U.S. panel of experts specializing in vitamin E
   d   all of the above
   e   none of the above.

7 Which of the following has/have been linked to significant toxicity in the United States and/or Europe?
   a   kava kava
   b   vitamin C
   c   ephedrine
   d   all of the above
   e   a and c.

8 Which of the following is/are true regarding vitamins?
   a   many are lost during the processing of certain foods
   b   some are used to treat certain sicknesses in megadoses
   c   both water- and fat-soluble vitamins are important
   d   deficiency syndromes lead to the discovery of many
   e   all of the above.

9 Which of the following is/are true of vitamins?
   a   all contain an amine group
   b   all are water soluble
   c   in general they have low toxicity
   d   Recommended Daily Allowance is a highly accurate expression
   e   all of the above.

10 Which of the following was first called "accessory factor(s)"?
   a   herbal drugs
   b   St John's wort
   c   vitamins
   d   a and c
   e   all of the above.

The history of drug abuse laws in the United States

> Sixty percent of most of our violent crimes are associated with alcohol or drug use. Many times they're robbing, stealing, and all of these things to get money to buy drugs, and I do feel that we would markedly reduce our crime rate if drugs were legalized. But I don't know the ramifications of this and I do feel that we need to do some studies. In some countries that have legalized drugs, and made it legal, they certainly have shown that there has been a reduction in their crime rate, and there has been no increase in their drug use rate.
>
> Surgeon General, Dr Joycelyn Elders, National Press Club, December 7, 1993

The political repercussions of that unexpected statement were not fully appreciated by Dr Elders at the time. However, on December 9, 1994, following the Republican Party's conservative-mediated victory at the polls, Dr Elders was fired by President Clinton, ostensibly for her views on sex education, but it was undoubtedly the controversial issue of drug legalization that began her political descent.

Despite the sensational headlines that followed Elders' comments, it should be remembered that there was a time, not so long ago, when many of the drugs against which we now wage an approximately $20 billion a year "war" were perfectly legal to use. At the turn of the century, for example, opium, morphine, heroin, cocaine, and marijuana were all either legal in the United States or subject to few restrictions. They were all present in patent medicines that were nonprescription drugs of secret composition. It has been estimated that millions of people were what we would today call "occasional" users at that time. The factors that have contributed to the evolution of extremely restrictive contemporary American drug laws have largely resulted from common problems, real or imagined, associated with nineteenth-century use of opiates (opium, morphine, and to some extent heroin) and cocaine, and the twentieth-century use of marijuana.

OPIUM (NINETEENTH CENTURY)

Although fines and public whippings were imposed for alcohol abuse as early as 1645 in New England, opium probably has the oldest history of use in this country among drugs usually considered illicit. Opium was available in America before 1800 in crude extracts with or without alcohol. One of the first written reports of opium use in the United States appeared in 1842, entitled "An opium-eater in America," a form of drug "confession" often mimicked by subsequent drug literature. This popularizing of a European fashion by Englishman Thomas De Quincey (the Timothy Leary of the 1840s) coincided with the introduction of legislation in the same year imposing a tariff upon the importation of crude opium into this country. Although the tariff legislation acknowledged, to some extent, a developing opium problem, it was designed as a tax, not a prohibition.

For a number of reasons (discussed later), the per capita, yearly consumption of crude opium continued to rise during the remainder of the century, reaching its peak in 1896 at a level of approximately 3.1 grams. In addition, the importation of opium for smoking was also substantial and opium dens were popular. Growing publicity at the turn of the century disclosing the contents of patent medicines, early state regulatory laws, and public opinion regarding opium smoking led to the importation of opium ultimately being prohibited in 1909 by the Opium Exclusion Act. Although domestic commercial sources of opium were never developed to any great extent in the United States, opium poppies were, in fact, legally grown in the United States until 1942 when the Opium Poppy Act was passed.

"Opium eating" was the phrase generally used throughout the latter half of the nineteenth century that actually referred to laudanum drinking. Laudanum (from the Latin, "something to be praised") of this period often contained "2 ounces of strained opium, 1 ounce of saffron, and a dram of cinnamon and cloves dissolved in 1 pint of Canary wine" and was the recipe of a seventeenth-century English physician, Thomas Sydenham. A dose of this concoction produced "a panacea . . . for all human woes, . . . equipoise to all the faculties" and could be ordered by mail from Sears, Roebuck, for $4 a pint. It has been estimated that no less than 1 percent of the population was addicted to opium at the time.

Opium also has a place in literature. Lewis Caroll, for example, made allusions to opium in his book *Through the Looking Glass*. During her journey, Alice found a small unlabeled bottle that she drank, knowing that something interesting was going to happen; it did. She subsequently met a large blue caterpillar sitting with its arms folded on a large mushroom quietly smoking a long *hookah* (opium pipe). Caroll is one of numerous nineteenth-century authors and notables who have been identified as chronic users of opium.

The importation of Chinese workers following the Civil War is generally associated with the introduction of smoking opium to Western Americans. Its practice spread widely among respectable young men and women, many of whom "were ruined morally and otherwise." Ironically, in 1875, the city of San Francisco, which today we associate with a liberal view toward drug use, enacted the first antidrug ordinance in the United States, forbidding opium smoking in opium houses or dens. This was soon followed by similar laws in New York City (1882) and the state of Ohio (1885). In addition to opium's alleged effect on the morals of the United States, Samuel Gompers, the industrial magnate, believed that its use by Chinese immigrants increased their productivity so substantially that whites were at a disadvantage in the labor market. As opium dens became less accessible, poorer addicts were forced to seek less expensive alternatives such as morphine, and later its derivative, heroin.

MORPHINE (NINETEENTH CENTURY)

Morphine is the most active component of crude opium (making up approximately 9 percent) and was first isolated in pure form in 1806 by a German pharmacist's assistant, Frederich Sertürner. It is easy to visualize the self-testing of morphine by Sertürner, which he did frequently, nearly dying of an overdose at one point, obliging him to name the substance after Morpheus, the god of dreams. The development of morphine use in the United States proceeded slowly over the next half-century, although both its medicinal and psychogenic properties were noted. However, with the general availability of the hypodermic syringe in the 1850s and its use in administering morphine during the American Civil War, a new form of addiction was created.

Pennsylvania, the home of morphine manufacturers of the day (Rosengarten and Company of Philadelphia—later merged into Merck, Sharpe and Dohme), enacted an antimorphine law as early as 1860, thus anticipating the start of the Civil War by 1 year. Morphine was used regularly, and probably indiscriminately, in large doses to treat many soldiers for the reduction of pain and relief from dysentery. As a consequence, a high proportion of men became addicted to morphine ("soldier's disease"). Despite the lessons learned during the Civil War, by the turn of the century morphine addiction was still quite prevalent. This fact was, in large part, due to questionable medical advocacy, such as "Advantages of Substituting the Morphia Habit for the Incurably Alcoholic," as well as being available OTC for 25 cents a day to sustain an addiction.

In 1874, C. R. Wright, of St Mary's Hospital in London, carried out a series of experiments that would have far-reaching repercussions in the twentieth century. Dr Wright prepared a series of acetylated derivatives of morphine. One of these (diacetylmorphine) was found to be three times as potent as morphine. It was given the brand name Heroin (from the German for "great" or "heroic") and placed on the market in the late 1890s by Bayer Laboratories. It was originally marketed in low doses to treat patients with tuberculosis, relieve cough, and induce sleep. It was considered a nonaddicting substance and viewed as having only minor problems with tolerance and addiction. Subsequent experience demonstrated quite dramatically, however, that heroin is, in fact, quite addicting when injected in higher doses and it was withdrawn from the market. Today, because of its potency, heroin has displaced both its forebears, opium and morphine, as the opiate of choice for illicit use.

COCAINE (LATTER HALF OF THE NINETEENTH CENTURY)

While opium and morphine were developing their own following into the second half of the nineteenth century, a new player was about to arrive on the scene. Although the chewing of coca leaves had been practiced for thousands of years in South America, it was not until 1859 that the purification of cocaine, the active ingredient, was achieved. The availability of pure cocaine allowed the creation of many innovative mixtures by patent medicine makers of the day. One of the most popular preparations that found favor in the United States during the 1870s and 1880s was imported coca-containing wines from Europe (a variation on Dr Sydenham's opium in Canary wine). The most famous wine of this type was manufactured by Angelo Mariani (Vin Mariani) and contained 6 mg of cocaine per ounce. These coca wines were used "for fatigue of mind and body" and sample bottles were often "free to medical men and clergymen on receipt of professional card."

Notables of that era who were said to be fond of Mr Mariani's coca wine included Queen Victoria, Sarah Bernhardt, Thomas Edison, Robert Louis Stevenson, Jules Verne, Alexander Dumas, and Pope Leo XIII—probably much the same people who indulged in opium. Robert Louis Stevenson, in fact, is believed to have used cocaine as the inspiration for the unnamed drug in *The Strange Case of Dr Jekyll and Mr Hyde*. Not all literary references to cocaine portrayed it in such a horrific light, however. Sir Arthur Conan Doyle's Sherlock Holmes realized that cocaine's influence was bad but could not resist its stimulating properties, as illustrated in the following excerpt from *The Sign of Four* (1890) as described by Dr Watson.

Sherlock Holmes took his bottle from the corner of the mantelpiece, and his hypodermic syringe from its neat morocco case. With his long, white, nervous fingers he adjusted the delicate needle and rolled back his left shirtcuff. For some little time his eyes rested thoughtfully upon the sinewy forearm and wrist, all dotted and scarred with innumerable puncture-marks. Finally, he thrust the sharp point home, pressed down the tiny piston, and sank back into the velvet-lined armchair with a long sigh of satisfaction.

Three times a day for many months I had witnessed this performance, but custom had not reconciled my mind to it . . .

"Which is it today," I asked, "Morphine or cocaine?"

He raised his eyes languidly from the old black-letter volume which he had opened.

"It is cocaine," he said, "a seven-per-cent solution. Would you care to try it?"

"No indeed," I answered brusquely. "My constitution has not got over the Afghan campaign yet. I cannot afford to throw any extra strain upon it."

He smiled at my vehemence. "Perhaps you are right, Watson," he said. "I suppose that its influence is physically a bad one. I find it, however, so transcendingly stimulating and clarifying to the mind that its secondary action is a matter of small moment."

"But consider!" I said earnestly. "Count the cost! Your brain may, as you say, be roused and excited, but it is a pathological and morbid process which involves increased tissue-change and may at least leave a permanent weakness. You know, too, what a black reaction comes upon you. Surely the game is hardly worth the candle. Why should you, for a mere passing pleasure, risk the loss of those great powers with which you have been endowed? Remember that I speak not only as one comrade to another but as a medical man to one whose constitution he is to some extent answerable."

He did not seem offended. On the contrary, he put his finger-tips together, and leaned his elbows on the arms of his chair, like someone who has a relish for conversation.

"My mind," he said, "rebels at stagnation. Give me problems, give me work, give me the most abstruse cryptogram, or the most intricate analysis, and I am in my own proper atmosphere. I can dispense then with artificial stimulants. But I abhor the dull routine of existence. I crave for mental exaltation."

During the latter decades of the 1800s, members of the medical community believed that cocaine, like opium and morphine before, was a new wonder drug. One of its original supporters was Sigmund Freud who asserted that "there is no danger of general damage to the body as is the case with the chronic use of morphine." Freud was later to repudiate that viewpoint. Early medical uses for cocaine included use as a local anesthetic (its most significant use), an antidepressant, and to relieve withdrawal symptoms of morphine addicts. It was also included in numerous tonics, elixirs, and patent medicines.

Parke-Davis and Company was among the first U.S. pharmaceutical companies to market extracts of cocaine in the early 1880s. These preparations were used by physicians for a wide variety of ailments including the "painless cure of opium and liquor habits" and provided the official remedy of the Hay Fever Association. Parke-Davis also appreciated the advantages of smoking cocaine by selling coca-leaf cigarettes and coca cheroots. Purveyors of patent medicines were also quick to jump on the bandwagon. Despite attempts by state regulations to curb cocaine abuse (Illinois enacted a law against cocaine sale without a prescription in 1897), patent medicine manufacturers were frequently able to obtain exemptions. In general, local laws were "chaotic," varied in severity, were difficult to enforce, and had little effect on the sale of drugs and patent medicines across state lines. In some drug stores, one could purchase a dime's or quarter's worth of cocaine or morphine.

One particular patent drug manufacturer of note at the end of the eighteenth century was John Styth Pemberton of Atlanta, Georgia. Unfortunately, Mr Pemberton's "French Wine Cola" version did not prove to be a successful competitor against Vin Mariani. However, he reformulated the cocaine with caffeine and named it "Coca-Cola," and the rest is history. Cocaine was present as an ingredient in Coca-Cola until 1903. In retrospect, it is fortunate that the cocaine content of patent medicine formulations containing alcohol was relatively modest. Today we know that when alcohol and cocaine are combined in the body, a new compound can be formed (cocaethylene) that is believed to contribute to cocaine's psychological and toxicological effects.

PURE FOOD AND DRUG ACT (1906)

By the beginning of the twentieth century, Americans had developed the facility to become addicted to drugs via swallowing, smoking, injecting, and snorting. Patent medicines had the broadest impact on drug use during the preceding 50 years due to their widespread distribution, extravagant claims, and popularity. Sales of patent medicines increased from $3.5 million in 1859 to $74 million in 1904. This increase in drug use occurred during a period of laissez-faire capitalism when the formulation, distribution, sales, and claims of many consumer products were not regulated. However, this open market was soon to change.

By the early 1900s, there was considerable governmental concern regarding the purity of not only drugs but food as well, the meat packing industry having performed just as irresponsibly as the makers of patent medicines during this era. The question of food and drug impurities received nationwide press coverage in books and periodicals and led President Theodore Roosevelt to recommend in 1905 "that a law be enacted to regulate interstate commerce in misbranded and adulterated foods, drinks, and drugs." Following relatively rapid congressional hearings, the Pure Food and Drugs Act was passed on June 30, 1906, providing an important stepping stone toward the eventual creation of the Food and Drug Administration (FDA). The government then had the responsibility for assessing drug hazards, prohibiting the sale of dangerous drugs, and requiring drug manufacturers to report adverse reactions associated with their products. It has been estimated that within a few years of the inclusion of these labeling changes, the sale of patent medicines containing a narcotic decreased by one-third.

The Pure Food and Drugs Act and its 1912 Sherley Amendment dealing with false and misleading advertising were primarily truth-in-labeling acts, and were not intended to criminalize the purchase and use of patent medicines, regardless of their content. The government, at that time, was principally concerned that the consumer be made aware of the possible presence of alcohol, morphine, opium, cocaine, heroin, and marijuana in what they were buying and to what extent. It was hoped that with this information the consumer would be more educated in assessing risk when consuming the patent medicines.

SHANGHAI OPIUM COMMISSION (1909)

In addition to the issues of purity and the advertising of its foods and drugs, early twentieth-century America, as well as other parts of the world, found itself with a drug dependency problem. The exact extent of the problem at that time is difficult to ascertain since estimates of the number of addicts range from 250,000 to 1,000,000, and more, in a population of approximately 76 million. Regardless of the number of addicts, between 1898 and 1902, while the population increased by only 10 percent, importation of cocaine rose 40 percent, opium 500 percent, and morphine 600 percent. By 1900, restrictive drug laws at the state level had been enacted, and reformers began to look to the federal government for effective national regulation.

In response to the apparent growing problem of domestic narcotic drug abuse, as well as attempting to assist China with its own international opium struggle, the United States organized the first international meeting in 1909 to consider international opium traffic (the Shanghai Opium Commission). Thirteen nations from the Far East, or who had possessions therein, were represented (the United States, Germany, Great Britain, the Netherlands, Portugal, Italy, France, Russia, Siam, Japan, Persia, China, and Austria-Hungary).

Most of the participants did not share the United State's zeal for prohibiting the nonmedical use of opium, since they had a vested interest in protecting their profits from this commodity. Britain, for example, feared that the suspension of the Indian opium trade would lead to an unbalanced budget. However, the attitude of the U.S. delegates at the meeting was that a worldwide prohibition of habit-forming drugs needed to be enacted. Despite the lack of enthusiasm by most of the participants, the commission did resolve that each country should take drastic internal measures to control morphine and other opium derivatives. With this admonition, the United States thus obtained a moral imprimatur to pursue strict federal legislation to compensate for the consistent failure of state and local laws.

Although the resolutions recommended by the Shanghai Commission were reassuring to U.S. interests, the United States still felt that more formal international commitments were desired. An early American proposal for a post-Shanghai conference was, however, not accepted as a commission resolution and, nearly 3 years would pass before the desired meeting finally took place. During this interval, attempts to enact exemplary domestic legislation were made in the United States for several reasons. First, many other nations already had more stringent legislation than the United States, and, second, the United States had, in fact, accepted an obligation to enact federal narcotic control at the Shanghai Commission. The most significant early attempt to establish significant narcotic control in the United States was the Foster Bill (the antecedent of the Harrison Act). This proposal contained sweeping regulations on narcotic use, but did not obtain the necessary congressional support to be enacted.

INTERNATIONAL OPIUM CONFERENCE (1911)

Despite delays by Germany, Great Britain, and the Netherlands, the United States succeeded in convening the first International Opium Conference on December 1, 1911, in The Hague. Twelve of the nations in attendance in Shanghai were represented (Austria-Hungary chose not to attend). The discussions were once again motivated by national interests, resulting in the convention ultimately placing the major burden of worldwide narcotic control on domestic legislation within each country itself. A mechanism was developed, however, for the signature and ratification of the convention by participants and "significant" nonparticipants alike. Although 44 nations signed, less than half of these ratified it and only seven nations implemented it within 5 years. Ratification by the U.S. Senate was officially deposited in The Hague on December 10, 1913; however, its own domestic bill was deadlocked in the Senate at that time.

HARRISON NARCOTIC ACT (1914)

Following the Hague Convention, it was imperative that the United States impress other signatories with the seriousness of its intent by passing its own domestic drug legislation. A bill had been introduced in 1912, primarily the creation of Dr Hamilton Wright (the "father of American drug laws"), who had been a representative at both the Shanghai Commission and the Hague Convention and had authored the previously defeated Foster Bill. Dr Wright's scientific claim to fame had been "proving" that beriberi (a thiamine deficiency) was a communicable disease.

Representative Francis Burton Harrison of New York introduced the new bill to Congress. This original Harrison Bill was basically designed to eliminate narcotic use except for medical purposes. On the face of it, it was a simple licensing law that simply required sellers to get a license if they were going to handle opiates and cocaine.

For various reasons, groups such as the American Association of Pharmaceutical Chemists, the National Association of Medicinal Products, and the National Association of Druggists had opposed the bill in its initial form and lobbied actively for a number of modifications resulting in submission of a "final" form in 1913. Following considerable debate between House and Senate committees over proposed amendments, the Harrison Narcotics Act was passed on December 14, 1914, and went into effect March 1, 1915. Enforcement was assigned to the Bureau of Internal Revenue within the Treasury Department.

The principal features of the enacted bill required record keeping by pharmacists and physicians, registration with the Treasury Department of anyone (physicians, dentists, or veterinarians) dealing with narcotics, except the consumer, and the yearly purchase of a $1 tax stamp by retail dealers and practicing physicians. Patent medicines containing small amounts of morphine, cocaine, opium, and heroin (chloral hydrate and cannabis were omitted) could continue to be sold by mail order or by retail dealers.

The purpose of the Act was to regulate the use of narcotics for "legitimate medical purposes." However, as a consequence, it became illegal to possess narcotics without a prescription. Eventually, in the 1920s it became illegal for addicts to obtain these drugs even from physicians. The main architect of the legislation, Dr Wright, was ironically not in government service at the time of its passage, having been summarily dismissed in June 1914 by Secretary of State Bryan for failing to take a pledge of abstinence from alcohol.

Since addiction was not considered a legitimate disease meriting a prescription for narcotics (the medical community itself was split), an increasing number of people subsequently resorted to criminal activity to obtain their drugs; the cost of heroin on the streets rose from $6.50/ounce to approximately $100. The increase in crime validated the Treasury Department's fear that deprived addicts would threaten the public order. Although passage of the Harrison Act did increase the price of street narcotics, it also resulted in a reduction of patent medicine narcotics as well as a decline in addiction rates.

By ignoring the physiological fact of addiction, American drug policy rejected the earlier experiences of clinics in Florida and Tennessee dealing with addict maintenance (which were available during the Harrison debate) and contributed in its own way to increased urban crime, escalation in the size of police agencies, and a diminution in civil liberties. Following a number of lower court decisions dealing with loopholes, the Supreme Court subsequently authenticated the constitutionality of the Harrison Act on March 3, 1919. In a five to four decision the court determined that maintenance of an addiction per se was illegal and that such use was a perversion of the meaning of the act such "that no discussion of the subject is required."

PROHIBITION (1919–1933)

Narcotics were, of course, not the only drugs of concern during the immediate post World War I era. If the use of narcotics could not be justified, then how could that of alcohol? The temperance movement, which had been active for years, now succeeded in having the use and distribution of alcohol banned. The Eighteenth Amendment

(National Prohibition), also known as the Volstead Act, was ratified on January 29, 1919, and became law on January 16, 1920. Immediately prior to ratification of the Prohibition Act, a Prohibition Unit was established on December 22, 1919. The Prohibition Unit was composed of Narcotic and Alcohol Divisions. An interesting question has been asked: "Why did the Supreme Court agree that a federal statute could outlaw narcotics, when the Constitution itself had to be amended to outlaw alcohol?"

The strength of the temperance movement in overcoming economic realities of the day is illustrated by the effect the Eightieth Amendment had on the collection of fees by the Internal Revenue Service (IRS). In 1916, gross receipts at the IRS were $513 million, of which $241 million were derived from distilled spirits and fermented liquors. Thus, 47 percent of IRS receipts were from alcohol-related income versus 13 percent from personal income tax. The movement's fervor also affected the medical profession. With the cynical belief that physicians would discharge their responsibilities under prohibition no better than they had under the Harrison Act, new legislation was created. The specific law, the Willis–Campbell Act of 1921, was enacted in order to restrict the number of liquor prescriptions permitted by each physician.

The Eightieth Amendment never, of course, achieved the same level of public support as the Harrison Act. This lack of public support forced its repeal on December 5, 1933. With the repeal of federal prohibition, the states assumed responsibility to regulate the distribution and sale of alcohol. In most states these regulatory units are referred to as alcoholic beverage control (ABC) agencies. They control the manufacture, distribution, and sale of alcoholic beverages. Vendors are required to obtain licenses from the ABC. In 1991, there were over 500,000 retail licenses issued nationally. In 39 states local communities regulate where and when alcohol can be sold. Although the National Minimum Drinking Age Act of 1984 required all states to raise their minimum alcohol purchase and possession age to 21, many state laws contain numerous loopholes.

POST HARRISON ACT (1920–1929)

During the 1920s, enforcement of prohibition of alcohol surpassed that of narcotics by the Harrison Act. However, despite disparate resources, the smaller Narcotic Division successfully closed 44 opiate-dispensing clinics by 1923. This hard-line attitude reflected the prevailing public mood of the day that narcotic maintenance served only to contribute to or create a menacing personality. Not much has changed in contemporary society.

The Harrison Narcotic Act, as enforced by the Narcotic Division of the Prohibition Unit, had, therefore, become the first significant drug policy in this country emphasizing a prohibitionist perspective while denying the concept of addiction as a disease. However, the prospect of a nation with 1 million narcotic addicts (contemporary estimates) in withdrawal was a sobering thought for the government. Therefore, a temporary supply of drugs was discretely provided at carefully selected clinics. Fortunately, the number of addicts estimated at the time appears to have been exaggerated. In New York City, for example, only 7500 addicts had been registered in city clinics before they were closed in early 1920. Previous estimates for the city had been in the 100,000 to 200,000 range. Nevertheless, critics alleged that narcotic clinics did nothing more than provide a destabilizing influence by sanctioning the indefinite maintenance of addiction.

Although the Narcotic Division was considerably smaller than the Alcohol Division of the Prohibition Unit, it was quite effective. By the end of 1923, the population of addicts in the New York state penitentiary at Sing Sing had risen from 1 to 9 percent. By mid-1928 one-third of all male and female inmates in federal prisons were there by virtue of violating the Harrison Act. Of the violators in federal prison, the majority were addicts and, therefore, presented a medical condition to wardens who did not wish to care for addicts. As a result of this situation, the Porter Narcotic Farm (as the facilities were originally known) bill was enacted on January 19, 1929, establishing the Lexington farm (opened in 1935) and the Fort Worth farm (opened in 1938). These hospitals, as they were eventually referred to, were institutions that provided additional prison space (complete with iron bars) and segregation of the addicts from the general prison population. It was not until the late 1960s that the bars were removed from the Lexington facility and the cells converted into rooms.

FEDERAL MARIJUANA TAX ACT (1930–1937)

In 1930 the Narcotics Division became a separate entity (Federal Bureau of Narcotics, FBN) within the Treasury Department. Harry J. Anslinger, then Assistant Commissioner of the Prohibition Bureau, became Acting Commissioner of Narcotics on July 1 and was appointed Commissioner on September 25 (a position he held for 32 years). Anslinger was free of any of the prior scandal associated with the Alcohol Division (during prohibition) and was considered to have desirable diplomatic skills developed during his years in the foreign service. He had, however, only sporadic experience with narcotics control. Anslinger's tenure in office was characterized by his belief that the most effective strategy of achieving public compliance with a law regulating a dangerous drug was a policy of harsh fines and severe mandatory prison sentences for first convictions. Anslinger had developed these proposals in the context of enforcing the Volstead Act (prohibition) but would refine them during the mid-1930s, with President Roosevelt's endorsement, in his attempt to enforce marijuana regulations.

The history of marijuana in the United States is not clear. However, it appears that hemp, hashish, and smokable marijuana were discovered at different times and were used in different contexts. The pilgrims, for example, brought hemp with them to Jamestown in 1611 and cultivated it for its fiber. The cultivation of hemp became so economically important that during the 1700s some states imposed penalties on those who did not produce it. In 1764 King George III offered American colonists a bounty of 8 pounds sterling for every bale of raw hemp delivered to London, to which Ben Franklin's reply was, "We have not yet enough for our own consumption." In 1788 the Viceroy of Mexico ordered the mission at Monterey to plant hemp, thus starting hemp cultivation in California. The hemp industry remained important up to the Civil War. Following the war, production declined as cheaper imported hemp became available and cotton and wool became less expensive alternatives.

Marijuana was first mentioned as a medicine in an American medical text in 1843 and in 1854 was listed in the U.S. Dispensatory. The latter year also marked the first written description by Bayard Taylor in *The Atlantic Monthly* of cannabis intoxication. In the 1850s, recommended medical uses for marijuana included the treatment of gout, rheumatism, tetanus, opiate and alcohol withdrawal, loss of appetite, dysmenorrhea, convulsions, depression, insanity, and asthma. Although its suggested uses were widespread, marijuana never actually achieved popular use in the medical community. The reasons for this include variations in potency of commercial preparations, variability in patients responses, slow onset of oral action, and lack of solubility preventing administration by injection. However, the drug was included in many patent medicine preparations and was officially recognized as a medicine in the *U.S. Pharmacopoeia* until 1937. In 1937 there were 28 pharmaceuticals that contained cannabis.

By 1906, the Pure Food and Drug Act required that the quantity of cannabis be clearly indicated on the label of any drug or food sold to the public. However, cannabis routinely escaped federal regulations including the Harrison Act. It was generally utilized in benign medical situations and its use was not considered a significant problem. For example, in 1894 the Indian Hemp Commission, appointed by the British Parliament, concluded that moderate use of cannabis was not injurious to the majority of users. In fact, cannabis was defended by the National Wholesale Druggists' Association and a pharmaceutical company (Lehn and Fink) during Congressional hearings in 1911 on a federal antinarcotic law. Testimony by their respective representatives described cannabis as not being habit-forming and without attraction to narcotic addicts as an alternative. Conflicting testimony was provided by Charles B. Towns, dedicated anti-addiction crusader and formulator of Towns' cure for addiction (1 part fluid extract of prickly ash bark, 1 part fluid extract of hyoscyamus, and 2 parts 15 percent tincture of belladonna; a tincture by definition contains alcohol).

Despite early passive views on cannabis use in the United States, however, a gradual accumulation of momentum in opposition to marijuana developed after World War I. Much of the antipathy was based on cultural fears relating to cannabis use by Syrians in New York, East Indians in California and, principally, Mexicans in the Southwest. Much of the pressure for federal legislation regulating marijuana arose not from the FBN but from local law enforcement agencies in the South and Southwest who saw it as a link to violent crime presumably committed by Mexican immigrants.

In response to the international aspect of marijuana's intrusion into the country, the United States succeeded at the Second Geneva Convention in 1925 in obtaining an agreement that international traffic in cannabis should be regulated. Although domestic fear of marijuana was minimal during the 1920s, the federal government's view was different. For example, in 1929 habitual cannabis users were deemed eligible for treatment in the newly approved narcotic "farms."

Continuing bad press occurred during the early 1930s describing marijuana as a "menace," a "developer of criminals" with the capacity to cause "intoxication" and facilitate prison "uprisings." Regardless of the extent of the marijuana "problem," the FBN believed, during its early years, that control should rest with state governments (particularly those with substantial Latin American populations). In fact, in their 1932 report the Bureau comments that the use of marijuana had been exaggerated in the press (the Hearst newspapers were particularly active in this regard) and that its use was not inordinately large. As late as 1937 the Bureau still advocated that controlling the distribution of marijuana lay in adoption of uniform state narcotic laws.

Despite the Bureau of Narcotics file on marijuana being less than 2 inches thick in 1931, all 48 states had, by the early 1930s, similar laws regulating the illegal use, sale, and/or possession of marijuana under the Uniform [state] Narcotic Drug Act. As mentioned earlier, the Bureau was still reluctant to seek a federal law directed at marijuana. Commissioner Anslinger felt it would be difficult to enforce, would probably be unconstitutional, and that the Bureau was better advised to concentrate on heroin. However, the enactment in 1934 of a "transfer tax" on firearms, and the subsequent finding of its constitutionality in 1937, provided a legal precedent that the Treasury Department felt could be applicable to marijuana. Therefore, in response to increasing pressure from local police forces, the Bureau somewhat reluctantly agreed to pursue a federal antimarijuana transfer tax statute.

Regardless of the ambiguous view that existed within the Bureau at that time, the Treasury Department opted to present a solid front before Congress. In the process, objectivity was not emphasized but, rather, bureaucratic excess in supporting the Tax Act, the goal being total prohibition. The only witness opposing the proposal to appear before the House Committee was an American Medical Association (AMA) spokesperson. He pleaded that the health professions did not need the burden of the bill's restrictions and that the evidence against marijuana was incomplete. The AMA's legislative activities committee did write to protest the impending legislation. Their solicitation read in part, "There is positively no evidence to indicate the abuse of cannabis as a medicinal agent or to show that its medicinal use is leading to the development of cannabis addiction. Cannabis at the present time is slightly used for medicinal purposes, but it would seem worthwhile to maintain its status as a medicinal agent . . . There is a possibility that a restudy of the drug by modern means may show other advantages to be derived from its medicinal use." Despite these protestations, the Federal Marijuana Tax Act was passed by Congress during a period of intolerance and came into effect on October 1, 1937.

The Marijuana Tax Act followed the regulation-by-taxation precedent set by the 1842 law taxing opium importation. In essence, the law stipulated that nonmedical use of marijuana and also the possession or sale of untaxed (i.e., unlicensed) marijuana were illegal. The courts were willing to accept the premise that it really was a tax violation when people were arrested for drugs. The fact that the government would not issue any licenses was not a defense. Furthermore, a legal "fiction" was created that whatever a person puts into their body must have come as a result of some form of interstate commerce. Because this form of enterprise is regulated by the federal government, in the form of taxes and licenses, the federal government should be allowed to regulate what anyone puts into their own body. Physicians and dentists, growers, and importer/manufacturers were required to pay $15, $25, and $50, respectively, in annual taxes. An interesting amendment to the act allowed the use of sterilized marijuana seeds in birdseed. From 1937 to 1971 the federal government referred to marijuana as a narcotic.

Controversy continues to surround *Cannabis sativa* as to whether marijuana laws should be changed. Proponents argue that marijuana is less harmful than tobacco, while opponents site undesirable behavioral effects. The dichotomy of viewpoints and legal status is illustrated by the conflict between state and federal officials regarding the medical use of marijuana. Despite the fact that voters in Arizona, Alaska, California, Colorado, Maine, Nevada, Oregon, and Washington have all approved ballot initiatives allowing the use of medical marijuana (Hawaii did so via legislative action), the U.S. Supreme Court in their wisdom concluded in 2001 that it is illegal to distribute marijuana for medical purposes.

In February 2002, agents of the DEA raided a medical pot club in San Francisco. Some 630 marijuana plants were seized and four arrests were made. If convicted, the sentences can range from 40 years to life in prison. An outspoken group in favor of changing marijuana laws is the National Organization for the Reform of Marihuana Laws (NORML).

POST WORLD WAR II (1945–1969)

It was once a patriotic duty for an American farmer to grow marijuana (hemp). In 1942 a film called *Hemp for Victory* was produced and distributed by the U.S. Department of Agriculture to encourage U.S. farmers to grow cannabis for much-needed hemp products, particularly rope. During World War II, narcotic drug use reached its twentieth-century low point in the United States. This was due to a continual decline in use as well as diminished supply due to disrupted international transportation.

Between 1945 and 1970 a transition occurred from the application of strict legal sanctions to narcotic drug use during the 1950s to more medically based treatment during the 1960s. For example, under the tutelage of Representative Hale Boggs, the Uniform Narcotic Drug Act was significantly empowered in 1951 to impose mandatory minimum sentences of 2 years for first-time narcotic offenders. However, even this was not deemed sufficiently severe. The high-water mark in punitive federal statutes against narcotics was reached in 1956. The Narcotic Control Act of that year (Little Boggs Act) authorized court verdicts to impose the death penalty on anyone over the age of 18 who sold heroin to anyone under the age of 18. The severity of these draconian sanctions ultimately elicited the opposition of the American Bar Association (ABA) as well as the AMA.

Now that the respectable institutions of law and medicine were beginning to question the merits of narcotic regulations, the FBN began to go on the defensive. It took umbrage, for example, at a Joint ABA–AMA Committee Report in 1958 advocating a lessening of criminal penalties and, significantly, the reestablishment of an experimental clinic. The Bureau attempted to discredit the report. However, the document's reasoned views began to permeate a more receptive Congress and initiated the transfer of narcotic control from the FBN to mental health professionals.

With the coincidental retirement in 1962 of Commissioner Anslinger and the Supreme Court's decision that addiction was a disease, and with the arrival of President Kennedy's New Frontier, the Bureau's approach was becoming anachronistic. The prevailing mood of the day encouraged reduced penalties, more medical treatment, possible development of maintenance clinics, and a reevaluation of drug laws. In 1962 a White House Panel on Narcotic and Drug Abuse reported that "It is the opinion of the Panel that the hazards of marijuana per se have been exaggerated and that long criminal sentences imposed on an occasional user or possessor of the drug are in poor social perspective."

In 1963 the Presidential Commission on Narcotic and Drug Abuse recommended relaxation of mandatory minimum sentences, increased appropriations for research, and the dismantling of the FBN. The Drug Abuse Control Amendments of 1965 further diminished the role of the FBN by establishing the Bureau of Drug Abuse Control within the Department of Health, Education, and Welfare (HEW). The Act also shifted the basis for drug control from taxation to interstate commerce regulation. One of the most significant results of the more liberal view of the time was the establishment of methadone maintenance clinics in the mid-1960s. This program is, of course, by its very nature the direct antithesis of earlier federal prohibition policy outlawing addiction maintenance (Supreme Court decision of 1919), since one addiction is substituted for another.

In 1968 the FBN was transferred to the Justice Department, fused with the Bureau of Drug Abuse Control of the HEW to become the Bureau of Narcotics and Dangerous Drugs. By this time, the budget for the National Institutes of Mental Health (NIMH) was 40 times that of the FBN. This funding reflected the successful persuasiveness of the mental health establishment in convincing Washington that addiction was a disease and, as such, should be treated by the medical profession. In addition to the reorganization of federal agencies concerned with regulation of narcotic drugs, an amalgamation of the vast number of regulations in effect at that time was also undertaken. They were repealed, replaced, or updated. In 1969, the United States Supreme Court ruled in the case of Timothy Leary that the Marijuana Tax Act could no longer be enforced because, had Dr Leary tried to pay the tax on cannabis required by federal law, he would have broken Texas law prohibiting possession of marijuana. This meant that federal drug laws had to be rewritten. The result was the framing of the Comprehensive Drug Abuse Prevention and Control Act (Controlled Substances Act, CSA) of 1970.

The CSA centralized federal regulations into one statute and separated marijuana from addicting drugs. At the federal level both simple possession and nonprofit distribution of small amounts of marijuana were changed from felonies to misdemeanors. In addition, first-time offenders could have their criminal records expunged. Many states copied these federal efforts, and within a few years all but Nevada had reduced simple possession of marijuana to a misdemeanor.

THE CONTROLLED SUBSTANCES ACT (1970)

The CSA was an attempt by the government to rank drugs into categories, called schedules, according to their level of dangerousness (i.e., potential for abuse and dependency). The final decision about which schedule a drug was put in was made not by medical experts but by the Justice Department and the Bureau of Narcotics and Dangerous Drugs, later named the Drug Enforcement Administration (DEA).

Schedule I includes drugs deemed to have no accepted medical use in the United States and cannot be prescribed (e.g., heroin, the hallucinogens dimethyltryptamine and psilocybin, and marijuana). The presence of marijuana in Schedule I is, of course, interesting because its inclusion is not consistent with either pharmacological data or the view of most qualified professionals in the medical field. This reality is dramatized by the DEA's own administrative law judge who ruled on September 6, 1988, that, "The evidence in this record clearly shows that marijuana has been accepted as capable of relieving the distress of great numbers of very ill people, and doing so with safety under medical supervision. It would be unreasonable, arbitrary and capricious for DEA to continue to stand between those sufferers and the benefits of this substance."

Schedule II contains dangerous prescribed drugs (e.g., morphine, cocaine, amphetamines, certain barbiturates, and methylphenidate); Schedule III contains drugs that have potential for abuse less than those in Schedules I and II (e.g., most barbiturates); Schedule IV drugs produce only limited physical and psychological dependence (e.g., chloral hydrate and meprobamate); and Schedule V drugs contain moderate quantities of certain opioid drugs (e.g., antitussives and antidiarrheals) that may be obtained without a prescription. In order to avoid innocent violations of the law, medical practitioners may obtain a manual of guidelines from the Drug Enforcement Administration, Registration Unit, PO Box 28083, Central Station, Washington, DC 20005.

To some degree the CSA was based upon the British Pharmacy Act of 1868, which attempted to accomplish a similar goal (though not related to abuse or dependency). The CSA was originally presented to Congress focusing on rehabilitation, research, and education. However, because of conflicting philosophies of the day (treatment/tolerance vs. Nixon's war on drugs), the act contained substantial law-and-order sentiment when passed. Nevertheless, this law has been viewed as a transition between reliance on law enforcement with severe penalties and a therapeutic approach. Significantly, it also de facto decriminalized marijuana to a certain extent by allowing first offenders possessing small amounts to be placed on probation for 1 year rather than mandatory incarceration. In the era from 1970 to 1980, law enforcement became more narrowly targeted on drug dealers.

THE 1970s

After the enactment of the CSA there followed a period of uncertainty as the use of illicit drugs increased. Because of conflicts between the philosophy of enforcement and that of treatment or toleration, a presidential National Commission on Marijuana and Drug Abuse (NCMDA) was established in 1972. Its task was to report within a year on marijuana, its highest priority, and within 2 years on drug abuse in general. The committee's first report recommended that possession of small amounts of marijuana should be decriminalized (i.e., a finable offense not subject to incarceration). The final report appeared in March 1973 and reconfirmed its original recommendation. Despite these recommendations, President Nixon remained opposed to decriminalization.

Nixon's successor, Gerald Ford, was less strident than Nixon on the question of recreational drug use. This is reflected in the White Paper on Drug Abuse prepared by the President's Domestic Council Drug Abuse Task Force and published in September 1975. The document acknowledged that elimination of drug abuse is unlikely but the government can contain the problem. Importantly, it also stated that all drugs are not equally dangerous and that priority should be given to reducing supply and demand for those drugs that pose a greater risk (e.g., heroin, amphetamines, and certain barbiturates). This softened position toward marijuana reflected the more relaxed attitude of the country, as evidenced by the decriminalization of marijuana by Oregon in 1973.

The election of Jimmy Carter as President in 1976 ensured a continuation of tolerance to drug use, particularly marijuana. In March 1977, the Special Assistant for Health Issues to the President, and high officials from the DEA, the State Department, the National Institute of Drug Abuse (NIDA), NIMH, the Customs Service, and the Justice Department appeared before the House Select Committee on Narcotics Abuse and Control to argue for the decriminalization of marijuana. The President himself repeated a similar theme before Congress later that year.

In 1977, publications of the DEA deemphasized the importance of the marijuana problem and argued that enforcement was a matter best left to the states. By 1978 11 states, with one-third of the U.S. population, had decriminalized marijuana use. Thirty others had provisions for conditional discharge (charges dropped or no penalty attached), and 12 allowed for the expungement of the record for first-possession offenders. The year 1978 became a watershed in the United State's relaxed view toward drug use. The decriminalization of marijuana possession was significant because approximately 90 percent of arrests during this period were for possession (360,000 per year). This brief era of relaxed federal and states attitude toward marijuana was about to change, however, as data emerged indicating a steep rise in marijuana and cocaine use particularly among young people.

THE 1980s AND 1990s

By 1980, the DEA had reversed its position and portrayed marijuana as the most serious drug problem facing the United States. The White House, occupied by Ronald Reagan, also shifted its stance to more of an uncompromising Nixonian position. The average penalty for convicted marijuana users in federal courts rose from approximately 30 months in 1975 to over 50 months in 1982 (thus approaching the 1961 average of 70 months). The impact of the late 1970s/early 1980s backlash in societal opinion is also reflected in the fact that since 1977 no additional states have decriminalized marijuana. On the contrary, states have been reinstituting criminal penalties (including Alaska and Oregon which were the most permissive).

In 1985, a new smokable form of cocaine ("crack") began to appear in certain parts of the United States. This new form of cocaine was cheap, highly effective, had a quick onset of action, did not require needle injection, and was less dangerous to manufacture than "freebase" cocaine. The violence and crime associated with this new, highly popular, and profitable drug had a significant impact on Americans. Because of the furor created, an Anti-Drug Abuse Act was signed into law in the autumn of 1986. This act authorized nearly $4 billion for an intensified battle against drugs. While most of the funding was destined for law enforcement, the law also provided some additional support for drug abuse research via NIDA.

In 1986, President Reagan also signed Executive Order Number 12564, the Drug Free Federal Workplace Act. This act initiated drug-testing programs for federal employees in safety-sensitive jobs. It also suggested procedures for drug-testing programs and plans for employee assistance programs to provide counseling and rehabilitation for workers with drug problems. In 1988 the drug-free policy act was extended to include all federal grantees and most federal contractors.

Drug use in the workplace is also a potential problem in nonfederal entities. According to an article in the *Houston Business Journal* in 2000, the American Management Association's Annual Survey on Workplace Drug Testing and Drug Abuse Policies found that workplace drug testing has increased more than 1200 percent since 1987. Virtually all companies that employ drug testing show steady decreases in drug use. Conversely, the number of employees trying to cheat or adulterate their tests is increasing. A quick search of the Internet reveals dozens of antidrug-testing websites where so-called "cleansing" aids are sold for the sole purpose of helping drug users produce a clean urine drug screen (e.g., http://www.testclean.com). Drug users can even purchase freeze-dried urine, or human urine that is purported to be "clean."

Laws pertaining to workplace drug testing in the United States are always changing, with courts, legislatures, and regulatory agencies at both the federal and state levels continually modifying their approach. Employers must keep abreast of these changes and regularly reevaluate their drug policies. An employer's right to implement drug and alcohol testing depends on several factors, including whether the employer is in the public or private sector, the employees are contract or "at will," and whether the company is covered by the U.S. Department of Transportation regulations. Collective bargaining agreements may also enter into the mix.

In addition to narcotics and marijuana, the nonmedical use of anabolic steroids became increasingly popular during the 1980s. This was particularly true for athletes seeking to increase skeletal muscle mass and performance, as discussed previously. The Omnibus Anti-Substance Abuse Act of 1988 made the unlawful distribution of anabolic steroids across state lines a felony under federal law, punishable by 1 to 3 years in prison and a fine of up to $250,000. State laws governing the possession and distribution of anabolic drugs vary, but a conviction in most states carries a stiff fine and imprisonment.

The subsequent Omnibus Crime Control Act (OCCA) of 1990 added certain anabolic-androgenic steroid substances to Schedule III of the CSA of 1970, which places them under the aegis of the DEA. Therefore, provisions for registration, reporting, record keeping, and prescribing, as well as investigation of and penalties for misuse, now apply to these drugs. Only registered clinicians can issue prescriptions for these drugs, and the prescriptions can be refilled a maximum of five times within 6 months. The OCCA also regulates human growth hormone distribution for nonmedical purposes, since this drug was being turned to as an alternative for anabolic steroids. Possession and distribution of steroids without a prescription is a federal crime punishable by up to a year in prison and a fine of at least $1000.

According to the Office of National Drug Control Policy (ONDCP), federal spending on drug control programs has increased from $1.5 billion in fiscal year 1981 to $18.1 billion (enacted) in fiscal year 2001 (a 12-fold increase). The budget is divided into three main categories: domestic enforcement (the largest), international/ border control, and demand reduction. The 1993 National Summit on U.S. Drug Policy has made five recommendations to modify future policy: (1) reduce spending

Table A.1 Federal drug control budget by function for fiscal years 2000 and 2001

	FY 2000 ($ million)	FY 2001 ($ million)
Total	17,940.3	18,053.1
Drug treatment	2915.2	3168.3
Drug prevention	2338.6	2515.7
Criminal justice system	8429.0	9357.7
International	1892.9	609.7
Interdiction	1965.9	1950.4
Research	89.6	106.1
Intelligence	309.1	345.2
International (U.S. Support for Plan Colombia and the Andean Region)	954.4	

Source: Office of National Drug Control Policy (ONDCP), *FY 2002 National Drug Control Budget*, April 2001.

Table A.2 State spending for substance abuse, 1998

	FY 1998 ($ billion)
Total	77.9
Justice	30.7
Education	16.5
Health	15.2
Child/family assistance	7.7

Source: National Center on Addiction and Substance Abuse at Columbia University, "Shoveling Up: The Impact of Substance Abuse on State Budgets," January 2001, press release.
Lesser amounts were budgeted for developmental disabilities (5.9) and public safety (1.5).

on international interdiction and eradication with corresponding increases for treatment and prevention; (2) fund only effective programs for drug dependence; (3) coerce hard-core users to get treatment; (4) continue strict law enforcement; and (5) avoid counterproductive prison terms for first-time offenders. A more specific breakdown of the federal budget for fiscal years 2000 and 2001 is shown in Table A.1. Table A.2 shows state spending for substance abuse in 1998. According to Bureau of Justice Statistics for 1990, U.S. law enforcement agencies now arrest more than 1.3 million citizens each year for the possession, distribution, and sale of prohibited drugs. More than a quarter of a million people are now incarcerated for drug offenses.

When he took office as the country's Drug Czar in 1996, Barry McCaffrey insisted there was not a shred of scientific evidence that smoking marijuana was useful or necessary. Nevertheless, McCaffrey commissioned yet another report to evaluate the scientific validity of marijuana for patients. The National Academy of Sciences' Institute of Medicine undertook an 18-month study of all available scientific evidence on medical marijuana. The 1999 report's authors found that the active components in marijuana appear to be helpful in treating pain, nausea, AIDS-related weight loss, and muscle spasms in multiple sclerosis. While there is currently no legal source for marijuana, patients can get access to a synthetic THC pill. In 1986, the FDA approved Marinol®.

THE NEXT MILLENNIUM

Unlike cocaine and opium, tobacco and its primary psychoactive ingredient, nicotine, are products of the New World, two species being in cultivation at the time of Columbus. The sale of tobacco to France helped finance much of our Revolutionary War. Thus, together with hemp, tobacco contributed to the young country's positive cash flow. Between the late eighteenth and early twentieth centuries, the primary forms of tobacco use in America were snuff and chewing. By 1911 smoking tobacco became the dominant form.

The government of the United States has supported the tobacco industry by various means for centuries. This support continues to this day, even though tobacco contributes to approximately 400,000 deaths annually. Beginning in the late 1980s, however, there were signs that the sacrosanct status of tobacco (i.e., nicotine) would be challenged. The warning shots were fired in 1988 when C. Everett Koop, then Surgeon General, testified before the Congress that nicotine should be listed as an addictive drug and should be regulated by the FDA.

In June 1988 the tobacco industry lost its first court case involving liability in the death of a smoker after heavy, chronic cigarette use. Although the decision was subsequently reversed in 1990, it represents a significant application of tort law. The question of addiction liability was the core of a landmark class action case against the tobacco industry in federal court in New Orleans (*Castano v. The American Tobacco Co.*). (This case was settled as part of the general settlement; see later discussion).

Tobacco companies have always denied that nicotine is addictive. However, there may be evidence that tobacco firms knew as long ago as 30 years that the opposite was true and went to great lengths to control the levels of nicotine. In any event, an advisory panel to the FDA found nicotine to be addictive, comparing it to cocaine and heroin. The FDA Commissioner Kessler indicated that the FDA would not back off from efforts to regulate tobacco (tobacco is not currently regulated by the FDA), labeling nicotine addiction a "pediatric disease" and asserting that cigarettes are, in fact, nicotine delivery devices and thus under the purview of the FDA. The Centers for Disease Control estimate that 3000 American teenagers start to smoke each day. Tobacco firms' intent may be the key to federal control if the FDA is correct in alleging that the tobacco companies deliberately alter nicotine levels (e.g., the development of a high-nicotine tobacco plant) in order to achieve dependency.

It is the long-standing denial of addiction by the tobacco industry that may render it more susceptible to recent court challenges. Alcohol manufacturers, on the other hand, have long acknowledged alcohol's potential for addiction. Thus, they have shielded themselves from claims now confronting the tobacco industry, such as fraud and intentional concealment. The industry's denial that nicotine is addictive is increasingly coming under scrutiny.

Some states began taking a more proactive position regarding smoking liability, independent of the government. In February 1995, in a state court in Indianapolis, five of six jurors rejected four tobacco companies' defense in a product defect claim that a man's smoking was wholly voluntary. The case ended in a mistrial. As reported in the April 16, 1995 edition of the *New York Times*, the Massachusetts House may ban all products containing nicotine. However, cigarette makers scored two big victories in West Virginia and Florida. In the West Virginia case the judge struck down eight of the 10 counts in the attorney general's suit. In Florida, massive lobbying resulted in the repeal of a new law allowing the state to litigate against third parties responsible for Medicaid costs.

Despite those victories, there was evidence of possible erosion of the tobacco industry's position. In a decision on December 8, 1995, by the Labor Department regarding liability for secondhand smoke, a claimant's position was vindicated. In the first worker's compensation case in the nation linking secondhand smoke to a cancer death, the Department of Veterans Affairs was ordered to pay the widower of a nurse $21,500 a year until his death. The decision was based upon his wife's 18-year exposure to secondhand smoke at a veterans hospital and expert testimony regarding causality. Although the worker's compensation ruling is not admissible in court, it may impact cigarette smoking by rendering employers susceptible to future claims.

Most significantly, in December 1995, Massachusetts became the fifth state to file a lawsuit against the tobacco industry (six major tobacco companies). The state was seeking more than $1 billion in damages to repay taxpayers for the money the state spent to fund medical care for poor people with tobacco-related maladies. The lawsuit alleged that "cigarette manufacturers and their trade associations have engaged in a conspiracy to mislead, deceive and confuse" the state and its citizens about "the overwhelming evidence that cigarette smoking causes fatal disease." In August 1996, Massachusetts passed a rigorous new cigarette disclosure law. If upheld, the bill will force tobacco companies to reveal additives in each brand, in descending order of weight, including ammonia-based compounds that critics say boost nicotine delivery and make cigarettes more potent. The tobacco industry responded by saying that "they wouldn't ask Coke, Pepsi or the Colonel to divulge their soft-drink or chicken recipe, so why should we be deprived of trade-secret privileges?"

By March 1996, the first real crack in the unified tobacco industry front became evident. Liggett Group, the smallest of the nation's five major tobacco companies, and five states (Florida, Massachusetts, Mississippi, West Virginia, and Louisiana) reached a settlement of the lawsuits seeking to recover the public health-care cost of treating illnesses linked to smoking (thus presaging the Master Settlement Agreement by two and a half years; see later). Simply getting a tobacco company to agree to pay plaintiffs anything is a watershed development in the 40-year history of tobacco litigation. Liggett became the first cigarette company ever to settle smoking-related lawsuits.

Liggett agreed to pay the five states $5 million over 10 years to defray the taxpayer costs of treating state Medicaid patients with smoking-related illnesses. If Liggett merges with RJR or another tobacco company, the settlement provides $160 million for all five states. The settlement also included annual payments of between 2 and 7 percent of Liggett's pretax profits for 24 years. At profit levels of the time, that amounts to approximately $250,000 per year for Liggett alone or $30 million annually if Liggett combines with RJR. The states estimated that, together, they spent in excess of $900 million on smoking-related health care costs. Significantly, Liggett also agreed to drop its opposition to the FDA proposal to regulate tobacco as a drug and to refrain from using various marketing and promotional gimmicks aimed at children.

The woes of the tobacco industry continued into the summer of 1996 when, on August 9, a Florida jury awarded a plaintiff and his wife $750,000 in their suit against Brown & Williamson Tobacco Corp. One document that was persuasive in the case was a 1963 memo from a former top counsel of the company. In that correspondence, the executive stated that "Nicotine is addictive. We are, then, in the business of selling nicotine, an addictive drug effective in the release of stress mechanisms."

SALES TO MINORS

It was also in August 1996 that a "final" rule on tobacco was published in the Federal Register. It identified the FDA as being in charge of regulating the sale and distribution of cigarettes and smokeless tobacco to children and adolescents. The action resulted from the FDA's assertion of jurisdiction over tobacco products. This was based on an extensive FDA investigation of the tobacco industry, tobacco use, and its health consequences. The rule prohibits the sale of cigarettes and smokeless tobacco to those under 18, while leaving the products on the market for adults.

Specifically, the rule made the sale of cigarettes and smokeless tobacco to children and adolescents, anyone younger than 18 years of age, a federal violation. In addition, the rule required manufacturers, distributors, and retailers to comply with certain conditions regarding the sale, distribution, and promotion of tobacco products. It prohibited all free samples and limits retail sales in most circumstances to face-to-face transactions. As a result, vending machines and self-service displays were prohibited, except in facilities where the retailer or operator ensures that no person younger than 18 is present or is permitted to enter at any time.

The rule limited advertising generally to a black-and-white, text-only format to ensure that advertising was not used to create demand for these products among young people and thus undermine the restrictions on access. Billboards and other outdoor advertising were prohibited within 1000 feet of schools and public playgrounds. The sale and distribution of nontobacco items, such as hats and teeshirts that carry cigarette logos, such as Joe Camel, were prohibited, and sponsorship of sporting and other events was limited to the corporate name only.

The FDA's authority, in its opinion, to carry out its mission to protect public health derives primarily from the Federal Food, Drug, and Cosmetic Act of 1906. This statute provides the agency authority to regulate a wide variety of consumer products, including drugs and devices. The FDA asserted that cigarettes were, in fact, combination products containing both an addictive drug (nicotine) and a delivery system (processed tobacco, ventilation system, and filters). (As a historical aside, it is interesting to note that at the beginning of the twentieth century, an atropine-like drug, stramonium, was put in cigarettes to be delivered by smoking to asthmatics.) The FDA determined that tobacco products are most appropriately regulated under the device provisions of the act and, thus, under its purview. The tobacco industry, of course, appealed. On August 14, 1998, the Fourth Circuit Court of Appeals ruled in the industry's favor stating that Congress had never intended to give the FDA the regulatory to regulate tobacco (2 to 1 decision) and overruled a lower court decision favoring the FDA.

As fate would have it, however, the tobacco industry had seen the writing on the wall and had been independently negotiating with a team of eight Attorney Generals to reach a substantial settlement. On November 23, 1998, a Master Settlement Agreement (MSA) was signed with the Attorney Generals of 46 states. The Attorney Generals said, "This is litigation, not legislation. Congress should pass legislation to provide essential reforms—including full Food and Drug Administration authority over tobacco."

The settlement, like the FDA proposal, has numerous provisions aimed primarily at protecting children. Under the settlement proposal, the tobacco industry would contribute $1.5 billion over the next 5 years for a national public education fund that would carry out a massive education and advertising campaign. It would also pay $250 million for a foundation dedicated to reducing teenage smoking. Like the FDA proposal, the settlement would ban cartoon characters in tobacco advertising, prohibit the industry from targeting youth in advertising and marketing, prohibit billboards and transit advertising, and ban the sale and distribution of apparel, backpacks, and other merchandise that bear brand-name logos and become, in effect, walking billboards.

Under the settlement, tobacco companies would pay the states more than $9 billion a year beginning in the year 2008. The industry will pay the states $12 billion in "up-front" money over 5 years. Total payments through to the year 2025 would be approximately $206 billion. This does not include settlements already reached with four other states (Florida, Mississippi, Minnesota, and Texas), totaling over $40 billion in the same period. To ensure the industry lives up to the agreement, the settlement would be enforceable through consent decrees that will be entered in each state court. In addition, the industry will provide $50 million for an enforcement fund, which states could use to pursue violations of the settlement. To cover the cost of this settlement manufacturers raised prices, between January 1998 and January 2000, the average U.S. wholesale price of cigarettes climbing from $1.31 per pack to $2.35, a 79 percent increase in 2 years.

The effect of the settlement directives may already have been manifested in 1999. In 1999, the five "leading" cigarette companies reported that they sold 47.2 billion fewer cigarettes than in 1998. This encouraging news suggests that perhaps the first substantive steps have been taken to arrest the single greatest preventable disease factor in the United States. The 400,000 lives claimed each year in the United States matches the number of Americans who died in World War II. Comparable figures in Britain are 120,000 fatalities per year. Yet, incredibly, a 2001 survey in Britain reveals that 54 percent of smokers and 61 percent of nonsmokers believe that smoking cigarettes is not dangerous to their health.

The Master Settlement Agreement assumed that a large portion of the money would pay for tobacco-use prevention programs. However, a 2001 report by the National Conference of State Legislatures found that the 46 states that joined in the settlement, plus the four that reached separate deals with the tobacco companies, had used only 5 percent of the money for smoking prevention and cessation programs. (The General Accounting Office has found similar data.) Many states appear to be using the money for other needs, such as public schools, elderly care, and balancing their budgets.

In conclusion, lest we be too harsh on the tobacco industry, we should be cognizant of a study on the financial cost of smoking carried out by the research company Arthur D. Little International commissioned by Philip Morris. Researchers looked at the Czech Republic and concluded that the government saved $30 million in 1999 because it did not have to support, house, and care for smokers who died prematurely from tobacco-related illness. The study also indicated that there were "indirect positive effects" of early deaths such as savings on health care, pensions, welfare, and housing for the elderly. The government's net gain from the tobacco industry was calculated to be $146 million. This reasoning was also actually argued at pretrial hearings in the Mississippi case in 1997. Citing a legal text on equity jurisprudence, the defendants wrote:

> A court of equity is a court of *conscience* [emphasis mine]; it seeks to do justice and equity between all parties; it seeks to strike a balance of convenience as between all litigants; and it looks to the whole situation. . . . Here, the Court's duty to look at the "whole situation" requires the Court to look at the full economic impact of the sale of cigarettes on the State.

The plaintiff's countered by characterizing the defendant's assertion as "ghoulish." Specifically, they wrote:

> Seeking a credit for a purported economic benefit from early death is akin to robbing the graves of Mississippi smokers who died from tobacco-related illness. No court of law or equity should entertain such a defense or counterclaim. It is offensive to human decency, an affront to justice, uncharacteristic of civilized society, and unquestionably contrary to public policy.

SELECTED BIBLIOGRAPHY

Baskys, A. and Remington, G. (eds) (1996) *Brain Mechanisms and Psychotropic Drugs*. Boca Raton, FL: CRC Press.

Bayer, R. and Oppenheimer, G. (eds) (1993) *Drug Policy: Illicit Drugs in a Free Society*. New York: Cambridge University Press.

Goldberg, R. (1994) *Drugs Across the Spectrum*. Minneapolis, MN: West Publishing Co.

Goldstein, A. (1994) *Addiction from Biology to Drug Policy*. New York: W. H. Freeman and Co.

Hardman, J. G., Limbird, L. L. and Gilman, A. G. (eds) (2001) *Goodman and Gilman's The Pharmacological Basis of Therapeutics*, 10th ed. New York: McGraw-Hill.

Karch, S. (1993) *The Pathology of Drug Abuse*. Boca Raton, FL: CRC Press.

Lidow, M. S. (ed.) (2000) *Neurotransmitter Receptors in Actions of Antipsychotic Medications*. Boca Raton, FL: CRC Press.

Moody, E. and Skolnich, P. (eds) (2001) *Molecular Basis of Anesthesia*. Boca Raton, FL: CRC Press.

Musto, D. F. (1987) *The American Disease*, 2nd ed. New York: Oxford University Press.

Niesink, R. J. M., Jaspers, R. M. A., Kornet, L. M. W. and van Ree, J. M. (eds) (1999) *Drugs of Abuse and Addiction: Neurobehavioral Toxicology*. Boca Raton, FL: CRC Press.

Orey, M. (1999) *Assuming the Risk: The Mavericks, the Lawyers, and the Whistle-Blowers Who Beat Big Tobacco*. Boston, MA: Little, Brown and Co.

Pinger, R. R., Payne, W. A., Hahn, D. B. and Hahn, E. J. (1995) *Drugs: Issues for Today*, 2nd ed. St Louis, MO: Mosby.

Ray, O. and Ksir, C. (1993) *Drugs, Society, and Human Behavior*, 6th ed. St Louis, MO: Mosby.

Redda, K., Walker, C. and Barnett, G. (1989) *Cocaine, Marijuana, Designer Drugs: Chemistry, Pharmacology, and Behavior*. Boca Raton, FL: CRC Press.

Snyder, S. (1996) *Drugs and the Brain*. New York: Scientific American Library.

Weil, A. and Rosen, W. (1993) *From Chocolate to Morphine*. Boston, MA: Houghton Miflin Co.

Weisheit, R. A. (1992) *Domestic Marijuana: A Neglected Industry*. New York: Greenwood Press.

Zernig, G., Saria, A., Kurz, M. and O'Malley, S. S. (eds) (2000) *Handbook of Alcoholism*. Boca Raton, FL: CRC Press.

QUESTIONS

1 Drug companies have been required to demonstrate both safety and efficacy of their compounds since which year?
   a   1906
   b   1926
   c   1933
   d   1962
   e   1970.

2 The Food and Drug Administration was created by legislation in which year?
   a   1906
   b   1910
   c   1947
   d   1958
   e   1976.

3 The Opium Exclusion Act was enacted in which year?
   a   1906
   b   1909
   c   1919
   d   1933
   e   1940.

4 Isolation of pure cocaine occurred in which year?
   a   1809
   b   1812
   c   1859
   d   1861
   e   1906.

5 The Harrison Narcotics Act was passed in which year?
   a   1906
   b   1911

   c   1914
   d   1915
   e   1919.

6 Prohibition (The Volstead Act) was ratified in which year?
   a   1906
   b   1911
   c   1914
   d   1915
   e   1919.

7 The Federal Marijuana Tax Act came into effect in which year?
   a   1906
   b   1911
   c   1919
   d   1937
   e   1938.

8 Which of the following years was probably the "watershed" in terms of America's relaxed view toward illicit drug use?
   a   1933
   b   1952
   c   1962
   d   1978
   e   1980.

9 The Master Settlement Agreement between the tobacco industry and 46 states was signed in which year?
   a   1989
   b   1991
   c   1993
   d   1996
   e   1998.

10 The Master Settlement Agreement between the tobacco industry and 46 states lasts until 2024 and includes a total payment of which of the following?
   a $200 million
   b $500 million
   c $200 billion
   d $500 billion
   e $1 trillion.

Glossary

Abbreviated new drug application (ANDA)   A simplified submission permitted for a duplicate of an already approved drug. ANDAs are for products with the same or very closely related active ingredients, dosage form, strength, administration route, use, and labeling as a product that has already been shown to be safe and effective. An ANDA includes all the information on chemistry and manufacturing controls found in an NDA, but does not have to include data from studies in animals and humans. It must, however, contain evidence that the duplicate drug is bioequivalent to the previously approved drug.

Accelerated approval   A highly specialized mechanism intended to speed approval of drugs promising significant benefit over existing therapy for serious or life-threatening illnesses. It incorporates elements aimed at making sure that rapid review and approval is balanced by safeguards to protect both the public health and the integrity of the regulatory process. This mechanism may be used when approval can be reliably based on evidence of a drug's effect on a "surrogate endpoint" (see Surrogate endpoint), or when the FDA determines an effective drug can be used safely only under restricted distribution or use. Usually, such a surrogate can be assessed much sooner than such an endpoint as survival. In accelerated approval, the FDA approves the drug on condition that the sponsor study the actual clinical benefit of the drug.

Acetylcholine   A chemical neurotransmitter released by nerve endings. Its effects include cardiac inhibition, increase in blood vessel diameter, and constricted pupils.

Acidosis/alkalosis   The condition when the pH of the blood falls/rises outside the normal acceptable limits.

Action letter   An official communication from the FDA to an NDA sponsor that informs of a decision by the agency. An approval letter allows commercial marketing of the product. An approval letter lists minor issues to be resolved before approval can be given. A not approvable letter describes important deficiencies that preclude approval unless corrected.

Active transport   Movement of materials across cell membranes that requires direct expenditure of metabolic energy.

Acute   Short-term exposure or response.

Acute toxicity   The short-term effects of a one-time exposure to a chemical substance.

Additive   When the therapeutic or toxic effect of several xenobiotics is equal to the sum of the individual components.

Adduct   Covalent binding of an exogenous chemical to a cellular macromolecule.

Adrenergic Nerves responding to the neurotransmitter norepinephrine.

Adverse effect A biochemical change, functional impairment, or pathological lesion that either singly or in combination deleteriously affects the performance of the whole organism, or reduces an organism's ability to respond to an additional environmental challenge.

Advisory committee A panel of outside experts convened periodically to advise the FDA on safety and efficacy issues about drugs and other FDA-related products. The FDA is not bound to make committee recommendations, but usually does.

Aerosol A colloidal system with a gas as the dispersion medium (such as a fog or mist of droplets or particles).

Agonist A drug that both binds to receptors and has intrinsic activity.

Alcohol See ethanol.

Allergen An antigenic substance capable of eliciting an allergic response.

Allergic reaction A reaction to a foreign agent giving rise to a hypersensitive state, mediated via an immunological mechanism and resulting in a particular series of responses.

Allosteric (change) Alteration of protein conformation resulting in alteration of function (e.g., noncompetitive receptor inhibition).

Amendment to an NDA A submission to change or add information to an NDA or supplement not yet approved.

Amino acid A component of every protein, in which up to 20 different amino acids are strung together into polymer chains.

Amphiphatic A molecule possessing both polar and nonpolar moieties.

Anaphylactic reaction A type I immunological response involving histamine and other mediator release.

Androgen Any substance that produces masculinization, such as testosterone.

Anoxia Absence of oxygen in the tissues.

Antagonism When the therapeutic effect of a drug is reduced in either a competitive or a noncompetitive manner.

Antagonist A drug that impedes the action of another drug (may be competitive or noncompetitive).

Anterior Situated in the front part of the organ or body.

Antibiotics Anti-infection drugs that inhibit the growth of or destroy microorganisms and are used extensively in treating bacteria-mediated disease.

Antibody A protein produced by B-lymphocytes in response to, and specific for, a foreign substance or antigen.

Anticoagulant A substance that prevents the normal process of blood clotting (e.g., heparin or courmarin).

Anticonvulsant A drug that counteracts or prevents convulsions caused by brain diseases, electric shock, and certain chemicals.

Antidote A substance that specifically blocks or reduces the toxic action of a drug or poison.

Antigen A protein or other macromolecule that is recognized as foreign by the immune system in an animal.

Antihistamine A drug that blocks the effects of histamine usually by competitive antagonism at the site. It can relieve symptoms such as sneezing, watery eyes, runny nose, and itching of the nose and throat.

Antihypertensive   A drug used for lowering blood pressure.

Antimetabolite   A chemical with a structure related to but not identical to a normal metabolite. If it counteracts the effects of the metabolite, it may be useful as a drug.

Antitussive   A drug that prevents coughing.

Apoptosis   Programmed cell death.

Area under the curve (AUC)   For example, a measure of how much drug reaches the bloodstream in a set period of time, usually 24 hours. AUC is calculated by plotting drug blood concentration at various times during a 24-hour or longer period and then measuring the area under the curve.

Arrhythmia   Irregularities in heart rate.

Astrocytes   Cells found in the central nervous system.

Atherosclerosis   Common form of arteriosclerosis with deposits of yellow plaques containing cholesterol, lipid material within the intima and inner media of arteries.

Atopic   Pertaining to genetic predisposition toward developing immediate hypersensitivity reactions to antigenic substances.

Atrial fibrillation   Rapid, irregular contractions of the atrial chambers of the heart.

Atrophy   Reduction in size of a structure or organ resulting from lack of nourishment or functional activity, death and reabsorption of cells, diminished cellular proliferation, ischemia, or hormone changes.

AUC   Area under the curve when the plasma (blood) concentration of a substance is plotted against time.

Autoimmune disease   Immune response in which antibodies are directed against the organism itself.

Autosomal   Pertaining to the ordinary paired chromosomes that can be distinguished from the sex chromosomes.

Axon   The process of a neuron that conducts impulses traveling away from the cell body.

Axoplasm   Cytoplasm of an axon.

Bactericidal   A drug that kills bacteria.

Bacteriostatic   A drug that slows or prevents the multiplication of bacteria.

Base pair   Unit of length for DNA work. Usually expressed as kb (kilobase) or kbp (kilo base pair). In the double-stranded molecule guanosine pairs with cytidine and adenosine with thymidine (or uridine in RNA).

Beta receptor   An autonomic receptor, of which there are three types.

Bioaccumulation   The accumulation of a substance in a biological organism, usually due to its lipophilicity.

Bioactivation   Metabolism of a xenobiotic to a chemically more reactive metabolite.

Bioavailability   A measure of the degree to which a dose of a substance becomes physiologically available to body tissues based upon blood levels. The standard of comparison is the intravenous dose.

Bioequivalence   Scientific basis on which generic and brand-name drugs are compared. To be considered bioequivalent, the bioavailability of two products must not differ significantly when the two products are given in studies at the same dosage under similar conditions. Some drugs, however, are intended to have a different absorption rate. The FDA may consider a product bioequivalent to a second product with a different rate of absorption if the difference is noted in the labeling and does not affect the drug's safety or effectiveness or change the drug's effects in any medically significant way.

Biotransformation An enzymatic chemical alteration of a substance within the body that generally leads to a more excretable metabolite, sometimes producing a more toxic form of the xenobiotic.

Blood–brain barrier The combination of tight endothelial junctions in cerebral capillaries together with their covering of astrocytes.

Bolus A single dose.

Bradycardia Slowing of the heart rate, usually below 60 beats per minute.

Bronchiole Smaller diameter, more distal branches of the bronchiole tree.

Bronchoconstriction Constriction of the smooth muscle in airways in the lungs due to exposure to irritant chemicals or to an immunological reaction involving release of inflammatory mediators.

Buccal Pertaining to the cheek.

Carcinogen/carcinogenic A substance/property of a substance that causes cancer when administered to an organism.

Cardiac arrythmias Abnormal beating rhythms in the heart.

Cardiac output The volume of blood pumped by the heart in one cycle.

Cardiomyopathy Pathological changes to heart tissue.

Catabolized Metabolically broken down.

Cathartic A chemical that stimulates intestinal peristalsis and relieves constipation.

cDNA A double-stranded copy of an RNA molecule that contains only the coding and flanking regions of the gene.

Cell culture Growth of living cells or microorganisms in a controlled, artificial environment.

Centrilobular The region of the liver lobule surrounding the central vein.

Chelation Binding of an inorganic ion (e.g., heavy metal) by an organic molecule.

Chiral The presence of asymmetry in a molecule giving rise to isomers.

Cholestasis Cessation of bile flow.

Cholinergic stimulation Stimulation of the nerve fibers utilizing acetylcholine as the neurotransmitter.

Chromosome A cellular structure composed of a long, folded DNA molecule and protein.

Chronic Long-term exposure to a xenobiotic.

Cirrhosis Liver disease characterized by loss of the normal microscopic lobular structure with fibrosis (collagen deposition). Usually the result of chronic exposure to a noxious agent such as ethanol.

Clearance The volume of plasma cleared of a drug in unit time.

Clinical trials Divided into three phases involving pharmacokinetc studies of the drug as well as studies designed to assess efficacy. Such studies conducted in the United States must be under an approved IND.

Cloning The insertion of foreign DNA into host plasmids or genomes.

CNS Central nervous system.

Coating, enteric Encapsulating a biologically active chemical in a layer such as wax or biodegradable plastic that delays and regulates the rate of release of a drug into tissues.

Cocaine   An alkaloid obtained from the dried leaves of the coca shrub. It is a Schedule I regulated drug with high addiction potential.

Codon   A group of three base pairs that code for a specific amino acid.

Cognitive   Brain functions related to sense perception or understanding.

Collagen   A fibrous protein.

Complement   A series of proteins found in extracellular fluids and involved in certain immunological reactions.

Cortex, cerebral   The outer layer (gray matter) of the brain.

Cyanosis   The pathological condition where there is an excessive concentration of reduced hemoglobin in the blood.

Cytochrome P448 and P450   Isozymes that are important in the detoxification by biotransformation of many xenobiotics. These enzymes are found primarily in the liver and, to a lesser extent, in the lungs and other tissues.

Cytosol   The internal part of the cell excluding the organelles.

Dalton   Unit of relative molecular mass, symbol Da.

Database   A computerized collection of information.

Deacetylation   Removal of an acetyl group.

Dealkylation   Removal of an alkyl group.

Deamination   Removal of an amine group.

Dechlorination   Removal of a chlorine group.

Deethylation   Removal of an ethyl group.

Dehalogenation   Removal of a halogen group.

Delaney amendment   Amendment to the Food, Drug, and Cosmetic Act of the Food and Drug Administration of the United States. The amendment states that food additives that cause cancer in humans or animals at any level shall not be considered safe and are, therefore, prohibited.

Demethylation   Removal of a methyl group.

Dendrites   Neuronal projections that usually convey impulses to the cell body.

Denervated   A tissue deprived of its nerve supply.

Dermatitis   Inflammation of the skin.

Desensitization   Loss of functional response. Can be short term (seconds or minutes) or long term (hours).

Detoxification   Reduction of a chemical's toxic properties by means of biotransformation processes, to form a more readily excreted or a less toxic chemical than the parent compound.

Developmental toxicity   Adverse effects on the developing organism. Adverse developmental effects may be detected at any point in the life span of the organism. Major manifestations of developmental toxicity include death of the developing embryo, induction of structural abnormalities (teratogenicity), altered growth, and functional deficiency.

Diabetes insipidus   Disease due to lack of antidiuretic hormone.

Diabetes mellitus   Disease with enhanced blood glucose levels due to lack of insulin.

Dimer   Subunit of a macromolecule (e.g., certain proteins exist as dimers).

Distal   Remote from the point of reference.

Diuretic   A drug that increases the flow of urine. Some diuretics also lower blood pressure.

DNA Deoxyribonucleic acid, the substance within cells that carries the "recipe" for the organism and is inherited from parents. A normally double-stranded molecule made up of deoxyadenosine, deoxycytidine, deoxyguanosine, and deoxythymidine.

Dopaminergic Receptors responsive to dopamine.

Dorsal Pertaining to the back.

Dose–response relationship The relationship between (1) the dose, actually based on "administered dose" (i.e., exposure) rather than actual absorbed dose, and (2) the extent of therapeutic or toxic effect produced by the xenobiotic.

Downregulation Loss of total receptor number due to agonist-induced endocytosis and subsequent degradation. Can become significant after an hour or more of agonist treatment.

Drug insert The paper in a drug package that contains a description of the drug, its main effects, toxicity, dosage form, and names.

Drug product The finished dosage form (tablet, capsule, etc.) that contains a drug substance—generally, but not necessarily, in association with other active or inactive ingredients.

Drug substance The active ingredient intended to diagnose, treat, cure, or prevent disease or affect the structure or function of the body, excluding other inactive substances used in the drug product.

Drugs, chiral Drugs with unsymmetrical molecular structure. Chiral drugs exist as enantiomers.

Duodenum First portion of the intestine between the pylorus and jejunum.

ED$_{50}$ The dose of a drug that is pharmacologically effective for 50 percent of the population exposed to the drug or a 50 percent response in a biological system that is exposed to the drug.

Edema Abnormal accumulation of fluid in cells, tissues, or body cavities resulting in swelling.

Effectiveness The desired measure of a drug's influence on a disease condition. Effectiveness must be proven by substantial evidence consisting of adequate and well-controlled investigations, including human studies by qualified experts, that prove the drug will have the effect claimed in its labeling.

Electrophile A chemical that is attracted to react with an electron-rich center in another molecule.

Elimination half-life The time it takes the body to eliminate or break down half the dose of a xenobiotic.

Elixir A solution, often an alcoholic tincture, of drugs.

Embolism Sudden blocking of an artery with a blood clot or foreign material.

Embryo In mammals, the stage in the developing organism at which organs and organ systems are developing. For humans, this involves the stage of development between the second and the eighth weeks from conception.

Emetic To induce vomiting.

Endocytosis Movement of receptor or ligand from the cell surface to an internal compartment. Usually occurs within minutes of agonist treatment. In the case of receptors there is a basal rate of endocytosis (usually slow, occurs without agonist ligand and is therefore constitutive) and an agonist-stimulating rate.

Endogenous Part of the internal environment of a living organism.

Endoplasmic reticulum (ER)   May be divided into rough ER with attendant ribosomes involved with protein synthesis and smooth ER where cytochrome P450 and many other drug-metabolizing enzymes are located.

Endothelium   The layer of endothelial cells lining the interior of blood vessels.

Endpoint   Refers to the point in an animal experiment when no more information can be obtained and the experiment is stopped.

Enteral   Refers to the gut.

Enterohepatic circulation   The recycling of a drug from the blood into the liver, then into the bile and gastrointestinal tract. This is followed by reuptake into the bloodstream from the gastrointestinal tract, possibly after chemical or enzymatic breakdown.

Epidemiology   The study of diseases in populations.

Epidural   Outside or directly above the dura mater covering the brain and spinal cord.

Epigenetic   Nongenetically mediated.

Epinephrine   Adrenaline.

Ethanol (alcohol)   The world's most popular drug, legally used in most countries. Ethanol is produced through the fermentation of fruits, vegetables, and grains.

Etiology   The study of the cause and/or origin of a disease.

Euphoria   A feeling of well-being. It can be induced by certain drugs.

Excretion   Elimination of chemicals from the body. Chemicals may be excreted through feces, urine, exhaled breath, etc.

Exocytosis   Cellular discharge of material; opposite of endocytosis.

Expression   Transcription and translation of a gene to protein.

Extrapolation   An estimate of response or quantity at a point outside the range of the experimental data. Also refers to the estimate of a measured response in a different species or by a different route than that used in the experimental study of interest (i.e., species-to-species, route-to-route, acute-to-chronic, etc.).

Extrapyramidal symptoms   Facial rigidity, tremors, and drooling.

Extrasystole   Premature heart contraction.

Feedback inhibition   Mechanism that maintains constant secretion of a product by exerting inhibitory control.

Fenestrations   Perforations.

Fetus   The postembryonic stage of the developing young. In humans, from the end of the second month of pregnancy up to birth.

Fibrillation, cardiac   Heart flutter and irregular beats.

Fibroblast   Connective tissue cell capable of producing collagen.

Fibrosis   The formation of fibrous tissue, which may be a response of tissue to injury resulting in increased deposition of collagen fibers.

Fick's law   At constant temperature the rate of diffusion of a substance across a cell membrane is proportional to the concentration gradient and the surface area.

First-order process   The rate of the process is proportional to the present concentration of the substance.

First-pass metabolism   Metabolism of a drug or other xenobiotic during the absorption process. Typically occurs in the liver or gastrointestinal tract after oral dosing.

Forced diuresis   Induced increased urine formation.

Free radical   An atom or molecule that has an unpaired electron. It may be uncharged or charged depending on the number of electrons. Free radicals are usually chemically very reactive.

Ganglion   A group of nerve cell bodies located in the peripheral nervous system.

Gastric lavage   Washing or rinsing the stomach.

Gene   The simplest complete functional unit in a DNA molecule. A linear sequence of nucleotides in DNA that is needed to synthesize a single protein and/or regulate cell function. A mutation in one or more of the nucleotides in a gene may lead to abnormalities in the structure of the gene product or in the amount of gene product synthesized. The gene is made up of coding regions (exons) and noncoding regions (introns).

Genetic code   The information contained in DNA molecules that scientists describe on the basis of a four-letter alphabet (A, C, G, and T).

Genetic engineering   The process of transferring DNA from one organism into another that results in a genetic modification; the production of a transgenic organism.

Genome   Complete set of hereditary factors found on chromosomes; all the genes of one organism.

Genotoxic   Toxic to the genetic material of an organism.

Glial cells   Support cells located adjacent to neurons in the central nervous system. May be a component of the blood–brain barrier.

Glomerulonephritis   Inflammation of the capillary loops in the glomerulus.

Glomerulus   A functional unit of the mammalian kidney consisting of a small bunch of capillaries projecting into a capsule (Bowman's capsule), which serves to collect the filtrate from the blood of those capillaries and direct it into the kidney tubule.

Glucuronidation   Addition of glucuronic acid to form a more water-soluble conjugate.

Glycosuria   The presence of glucose in the urine.

Good laboratory practice (GLP)   A system of protocols (standard operating procedures) recommended to be followed so as to avoid the production of unreliable and erroneous data. Accurate record keeping and careful forethought in the design of the study are important aspects of GLP.

Gray baby syndrome   Cyanosis of the newborn due to inadequate capacity for glucuronidation of chloramphenicol.

GSH   Reduced glutathione (the tripeptide glutamyl-cysteinyl-glycine). Found in most tissue, particularly the liver. Plays a major role in detoxification of electrophiles and cellular protection against oxidative damage.

GSSG   Oxidized glutathione.

Half-life   The time taken for the concentration of a xenobiotic in a body fluid to decrease by half.

Hapten   A molecule (e.g., a drug metabolite) that becomes attached to an endogenous protein or other tissue macromolecule and so renders it antigenic.

Hashish   Cannabis preparation more concentrated than marijuana. It comes from the resinous secretions of the marijuana plants' flowering tops.

Hemodialysis   The process by which a drug is removed from the blood of a poisoned patient by allowing it to diffuse across a semipermeable membrane while the blood is pumped through a dialysis machine.

Hemolysis   Destruction of erythrocytes with the release of hemoglobin.

Hemolytic anemia   The pathological condition where red blood cells undergo uncontrolled destruction.

Hemoperfusion   The process by which a drug is removed from the blood of a poisoned patient by allowing it to be absorbed by activated charcoal or a resin while the blood is pumped through a special machine.

Henderson–Hasselbach equation $pH = pK_a + \log A^-/HA$.

Heparin   Endogenous compound that prevents blood clotting.

Hepatocellular   Relating to hepatocytes.

Hepatomegally   Increase in liver size.

Heroin   Acetylated morphine.

Histamine   A mediator of inflammatory reactions in the body, which may be part of an allergic reaction. Present in preformed granules in mast cells and basophils.

Homeostasis   Maintenance of normal, internal stability in an organism by co-ordinated responses of the organ systems, particularly the endocrine.

Homogenate   The mixture resulting from the homogenization of tissue.

Hormone   A chemical (usually peptide, amino acid derivative, or steroid) produced by an endocrine gland and affecting the function of target cells.

Hydrophobic/hydrophilic   A substance that repels/attracts water.

Hyper   Prefix indicating an increase.

Hyperkinesis   Hyperactivity.

Hyperplasia   An abnormal increase in the number of cells in a tissue.

Hypo   Prefix indicating a decrease.

Hypoglycemia   The physiological state where there is a low blood glucose concentration.

Hypothalamus   The region of the brain lying immediately above the pituitary gland and responsible for coordinating and controlling the autonomic nervous system.

Hypoxia   The physiological state where there is a low oxygen concentration.

Icterus   Jaundice.

Idiopathic   Of unknown origin or cause.

Idiosyncrasy   In pharmacology this is an adverse reaction to a drug occurring in small numbers of individuals in a distinct frequency distribution as a result of a genetic abnormality.

Immune complex   A complex of antibody(ies) and antigen(s) that may lead to pathological consequences such as inflammation or blockage of a vessel (i.e., a type III reaction).

Immunoglobin (Ig)   One of five classes of antibody protein involved in immune responses (i.e., IgA, IgD, IgE, IgG, and IgM).

Infarction   Loss of blood supply due to obstruction (e.g., myocardial infarct due to the blockage caused by a blood clot).

Inflammation   A protective tissue response to injury that serves to destroy, dilute, or wall off both the injurious agent and the injured tissue. It is characterized by symptoms such as pain, heat, and redness and is the result of the combined effects of numerous inflammatory mediators (e.g., prostaglandins, histamine, cytokines, etc.).

Interferon   A protein produced by the body in response to a stimulus such as an infection.

Internalization   Loss of surface receptor number determined by a combination of the effects of endocytosis and recycling.

Interstitial   Between cells in tissue.

Intraperitoneal (IP)   A route of drug administration for a drug to an animal by direct injection into the peritoneal cavity.

Investigational New Drug Application (IND)   An application that a drug sponsor must submit to the FDA before beginning tests of a new drug on humans. The IND contains the plan for the study and is supposed to give a complete picture of the drug, including its structural formula, animal test results, and manufacturing information.

In vitro   From the Latin meaning in glass; in an artificial environment such as a test tube.

In vivo   Tests conducted within the whole living body.

Ischemia   The condition where there is reduced or blocked blood flow to a tissue, which will lead to ischemic tissue damage.

Isoenzyme   One of several forms of an enzyme with identical function but different structure.

Isotonic   Having the same osmotic pressure and salt concentration as blood.

Kernicterus   Central neuropathy associated with high bilirubin levels and characterized by yellow staining of the basal ganglia.

Latency   The period of time between exposure to an injurious agent and the manifestation of a response (e.g., sensitization period following initial exposure to an antigen).

LD$_{50}$ The lethal dose of a compound for 50 percent of the animals exposed.

L-Dopa   Dihydroxyphenylalanine, a drug used to treat Parkinson's disease.

Ligand   A substance that binds specifically to a receptor.

Ligation   The rejoining of restriction digested DNA fragments using the enzyme T4 DNA ligase.

Lipid peroxidation   Oxidative breakdown of lipids usually involving a free radical mechanism or active oxygen species and giving rise to reactive products that may be responsible for cellular damage.

Lipid solubility   See lipophilicity.

Lipophilicity   A term used to describe the ability of a substance to dissolve in or associate with fat and therefore living tissue. This usually applies to compounds that are nonionized or nonpolar or have a nonpolar portion. Therefore, high lipid solubility usually implies low water solubility.

Local toxicity   Toxicity that affects only the site of application or exposure.

LSD, D-lysergic acid diethylamide   This chemical was synthesized from ergot in 1938 by Albert Hoffman of the Sandoz Laboratories in Switzerland. It is a potent hallucinogen in the microgram range.

Lupus erythematosus   Autoimmune disease characterized by inflammation and localized skin discoloration.

Lymphocyte   Type of white blood cell produced in the thymus and bone marrow. Two types, T and B.

Lysis   Breakdown of a tissue or macromolecule.

Macrophage   Large phagocytic cells that are components of the reticuloendothelial system.

Mast cell A granulated cell containing numerous preformed and formed mediators of inflammation. Distributed within the body but particularly concentrated in the lungs.

Metastasis Migration and relocation of malignant cancer cells.

Microflora Microorganisms such as bacteria that normally inhabit the gastrointestinal tract.

Microsomes/microsomal The subcellular fraction containing the fragments of the smooth endoplasmic reticulum (ER) after ultracentrifugation of a cellular homogenate.

Mitochondria The intracellular organelle in which respiration and other important metabolic reactions take place.

Monooxygenase Enzyme system (such as cytochrome P450) involved in the oxidation of xenobiotics.

Mucosa Membrane containing mucus-secreting cells.

Muscarinic receptors Receptors for acetylcholine found in smooth muscle, heart, and exocrine glands. Named after the substance muscarine, which was used in the early experiments.

Mutagen/mutagenic A substance/property of a substance that causes some type of mutation in the genetic material of an organism exposed to it.

Mutation A change of one of the "letters" in the DNA "recipe" caused by chemicals, ultraviolet light, X-rays, or natural processes.

Mydriasis Dilation of the pupil of the eye.

Myesthenia gravis Progressive disease with skeletal muscle weakness associated with neuromuscular junction cholinergic receptor autoantibodies.

Myocardium The middle and thickest layer of cardiac muscle in the heart wall.

NADH The coenzyme nicotinamide adenine dinucleotide.

NADPH The coenzyme reduced nicotinamide adenine dinucleotide phosphate.

Necrosis The process of cell death within a living organism and the end result of irreversible changes following cellular injury.

Neonatal Newly born; in humans up to 6 weeks of age.

Neoplasia The pathologic process that results in the formation and growth of a tumor.

Nephritis Inflammation of the kidney.

Nephron The functional unit of the kidney that produces urine. It consists of a long tubule divided into sections in which reabsorption into the bloodstream of certain solutes filtered by the glomerulus from the blood takes place.

Nephropathy Pathological damage to the nephrons of the kidney.

Neuronal Relating to nerve cells.

Neurotransmission Passage of nerve impulses between neurons mediated by chemical neurotransmitters (e.g., norepinephrine and acetylcholine).

Neutrophil A phagocytic white blood cell that plays an important role in the inflammatory process.

New Drug Application (NDA) An application requesting FDA approval to market a new drug for human use in interstate commerce. The application must contain, among other things, data from specific technical viewpoints for FDA review—including chemistry, pharmacology, medical, biopharmaceutics, statistics, and, for anti-infectives, microbiology.

Nodes of Ranvier   Areas in peripheral nerves between myelin sheaths occurring at regular intervals of approximately 1 mm.

Nonsteroidal anti-inflammatory drug (NSAID)   A drug useful in arthritis and other inflammatory conditions, such as salicylates, indomethacin, and ibuprofen.

Occlusion   Constriction or blockage as can occur in a blood vessel.

Opiates   Compounds derived from, or similar in action to, potent analgesic opium alkaloids.

Organelle   A subcellular structure such as the mitochondrion or nucleus of a cell.

Organogenesis   The development of specific body structures or organs from undifferentiated tissue. In humans, this corresponds to weeks 2 through 8 postconception.

Orphan drug   A drug for which the target population is limited or for which the disease it treats occurs only rarely.

Parallel Track Mechanism   A U.S. Public Health Service policy that makes promising investigational drugs for AIDS and other HIV-related diseases more widely available under "parallel track" protocols while the controlled clinical trials essential to establish the safety and effectiveness of new drugs are carried out. The system established by this policy is designed to make drugs more widely available to patients with these illnesses who have no therapeutic alternatives and who cannot participate in the controlled clinical trials.

Parathesias   Abnormal sensations such as tingling.

Parenteral   Routes of drug administration other than via the gastrointestinal tract.

Parkinson's disease   Neurological disorder accompanied by dopamine deficiency. Patients exhibit extrapyramidal symptoms.

PCR   The polymerase chain reaction that utilizes a thermostable DNA polymerase to make many copies of the same piece of DNA. This allows specific amplification of rare pieces of DNA.

Percutaneous   Through the skin.

Peripheral neuropathy   Damage to nerves of the peripheral rather than the central nervous system.

Peroxidases   Enzymes that catalyze oxidation utilizing hydrogen peroxide. Found in many tissues including certain types of white blood cells (e.g., neutrophils).

Pesticide   An agent used to exterminate pests of various types. Includes insecticides, herbicides, and fungicides.

pH partition theory   This states that a foreign compound in the nonionized state will pass across a cell membrane by passive diffusion down a concentration gradient.

Phago/pinocytosis   The uptake of a solid substance (phago) or solution (pino) into a cell by invagination of the cell membrane, eventually forming a vesicle inside the cell.

Pharmacodynamic   Relating to the effects of drugs on living systems.

Pharmacokinetics   The field of study concerned with defining, through measurement or modeling, the absorption, distribution, metabolism, and excretion of drugs or other xenobiotics in a biological system as a function of time.

Pharmacopoeia   An official compendium listing medicinal drugs, their properties, standards of purity, and other useful information.

Phase I   The term applied to the first stage of drug metabolism, commonly involving either oxidation, reduction, or hydrolysis of the molecule.

Phase II The term applied to the second stage of drug metabolism, usually involving conjugation of a functional group with a moiety available endogenously and conferring water solubility on the molecule.

Phenotype The expression of the genotype or genetic makeup of an organism.

Phocomelia The syndrome of having shortened arms and legs due to an adverse effect on the embryo such as caused by thalidomide.

Phospholipid A lipid in which one of the hydroxyl groups of glycerol or sphingosine is esterified with a phosphorylated alcohol.

Phosphorylation The process of adding phosphate groups to a compound. Particularly important in the transduction processes of G-protein receptors.

"Pill", the (contraceptive) A mixture of synthetic estrogen and progestin that controls menstrual cycles and produces a state of pseudopregnancy.

Placebo An inactive compound having no physiological effects; an inert substance identical in appearance to the treatment drug used in clinical studies.

Plasma Blood from which the cells have been removed by centrifugation but distinct from serum in which the blood is first allowed to clot.

Plasmid An extrachromosomal circle of DNA found in bacteria and yeast that can confer antibiotic resistance to a bacterial host and can be transferred from one cell to another. Capable of self-replicating and can exist in multicopy numbers within a cell. Used as the main vector for gene cloning.

Pneumonitis Inflammation of the lungs.

Polar A term used to describe a molecule that is charged or has a tendency to become polarized.

Polydipsia Excessive thirst.

Polymer A molecule formed by the joining of many smaller molecules; a protein, for example, is a polymer of amino acids.

Polymerase An enzyme that forms long-chain polymers from simple molecular components; DNA polymerase, for example, forms DNA strands from nucleotides.

Polypeptide A chain of amino acids joined by peptide bonds.

Population variability The concept of differences in susceptibility of individuals within a population to drugs or toxicants due to genetic variations in metabolism, for example, or differences in biological responses.

Portal The term applied to the venous circulation draining the tissues of the gastrointestinal tract into the liver.

Postmarketing surveillance The FDA's ongoing safety monitoring of marketed drugs.

Potency A comparative expression of drug activity measured in terms of the relationship between the intensity or incidence of a particular effect and the administered dose. Most appropriately used when comparing drugs that interact with the same population of receptors.

Potentiation When an effect due to two drugs with different modes of action is greater than expected from the effects of the individual drugs.

ppm A measure of concentration of a substance in which the units of the substance are one millionth of the solvent (e.g., μg per gram).

Preclinical studies Studies that test a drug on animals and other nonhuman test systems. They must comply with the FDA's good laboratory practices. Data about a drug's activities and effects in animals help to establish boundaries for safe use of the drug in subsequent human testing (clinical studies). Also, because animals have a much shorter life span than humans, valuable information can be gained about a drug's possible toxic effects over an animal's life cycle and on offspring.

Prodrugs Inactive drugs that undergo metabolic activation.

Promoter Region of DNA close to the 5' end of the gene where transcription factors bind and help the binding of RNA polymerase at the start of transcription.

Prospective, randomized, double-blind trial A clinical trial in which the method for analyzing data has been specified in the protocol before the study has begun (prospective), the patients have been randomly assigned to receive either the study drug or alternative treatment, and neither the patient nor the physician conducting the study know which treatment is being given to which patient.

Prostaglandins Endogenous chemical mediators involved in inflammation derived from the cellular membrane unsaturated fatty acid arachidonic acid.

Proteinuria Presence of protein in the urine above normal limits.

Psychoactive drugs Drugs that produce behavioral changes.

Psychotomimetic A chemical that produces symptoms similar to pathologic psychoses, such as amphetamine, LSD, and mescaline.

Quantal response A response that is all-or-none rather than graded.

Racemate A mixture of stereoisomers.

Raw data Researcher's records of patients, such as patient charts, hospital records, X-rays, and attending physician notes. These records may or may not accompany an NDA, but must be kept in the researcher's file. The FDA may request their submission or may audit them at the researcher's office.

Receptor cycling Continual agonist-stimulated endocytosis and constitutive recycling of receptors.

Recombinant DNA DNA formed by joining pieces of DNA from two or more organisms.

Recycling Movement of receptor or ligand from an internal compartment to the cell surface. Recycling is assumed to be constitutive.

Renal elimination Excretion of a substance via the kidneys.

Resensitization Recovery of functional response after desensitization.

Restriction enzyme An enzyme that cuts DNA at a specific sequence leaving a complimentary "sticky end."

Retrovirus A type of virus whose genetic material consists of RNA rather than DNA.

Reverse transcriptase A retroviral enzyme that copies RNA into DNA.

Rhinitis Inflammation of the mucous membranes of the nose.

Ribosomes The intracellular organelles attached to the rough endoplasmic reticulum and involved with protein synthesis.

RNA A single-stranded copy of DNA consisting of adenosine, cytidine, guanosine, and uridine. Most commonly found as messenger RNA (mRNA), transfer RNA (tRNA), or ribosomal RNA (rRNA).

RNA processing The removal of the introns from the coding (exon) sequence to give the mRNA.

Safety No drug is completely safe or without the potential for side effects. Before a drug may be approved for marketing, the law requires the submission of results of tests adequate to show the drug is safe under the conditions of use in the proposed labeling. Thus "safety" is determined case by case and reflects the drug's risk-versus-benefit relationship.

Safety update reports   Reports that an NDA sponsor must submit to the FDA about new safety information that may affect the use for which the drug will be approved, or draft labeling statements about contraindications, warnings, precautions, and adverse reactions. Safety update reports are required 4 months after application is submitted, after the applicant receives an approval letter, and at other times upon FDA request.

Schwann cells   Large nucleated cells that wrap around myelinated peripheral neurons to form the myelin sheath.

Sensitization   A term used in reference to the period following exposure to an antigen when the body begins to produce antigens.

Sequencing   The determination of the nucleotide sequence of a DNA fragment.

Sequestration   Synonymous with internalization.

Sinsemilla   There are male and female marijuana plants. The flowers of the female plant contain the highest concentration of THC. Growers have learned that if the female plants are not allowed to be pollinated, the flowers cluster and excrete greater quantities of resin. Marijuana grown in this fashion is called Sinsemilla, which means "no seeds."

Splanchnic   Pertaining to the internal organs.

St Anthony's Fire   Ergotism or toxicity from ingesting ergot alkaloids with cerebrospinal symptoms, spasms, cramps, and gangrene in the extremities.

Structure–activity relationship   Relationship of pharmacological activity or toxicity of a xenobiotic to its chemical structure.

Subchronic   An exposure of duration intermediate between acute and chronic (e.g., 28 or 90 days) or approximately 10 percent of the lifetime of an organism.

Subcutaneous   Below the skin.

Sublingual   Below the tongue.

Superoxide   The oxygen molecule with an extra unpaired electron. It is thus a charged free radical and highly reactive.

Supplement   A marketing application submitted for changes in a product that already has an approved NDA. The FDA must approve all important NDA changes (in packaging or ingredients, for example) to ensure that the conditions originally set for the product are not adversely affected.

Surrogate endpoint   A laboratory finding or physical sign that may not, in itself, be a direct measurement of how a patient feels, functions, or survives, but nevertheless is considered likely to predict therapeutic benefit. An example would be CD4 cell counts, used to measure the strength of the immune system in AIDS.

Synergism/synergistic   When effects of two or more drugs are greater than the sum of their individual effects.

Synovial   Relating to the lubricating fluid in joints.

Synovitis   Inflammation of the joints; arthritis.

Systemic toxicity   Toxicity that affects a system in the organism other than and probably distant from the site of application or exposure.

Tachycardia   Excess rapid heart rate.

Tachyphylaxis   Rapid decrease in physiological response to a drug after administration of a few doses (i.e., acute tolerance).

TD$_{50}$ The dose that is toxic to 50 percent of the population exposed to the substance or a 50 percent toxic response in a biological system exposed to the substance (i.e., nausea).

Teratogen/teratogenicity A substance/property of a substance causing abnormalities in the embryo or fetus when administered to the maternal organism.

Therapeutic index The ratio of LD$_{50}$ to ED$_{50}$.

Thiol SH or sulfhydryl group.

Thromboembolism Obstruction of a blood vessel by a broken thrombus (blood clot) that was transported to the occluded vessel from another site of formation.

Thrombosis Formation of blood clots causing vascular obstruction.

Tinnitus A "ringing" in the ears.

Tolerance When repeated administration of or dosing with a drug leads to a decrease in the potency in the biological activity of that drug. May have a metabolic or cellular basis. Acute tolerance is referred to as tachyphylaxis.

Toxic effect Any change in an organism that results in impairment of functional capacity of the organism (as determined by anatomical, physiological, biochemical, or behavioral parameters); causes decrements in the organism's ability to maintain its normal function; or enhances the susceptibility of the organism to the deleterious effects of other environmental influences.

Toxicology The multidisciplinary study of toxicants, their harmful effects on biological systems, and the conditions under which these harmful effects occur. The mechanisms of action, detection, and treatment of the conditions produced by toxicants are studied.

Transcription The process of copying DNA to RNA performed by RNA polymerases.

Transdermal Through the skin.

Transfection Introduction of a foreign gene into a cell's genome.

Transgenic An organism that has been modified by genetic engineering to contain DNA from an external source.

Transgenic animals Animals in which a gene from a different species has been inserted.

Translation The process of copying mRNA into protein performed by ribosomal RNA.

Treatment IND A mechanism that allows promising investigational drugs to be used in "expanded access" protocols—relatively unrestricted studies in which the intent is both to learn more about the drugs, especially their safety, and to provide treatment for people with immediately life-threatening or otherwise serious diseases for which there is no real alternative. But these expanded protocols also require researchers to formally investigate the drugs in well-controlled studies and to supply some evidence that the drugs are likely to be helpful. The drugs cannot expose patients to unreasonable risk.

Trimodal Frequency distribution that divides into three groups.

Ultrafiltrate The fluid formed in the renal tubule from blood passing through the glomerulus/Bowman's capsule in the kidney.

Urticaria A vascular reaction of the skin marked by the appearance of wheals; may be caused by direct or indirect exposure to a toxic substance. Also known as hives.

User fees   Charges to drug firms for certain NDAs, drug products, and manufacturing establishments. The FDA uses these fees to hire more application reviewers and to accelerate reviews through the use of computer technology.

Vasculitis   Inflammation of a blood vessel.

Vasoconstriction   Constriction of blood vessels.

Vasodilatation/vascular dilatation   Dilation of blood vessels.

Vector   Any DNA structure that is used to transfer DNA into an organism; most commonly used are plasmid DNA vectors or viruses.

Vivissection   Originally the surgical cutting of a living animal in scientific research; often used today as a synonym for any type of animal research.

Volume of distribution (V_d)   The volume of body fluid in which a xenobiotic is apparently distributed when administered to an animal.

Wheals   Raised patches on the skin; usually an immunological response.

Xenobiotic   A chemical foreign to the body.

Zero-order process   The rate of the process is independent of the concentration of the substance (e.g., liver metabolism of ethyl alcohol).

ANSWERS TO QUESTIONS

Chapter 1	Chapter 2	Chapter 3	Chapter 4
1-c	1-d	1-a	1-c
2-b	2-a	2-e	2-e
3-d	3-c	3-e	3-e
4-e	4-b	4-e	4-d
5-e	5-a	5-c	5-e
6-e	6-c	6-d	6-d
7-d	7-c	7-e	7-c
8-b	8-d	8-e	8-b
9-d	9-a	9-a	9-a
10-e	10-a	10-d	10-e

Chapter 5	Chapter 6	Chapter 7	Chapter 8
1-c	1-b	1-d	1-a
2-e	2-c	2-a	2-e
3-e	3-c	3-c	3-d
4-e	4-c	4-e	4-e
5-e	5-e	5-b	5-e
6-d	6-e	6-d	6-e
7-d	7-d	7-c	7-e
8-e	8-e	8-a	8-c
9-b	9-e	9-c	9-c
10-d	10-c	10-e	10-e

Chapter 9	Chapter 10	Chapter 11	Chapter 12
1-e	1-e	1-e	1-b
2-d	2-c	2-e	2-b
3-e	3-b	3-e	3-a
4-d	4-b	4-c	4-b
5-c	5-d	5-e	5-d
6-e	6-d	6-d	6-a
7-e	7-e	7-c	7-a
8-e	8-e	8-d	8-a
9-c	9-e	9-d	9-d
10-b	10-e	10-d	10-d

Chapter 13	Chapter 14	Chapter 15	Chapter 16
1-d	1-e	1-c	1-e
2-e	2-c	2-e	2-b
3-e	3-d	3-d	3-e
4-e	4-c	4-c	4-a
5-c	5-a	5-e	5-c
6-e	6-a	6-b	6-a
7-e	7-e	7-c	7-e
8-b	8-e	8-e	8-e
9-e	9-c	9-e	9-c
10-b	10-e	10-b	10-c

Appendix

1-d
2-a
3-b
4-c
5-c
6-e
7-d
8-d
9-e
10-c

Index

Note: page numbers in *italics* refer to figures and tables. All legislation and government departments and organizations are US unless indicated otherwise by country name in parentheses.